Human Semen Analysis

Ashok Agarwal • Florence Boitrelle
Ramadan Saleh • Rupin Shah
Editors

Human Semen Analysis

From the WHO Manual to the Clinical Management of Infertile Men

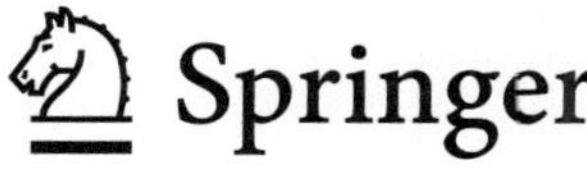

Editors
Ashok Agarwal
Global Andrology Forum
Moreland Hills, OH, USA

Ramadan Saleh
Dermatology, Venereology, & Andrology
Sohag University
Sohag, Egypt

Florence Boitrelle
Reproductive Biology, Andrology
CECOS, Centre Hospitalier Intercommunal
de Poissy
Poissy, France

Rupin Shah
Department of Urology
Lilavati Hospital & Research Centre
Mumbai, India

ISBN 978-3-031-55339-4   ISBN 978-3-031-55337-0   (eBook)
https://doi.org/10.1007/978-3-031-55337-0

This Springer imprint is published by the registered company Springer Nature Switzerland AG
The registered company address is: Gewerbestrasse 11, 6330 Cham, Switzerland

If disposing of this product, please recycle the paper.

In memory of my father, Professor RC Aggarwal, whose legacy of integrity, dedication, and hard work remains a guiding light. To my wife, Meenu, and sons, Rishi and Neil-Yogi, whose unwavering love sustains me. Gratitude to Professor Kevin Loughlin (Harvard Medical School), the late Professor Anthony Thomas (Cleveland Clinic), and Dr. Rupin Shah (India) for their invaluable friendship, guidance, and profound impact on my journey. To over thousand researchers, students, and the countless patients who entrusted me over four decades—your collaboration and trust have been my greatest inspiration.

—Ashok Agarwal, MSc, PhD, HCLD (Andrology)

The idea for this book was born a few years ago. While the WHO manual is part of our day-to-day work as andrologists, we felt it was important to understand it better in order to use it more effectively. To improve international research in Andrology, Prof. Agarwal created the

Global Andrology Forum. For me, becoming a member of this group has enabled me to get to know andrologists who are passionate about their profession, whether they live in France, Europe, or the rest of the world. I would like to thank him warmly for inviting me to edit this book with him. Dear Ashok, dear co-editors (Rupin and Ramadan), thank you for this wonderful adventure.

—Florence Boitrelle (MD, PhD, France)

To my family for your constant love and support. You have always been there for me.

To Professor Ashok Agarwal (Global Andrology Forum, USA) for your guidance and support. Thank you for believing in my dream. You were the first person to encourage me to be part of this achievement.

To the late Professor Kamal Abdel Hafez (Assiut University, Egypt) for his mentorship and guidance.

—Ramadan Saleh, MD

This book is dedicated to my wife Urvashi, for her patient understanding; to my patients, who have been my true teachers; to my co-editors, Florence and Ramadan, who have been wonderful partners in this journey; and to Ashok Agarwal, who made this book possible and has been a great friend and inspiration in my academic journey.

—Rupin Shah

Foreword

This is much more than a reference book. Many experts have collaborated to explain why such a fundamental biological test (semen analysis) fails to define the most important of human conditions—fertility.

Previous editions of the WHO manual sought to define reference limits, but the sixth edition describes a continuum of parameters which, at the extremes, predict either a fertile or an infertile state. Once reference values have been removed, semen analysis can no longer be used as a gateway to some kind of artificial reproductive technology (ART) because abnormalities require explanation by further tests and most significantly, as nearly every chapter states, by clinical examination and scrutiny.

Male fertility has moved from a largely laboratory-based definition to the more traditional realm of clinical input and further clinically directed tests. Diagnosis therefore replaces diktat, and proper treatment with measured improvement replaces the former solution, which was so often some form of ART.

Overall, this excellent commentary has recalibrated the status of male infertility, which can now be regarded as a disease, a major health issue, with many associations with significant other medical conditions.

Considering that repeated studies have shown that standard semen analysis, according to WHO guidelines, is very limited in predicting male fertility potential, and leaves a large proportion of men either undiagnosed or not correctly diagnosed, situations which lead to inappropriate treatment. Therefore, by elegantly combining clinical aspects and future developments, clinicians and researchers are provided with directions for further developments in how andrological diagnostics will improve in the years to come.

This book highlights the implementation of artificial intelligence (AI) into automated CASA systems to improve the determination of sperm count, motility, and normal morphology to make semen analysis faster, more accurate, and reliable. Other areas of research include the better understanding and determination of redox stress and sperm DNA fragmentation with robust clinical cut-off values since these fields have recently been recognized by the WHO as important and recommended for advanced examination. The book also underscores the importance of genetic screening for sperm aneuploidy as many aspects of male infertility have genetic causes.

This book explains why, and how, semen analysis is merely the first step in a diagnostic journey which may lead us to understand the basis of disordered spermatogenesis.

Eventually, all these research efforts must lead not only to a better understanding of male fertility with better diagnostic and treatment, and improved pregnancy rates in vitro and in vivo, but also to novel methodologies for male contraception. In this sense, this book will also lead the way to change the perception by recognizing the man as a patient who should be treated, rather than his sperm.

Berkshire, UK   Prof. Ralf Henkel

London, UK

Bellville, South Africa

London, UK   Mr. Jonathan Ramsay MS., FRCS(Urol)

Preface

The *WHO laboratory manual for the examination and processing of human semen* is the most widely referenced document in the evaluation of male infertility. It provides a detailed description of a variety of semen tests that are considered relevant to the evaluation and management of an infertile male. However, its clinical utility is severely limited by the fact that it is, indeed, as its name suggests, a laboratory manual and does not provide a clinical context for the various tests described.

Hence, the clinician is left with a range of tests to prescribe but with no guidance as to when to ask for a specific test, how to interpret the test results, and what subsequent clinical action to take. As a result, many of the tests described in the manual, especially the extended and advanced tests, remain underutilized, and even the interpretation of some components of the basic semen analysis is unclear.

The purpose of this book is to bridge this gap between the laboratory manual and the clinician by explaining in detail the test indication, its clinical utility, interpretation of results, and presenting a decision algorithm based on the test results. Even the cost-effectiveness and future perspectives of the tests are discussed where relevant.

The book has 19 chapters grouped under seven parts that follow the chapters of the sixth edition of the WHO manual. Each chapter is written and reviewed by a team of senior clinicians, thus bringing a perspective that is truly clinically relevant. This book will be of great value to all clinicians involved in the management of male infertility and will also be of interest to laboratory scientists involved in semen testing by providing them with clinical perspectives of the test they perform.

Our book is poised to become an indispensable guide for clinicians, medical laboratory technologists, scientists, embryologists, researchers, and healthcare professionals dedicated to the care of infertile couples. It also stands as a valuable resource for students and residents eager to deepen their understanding of this critical subject, making it a significant addition to the realm of male infertility literature.

A heartfelt appreciation goes out to the impressive collaboration of experts—35 authors from 20 countries—who have dedicated their efforts to provide the latest, well-written, and meticulously researched manuscripts. Without their unwavering support, this book would not have been possible. Special thanks are extended to the organizational prowess of Lillie Mae Gaurano, Springer Editor, Clinical Medicine (Books), and the day-to-day support of Production Editor Janakiraman G.

In honor of our families, mentors, and patients, this book is a dedication to those who inspire and motivate us in the pursuit of advancing knowledge in the field of male infertility.

Moreland Hills, OH, USA   Ashok Agarwal
Poissy, France   Florence Boitrelle
Sohag, Egypt   Ramadan Saleh
Mumbai, India   Rupin Shah

Contents

About the Editors

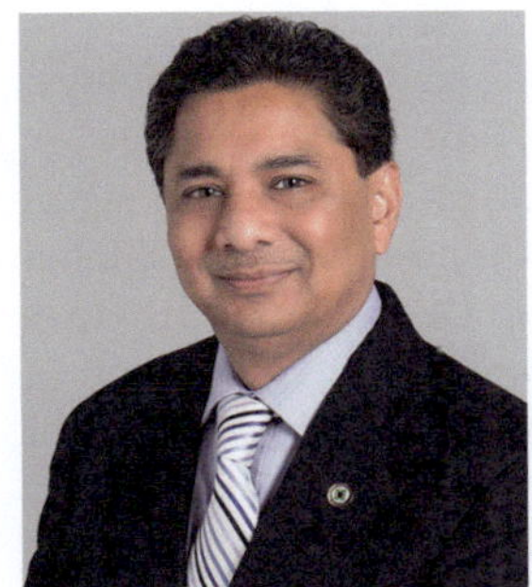

Ashok Agarwal is a highly regarded andrologist and researcher who has made significant contributions to the field of male infertility. As the founder and current President of the Global Andrology Forum (GAF) headquartered in Moreland Hills, Ohio, he leads an international coalition of 700 members from 84 countries, tirelessly propelling the advancements in male reproductive health. For nearly three decades (1993–2022), Ashok served as the Director of the Andrology Laboratory and Research in Urology at Cleveland Clinic, concurrently holding the position of Professor of Surgery at Case Western Reserve University, Cleveland. His prolific contributions encompass over 950 scientific articles and the editing of 55 medical textbooks, earning him numerous accolades in andrology and male infertility research. Beyond his groundbreaking research and clinical expertise, Ashok's dedication extends to education and mentorship. He has shared his knowledge with over 1000 clinicians and scientists from 65+ countries, shaping the future of andrology. Recognized as a foremost authority in male infertility research, Ashok has been a featured speaker at countless national and international conferences, showcasing his leadership in the global dialogue on male reproductive health.

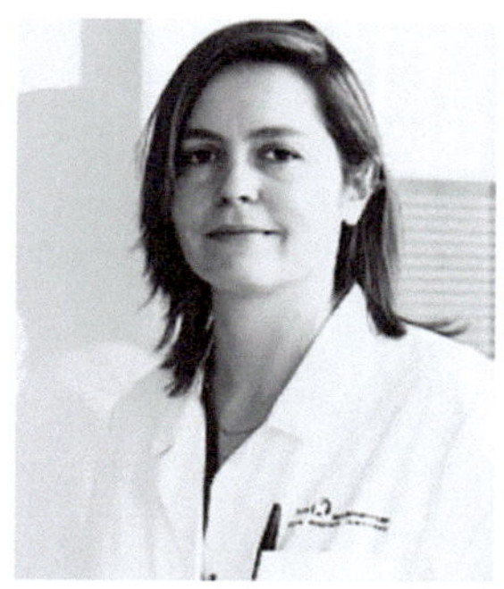

Florence Boitrelle is a doctor specializing in andrology and assisted reproduction. She is head of department, head of a MPA center, former president of the Société d'Andrologie de langue Française, and a member of various learned societies in France and internationally (ESHRE, Global Andrology Forum…). Passionate about clinical andrology and research, she is the author of over 100 articles referenced in Pubmed and has participated in over 80 communications in France and abroad.

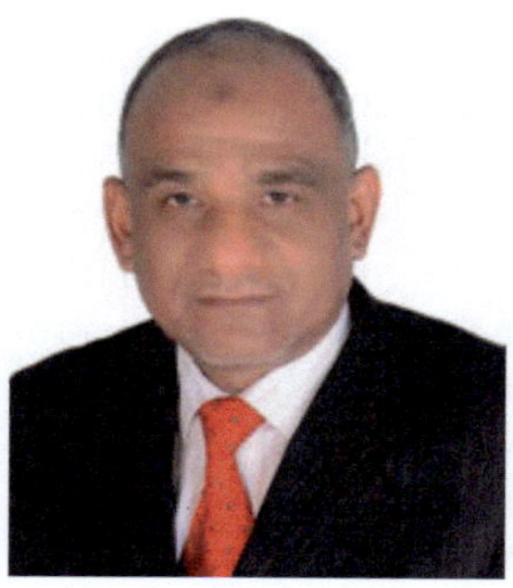

Ramadan Saleh is a Professor of Dermatology, Venereology and Andrology, in Sohag University, Egypt. He is the founder of Ajyal IVF Center, Ajyal Hospital, Sohag, Egypt. He is a co-founder of Global Andrology Forum established in December 2021. He is a member of several professional societies and a reviewer in many international journals in the field of reproductive medicine. He has published more than 150 research articles in peer-reviewed scientific journals and co-edited three books.

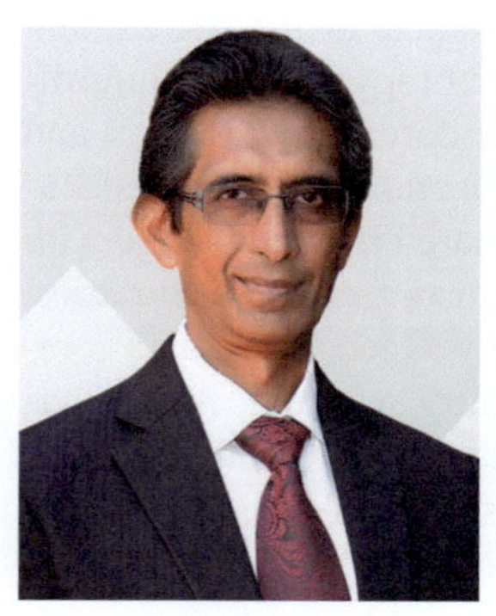

Rupin Shah is a senior uro-andrologist practicing male infertility and sexual dysfunction in Mumbai at the Lilavati Hospital & Research Centre. He is Founder-President of the South Asian Society of Sexual Medicine, Chairman of the Post-Doctoral Fellowship in Andrology of the National Board of Examinations of India, Co-Chair of the International Consultation on Sexual Medicine-2024, Associate Editor of the journal *Fertility and Reproduction*, and Senior advisor to the Global Andrology Forum.

Part I

WHO Manual for Human Semen Analysis

Historical View: From First to the Sixth WHO Manual

Eric Chung and Hyun Jun Park

Introduction

Semen analysis remains the cornerstone of male infertility evaluation and the presence of abnormal semen parameters is estimated to play a role in up to 50% of all cases of infertility. The first edition of the World Health Organization (WHO) *Laboratory Manual for the Examination and Processing of Human Semen* was released in 1980 [1] and has undergone five more revisions, culminating in the current sixth edition published last year. The WHO "semen manual" is developed under the coordination of the United Nations Development Programme/United Nations Population Fund/United Nations Children's Fund/WHO/World Bank Special Programme of Research, Development and Research Training in Human Reproduction (HRP) within the WHO Department of Reproductive Health and Research, with the aims to standardize the procedures for the examination of human semen and provide guidance in the diagnosis and management of reproductive function in men [2]. Before the WHO manual, the preparation and examination of various semen parameters have been largely unregulated and subjective to individual laboratory processes.

The first edition called the *Laboratory Manual for the Examination of Human Semen and Semen-Cervical Mucus Interaction* was produced following consultations with various international experts and provided the first attempt to standardize and validate the laboratory procedures for semen analysis scientifically [1]. The

E. Chung (✉)
Department of Urology, Princess Alexandra Hospital, The University of Queensland, Brisbane, QLD, Australia

AndroUrology Centre, Brisbane, QLD, Australia

H. J. Park
Department of Urology, Pusan National University School of Medicine/Pusan National University Hospital, Busan, South Korea

second [3], third [4], and fourth [5] editions of the WHO semen manual were produced in response to the rapid development of assisted reproductive techniques and increased understanding on male reproduction, coupled with increasing awareness of the importance of the objective assessment of the quality and functional characteristics of human spermatozoa. Expansive commercialization of andrology laboratories in infertility treatment centers and scientific advances in the genetics of male infertility and the hormonal manipulation of spermatogenesis have created a need to achieve better standardization and improved procedures for semen analysis. The fifth edition of the laboratory manual's name was changed to *WHO Laboratory Manual for the Examination and Processing of Human Semen* [6] and established the manual as global guidance that will set standards across various laboratory settings and resources. The WHO manual became widely available in free print, and as an electronic version downloadable from the WHO website.

The latest edition was published more than a decade later and expanded its content to cover areas on semen examination and preparation for clinical evaluation, cryopreservation, and quality control in the semen analysis laboratory, as well as in-depth laboratory examination techniques in the evaluation of male sexual and reproductive health [7].

Major Advances in Each of the WHO Editions

The World Health Organization (WHO) laboratory manual for the examination and processing of human semen was first published in 1980. Since then, it has been revised and updated five times and has become an essential and useful guideline for researchers worldwide majoring in reproductive medicine.

First Edition (1980): This was published under the title "Laboratory Manual for the Examination of Human Semen and Semen-Cervical Mucus Interaction." This manual aimed to provide standardized, precise, reproducible, sensitive, and validated laboratory procedures for semen analysis. The main sections were about semen sample collection, initial examination, and assessment of sperm motility, concentration, morphology, and viability.

Second Edition (1987): The title of the manual was the same as in the first edition. Semen analysis was divided into standard and optional tests. It started to provide normal values obtained from large-scale studies of sperm variables.

Third Edition (1992): The title has been changed to the "WHO Laboratory Manual for the Examination of Human Semen and Sperm-Cervical Mucus Interaction." Semen analysis was divided into three sections: standard procedures, optional tests, and research tests. As in the previous edition, reference limits of sperm variables were provided, and empirical cutoff points of 30% normal forms were introduced.

Fourth Edition (1992): The fourth edition was revised mainly based on changes in trends, such as the genetics of male infertility and the success of intracytoplasmic sperm injection. The multiple sperm defect index and hypoosmotic swelling test were added to the optional tests, and the measurement of reactive oxygen species was added to the research test. Referring to reference values for semen variables, a percent normal morphology of <15% may be associated with a lower in vitro fertilization rate. The description and standardization of techniques were considered significant improvements over the previous edition.

Fifth Edition (2010): The title of the fifth edition was changed to the "WHO Laboratory Manual for the Examination and Processing of Human Semen." The revision was made based on the principles of "Evidence-Based Medicine." The fifth edition has been published on the WHO website and can be accessed and downloaded for free. Reference ranges of semen variables were provided from studies on fertile men with partners who conceived within 12 months. The lower fifth percentile was used as the lower reference range, with a clear statement indicating that this lower limit does not distinguish subfertile and fertile men and that clinical information must be used together with semen analysis data.

Sixth Edition (2021): The preparatory process took approximately 3.5 years and was partially affected by the coronavirus disease 2019 pandemic. On July 20, 2021, a webinar introduced a new edition of the WHO Laboratory Manual for the Examination and Processing of Human Semen. The final form can be downloaded from the WHO website.

What Is New in the Sixth Edition of the WHO Manual of Semen Analysis?

The sixth edition introduces the methodology used by the WHO to prepare this new edition. When published via webinar, the WHO declared that high-quality laboratory services are crucial for ensuring the value of health research. Effectively analyzing and comparing results across various laboratories helps to ensure that healthcare workers receive high-quality information, which in turn helps them provide the best quality care. The sixth edition of the WHO Laboratory Manual for the Examination and Processing of Human Semen replaced the 2010 version. It provides important information on semen examination and preparation for clinical evaluation, assessment, cryopreservation, quality control in the semen analysis laboratory, and laboratory examination in the investigation of male sexual and reproductive health.

The sixth edition was intended to provide a "step-by-step, easy-to-follow procedure." It consists of a basic examination, an extended examination, an advanced examination, and emerging methods of semen analysis without a microscope. The major changes are as follows.

- Basic examination—Standard tests, slow progressive motility reintroduction
- Extended examination—Optional tests like leukocytes, immature germ cells, added sperm aneuploidy, sperm genetics, and DNA fragmentation
- Advanced examination—Research tests, added membrane ion channels
- Emerging methods of semen analysis without a microscope

- Eliminate the hamster zona-free penetration test, human zona binding test, and section on sperm-cervical interaction

Reference ranges of semen variables were more elaborately modified from data from approximately 3500 fertile men from 12 countries across five continents. The new edition is different from older ones because it only recommends one method of assessing semen volume, sperm concentration, motility, and morphology. This simplifies the recommended procedures for laboratories.

Practical Considerations and Expert Opinion

The new sixth edition of the WHO manual aims to provide not only an update of the current methods and thresholds but also an insight into contemporary advances in semen examination, sperm preparation, and cryopreservation, as well as quality control and assurance [8]. Consistent with previous editions, the current sixth edition includes basic examination, semen volume, sperm motility, concentration, morphology, and vitality assessments as well as estimation of sperm numbers in samples with very low sperm concentration. But unlike prior manuals, the sixth edition proposed only one recommended method to standardize the various complex laboratory procedures for quality assurance and reproducibility of results across different laboratories worldwide. Importantly, the reference ranges and limits on various sperm parameters have been revised to remove the present dichotomy separating "fertile" and "infertile" men, so that values of semen parameters are considered as a continuum spectrum of normality, borderline or pathological instead [9].

Furthermore, future expansion of various methodologies on sperm preparation techniques for clinical use or specialized sperm function assays, sperm cryopreservation, and sperm DNA fragmentation will need to be standardized in assisted reproductive technology. Dedicated chapters on extended semen examination that involves specific tests related to immunology and immunological methods to quantify the leukocyte population in semen as well as assessment of interleukins invariably serve as important highlights into the emerging role of biomarkers for male genital tract inflammation and new potential avenues for therapeutic interventions.

Given the significant scientific advances in our reproductive knowledge and modern technology in functional assessment of male infertility, advanced examination with (novel) computer assisted sperm analysis, seminal oxidative stress, and reactive oxygen species as well as sperm chromosomal abnormalities and genetic studies have been highlighted in this new edition although it will require further scientific validation as the evidence is accruing [10]. Epigenetic profiling of spermatozoa is an exciting and rapidly evolving field that will require the formulation of a consensus guideline by the WHO since it has significant bioethical and medicolegal implications [11].

The sixth edition WHO manual functions both as an aid as well as a foundation for human semen examination and processing but is not intended to replace actual clinical management of male infertility. It is anticipated that this latest edition will be widely used as a teaching guide for both basic and more advanced semen analyses workshops and andrology training programs. Although there have been significant advances in the understanding of male reproductive health, the translation from basic science to clinical practice in the management of male infertility is still limited. Men with fertility risk factors or abnormal semen parameters should be referred to a male reproductive specialist for a comprehensive clinical evaluation, informed counseling, and evidence-based therapeutic interventions.

References

1. World Health Organization. Laboratory manual for the examination of human semen and semen-cervical mucus interaction. Singapore: Press Concern; 1980.
2. Barratt CLR, Björndahl L, De Jonge CJ, et al. The diagnosis of male infertility: an analysis of the evidence to support the development of global WHO guidance challenges and future research opportunities. Human Reprod Update. 2017;23:660–80.
3. World Health Organization. WHO Laboratory manual for the examination of human semen and semen-cervical mucus interaction. 2nd ed. Cambridge: Cambridge University Press; 1987.
4. World Health Organization. WHO Laboratory manual for the examination of human semen and sperm-cervical mucus interaction. 3rd ed. Cambridge: Cambridge University Press; 1992.
5. World Health Organization. WHO Laboratory manual for the examination of human semen and sperm-cervical mucus interaction. 4th ed. Cambridge: Cambridge University Press; 1999.
6. World Health Organization. WHO laboratory manual for the examination and processing of human semen. 5th ed. Geneva: World Health Organization; 2010.
7. World Health Organization. WHO laboratory manual for the examination and processing of human semen. 6th ed. Geneva: World Health Organization; 2021.
8. Wang C, Mbizvo M, Festin MP, Björndahl L, Toskin T, et al. Evolution of the WHO "Semen" processing manual from the first (1980) to the sixth edition (2021). Fertil Steril. 2022;117(2):237–45.
9. Chung E, Arafa M, Boitrelle F, Kandil H, Renkel R, Saleh S, et al. The new 6th edition of the WHO laboratory manual for examination and processing of human semen: is it a step toward better standard operating procedure? Asian J Androl. 2022;24(2):123–4.
10. Boitrell F, Shah R, Saleh R, Henkel R, Kandil H, Chung E, et al. The sixth edition of the WHO manual for human semen analysis: a critical review and SWOT analysis. Life (Basel). 2021;11(12):1368.
11. Thirumavalavan N, Gabrielsen JS, Lamb DJ. Where are we going with gene screening for male infertility? Fertil Steril. 2019;111:842–50.

Basic Semen Examinations in Clinical Practice

Role of Semen Examination in the Couple's Fertility Assessment

2

Amarnath Rambhatla and Florence Boitrelle

Introduction

Infertility affects approximately 15% of couples world wide and 50% of the time a male factor is involved [1]. When a couple presents with infertility, it is important to evaluate both the male and female partner. The cornerstone of the male infertility evaluation is the conventional semen analysis, which provides a basic measure of the male reproductive system. This is usually the first test ordered for the male partner as it is non-invasive and relatively inexpensive.

Since the 1980s the World Health Organization (WHO) has standardized the process of the conventional semen analysis and continues to update its manual on how the test should be performed [2]. In 2021, the WHO published the sixth edition of the "Manual for the Examination and Processing of Human Semen". Essentially, the new manual comprises three parts: semen examination; sperm preparation and cryopreservation; and quality control/assurance. The procedures for semen examination (analysis) include basic (routine) examinations, extended examinations (which may be used by laboratories or clinicians in certain situations), and advanced tests (which are not currently recommended for routine use and are primarily for research purposes). The sections on extended and advanced examinations have been written in concordance with current clinical practice, with many older tests being abandoned and new tests being adopted. Furthermore, in this current edition, normal reference ranges have been removed and it is up to the clinician to interpret the results of the semen analysis in the context of fertility potential.

A. Rambhatla
Department of Urology, Vattikuti Urology Institute, Henry Ford Health, Detroit, MI, USA
e-mail: arambha1@hfhs.org

F. Boitrelle (✉)
Reproductive Biology, Andrology, CECOS, Centre Hospitalier Intercommunal de Poissy, Poissy, France

A. Agarwal et al. (eds.), *Human Semen Analysis*,
https://doi.org/10.1007/978-3-031-55337-0_2

It should be noted that conventional semen analyses does not measure the functional capacity of spermatozoa which need to undergo an arduous journey in the female reproductive tract before fertilization can occur. The diagnostic and clinical value of the conventional semen analysis is modest at best as individual semen parameters can exhibit significant variability [3]. Extended and advanced semen examinations have been developed to help more reliably predict a male partner's fertility potential. These tests are not routinely utilized but are indicated in certain clinical and research scenarios. They can help identify dysfunction of sperm, abnormalities of internal sperm components, as well as markers of male reproductive tract inflammation, all of which can reduce fertility capabilities in the male.

In this chapter, we will detail the recommendations for infertility management, explain the place of semen testing in the infertility workup, and review basic semen testing and expanded and advanced sperm function tests. We will also review the recommendations of the three major male infertility guidelines, the American Urologic Association/American Society of Reproductive Medicine (AUA/ASRM), the European Association of Urology (EAU), and the European Academy of Andrology (EAA), regarding when to use these tests.

Semen Analysis in the Initial Work-Up of the Infertile Couple

According to the latest recommendations for the management of infertile men and couples [4], the basic sperm examination is the first analysis to prescribe for men who consult for infertility. This examination is prescribed after questioning the man about his history, symptoms, sexual and reproductive history, but it is prescribed before the man's clinical examination [4]. The decision tree below summarizes the recommendations for prescribing semen analysis and clinical examination in the man consulting for infertility (Fig. 2.1).

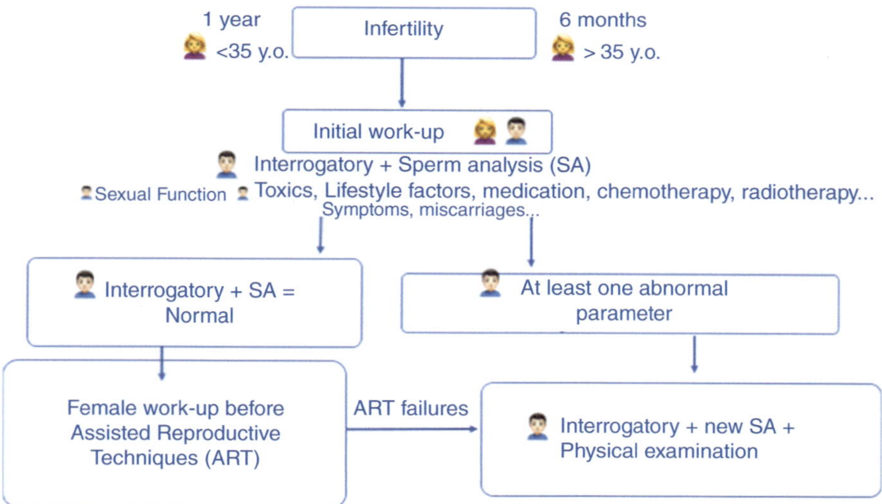

Fig. 2.1 Decision tree for the initial assessment of couples and men consulting for infertility, according to international recommendations [4]

Basic Semen Parameters

Basic semen examination is a panel of tests that are combined to provide an estimate of the male partner being able to contribute to conception. Parameters include semen volume, coagulation, liquefaction, consistency, sperm count, sperm motility, sperm morphology, sperm viability, presence of round cells, and leukocyte concentration. Since the 1980s, the WHO has published a reference manual every 10 years that serves as a technical reference guide to the performance of sperm analysis; the latest manual was published in July 2021 [5]. The purpose of performing sperm analysis is to obtain information on spermatogenesis and the proper functioning of the male accessory glands. The main purpose of the semen analysis is to identify patients at risk of infertility and to distinguish them from fertile patients. This methodology consisting of studying and comparing the spontaneous fertility of couples, according to sperm parameters has allowed a change in the WHO manual in 2010 (fifth edition). Standards and reference intervals of sperm parameters were defined according to the statistical method of the fifth percentile. This methodology was also used in the sixth and last edition of the manual, though with the caveat that this has limitations. Between the fifth and sixth editions of the WHO manual, these fifth percentile values changed only slightly [2]. The addition of data collected from 1789 men in couples, together with data collected from 1800 other couples before 2010, allowed the establishment of percentile values for each sperm parameter (Table 2.1).

Sperm analyses allow the diagnosis of infertility due to azoospermia (total absence of sperm in the ejaculate) and contribute to the diagnosis of other causes of male infertility. In case of normal sperm parameters, then the female partner needs to undergo evaluation for female factor infertility. If both the male and female evaluation are normal, then the couple is classified as having unexplained infertility. In case of normal sperm parameters and in the absence of elements suggestive of male infertility, it is not necessary to re-check the sperm results in a couple consulting for an initial fertility assessment. In the case of abnormal sperm parameters, the results of a single ejaculate examination may be sufficient to decide the next steps in a male infertility investigation [6–12]. However, due to the variability of sperm parameters from one ejaculate to another, repeated sperm analysis (examination of two or three different ejaculates) can provide accurate averaged values of sperm parameters [7–17]. Thus, if one or more sperm parameters are abnormal (below the fifth percentile values) [5], or if any element of the history is suggestive of male infertility, the

Table 2.1 Fifth percentile values obtained in fertile men ($n = 3589$ men), according to [5]		
Semen volume (mL)		1.4 (1.3–1.5)
Total sperm count (10^6 per ejaculate)		39 (35–40)
Total sperm motility (%)		42 (40–43)
Progressive sperm motility (%)		30 (29–31)
Sperm vitality (%)		54 (50–56)
Normal sperm forms (%)		4 (3.9–4)

couple should be referred for specialist management. A full history, clinical examination and sperm analysis are then recommended [4].

Extended Tests

The WHO sixth edition has grouped together a series of extended semen tests that are not part of the routine semen analysis but can be used to better evaluate sperm function and male fertility potential in certain clinical scenarios. These tests include indices of multiple sperm defects, sperm DNA fragmentation (SDF), genetic and genomic tests, tests related to immunology and immunological methods, assessment of interleukins, assessment of immature germ cells, testing for antibody coating of spermatozoa, biochemical assays for accessory gland function, and assessment of sequence of ejaculation [5].

Indices of multiple sperm defects consist of a detailed assessment of the incidence of morphological abnormalities compared to an evaluation of the percentage of morphologically normal sperm reported in the basic semen evaluation. This consists of three indices known as the teratozoospermia index (TZI), multiple anomalies index (MAI), and sperm deformity index (SDI) which evaluate the sperm head, mid-piece, and principal piece [5]. The AUA/ASRM, EAU, and EAA male infertility guidelines suggest Kruger morphology assessment of spermatozoa as part of a semen analysis and do not mention use of indices of multiple sperm defects [4, 18, 19]. This is due to poor sensitivity and specificity of indices of multiple sperm defects, and morphology in general, in male infertility except in specific situations that have a genetic basis for abnormal morphology such as macrocephaly, globozoospermia, or fibrous sheath dysplasia [20]. However, indices of multiple sperm defects can be considered in situations where a detailed assessment of morphology is needed.

SDF can occur when there is damage to base pairs or a break in one or both DNA strands in chromosomes within spermatozoa [21, 22]. SDF can be caused by both intrinsic and extrinsic factors and an increase in SDF is associated with male infertility [23]. Abnormal SDF may affect embryo development, implantation, and clinical pregnancies in both natural and assisted reproduction [5]. Four assays that assess SDF are described in the WHO sixth edition: terminal deoxynucleotidyl transferase biotin-dUTP nick end labeling (TUNEL), sperm chromatin dispersion test (SCD), Comet assay, and acridine orange flow cytometry. It is unclear which of the tests best evaluates SDF and there is no consensus on thresholds for normal limits. The AUA/ASRM male infertility guideline suggests that SDF should be checked in male partners of couples with recurrent pregnancy loss (RPL) [4]. The EAU guideline is in concordance with this and also includes testing for men with unexplained infertility as well as instances when assisted reproductive technology (ART) has failed [19]. The EAA guideline states that SDF should be evaluated prior to consideration of ART [18]. This would lead to an opportunity to correct reversible causes of elevated SDF such as cessation of smoking and other lifestyle modifications, repair of varicocele, and treatment of male accessory gland infections. All indications of these tests will be discussed in the chapter "Sperm DNA fragmentation."

Sperm fluorescence in situ hybridization (FISH) is a cytogenetic test that can detect sperm aneuploidy. Gonodotoxic therapies, such as chemotherapy and radiation, or advanced paternal age can lead to aneuploidy in sperm [19]. If an aneuploid sperm fertilizes an euploid egg, it can lead to chromosomal abnormalities in the offspring such as trisomy of an autosome, sex chromosome abnormalities such as 47 XXX or 47 XXY, or Robertsonian translocations [5] The indications for spermatozoa FISH testing are not detailed in the WHO manual and remain unclear but it has been applied for couples with recurrent pregnancy loss and repetitive implantation failure [24]. The AUA/ASRM, EAU, and EAA male infertility guidelines do not indicate when this test should be utilized.

Leukocytes are normally present in most semen samples but an abnormally high concentration is known as leukocytospermia and can increase reactive oxygen species (ROS) leading to elevated SDF. Leukocytospermia has several causes including infection or inflammation in the male genitourinary tract, varicoceles, urethral strictures, infrequent ejaculation, smoking and alcohol use, and autoimmune conditions. The WHO sixth edition describes two tests to identify neutrophils in semen: staining cellular peroxidase using ortho-toluidine and pan-leukocyte immunocytochemical staining (see Chap. 9). In addition there are protocols for the assessment of interleukins, which are a marker of male genital tract inflammation, as well as round cells in the semen. The AUA/ASRM, EAU, and EAA guidelines suggest that if leukocytospermia is identified on semen analysis then consideration should be made for obtaining a semen culture and treatment as it can impact fertility status.

Antisperm antibodies (ASA) are antibodies derived from an immune response that are directed towards sperm antigens. IgA and IgG ASA can be detected in semen, cervical mucus, and blood while IgM are usually detected in blood. These can be identified following a vasectomy, trauma, or infection involving the male reproductive tract. The presence of ASA can impair sperm motility, transit through cervical mucus, and the acrosome reaction [5]. The WHO sixth edition has described direct (mixed antiglobulin reaction and immunobead assay) and indirect (indirect immunobead test) protocols to identify ASA. The AUA/ASRM and EAU guidelines recognize ASA as an immunologic cause of male infertility but testing should only be carried out if it is clinically relevant and will change patient management [4, 19].

Measurement of zinc, fructose, and alpha-glucosidase in the semen can provide important insight into the secretory health of the prostate, seminal vesicles, and epididymides. The WHO sixth edition outlines protocols to measure levels of these substances to aid in making a clinical diagnosis of infection or obstruction. Neither the AUA/ASRM or EAU guidelines mention the clinical usefulness of these tests. The EAA guideline only discusses the utility of the seminal fructose evaluation [18]. History and physical exam, endocrine evaluation, and acidic semen pH with low ejaculate volume are increasingly being used to help identify obstructive causes of male infertility leaving these tests that evaluate the secretory health of the male accessory glands to have limited utilization.

Assessment of sequence of ejaculation is an extended semen test relying on the fact that the initial one third of the ejaculate contains spermatozoa along with prostatic secretions and the latter two thirds contains seminal vesicular fluid [5]. This assessment is not recommended by any of the major male infertility guidelines. The practicality for this test is low due to the specimen collection process which makes this test mostly utilized for research purposes.

Advanced Tests

The WHO sixth edition has identified that male factor infertility may be due to functional defects of sperm rather than due to insufficient production or impaired motility. Advanced semen examinations have been developed to further evaluate how well sperm would function in performing tasks that are required of them to fertilize an egg in the female reproductive tract. These tests include seminal oxidative stress and reactive oxygen species testing, assessment of the acrosome reaction, assessment of sperm chromatin, transmembrane ion flux and transport in sperm, computer aided sperm analysis (CASA), and other emerging technologies [5].

There is increasing evidence that seminal oxidative stress and reactive oxygen species (ROS) play a significant role in male infertility [25–27]. Seminal ROS are produced by leukocytes, immature sperm, and also as a normal byproduct of ATP production [28–30]. A balance between ROS and antioxidants is necessary for optimal sperm function. When there is an imbalance between ROS and antioxidants, a state of oxidative stress (OS) occurs [31] OS can damage the sperm plasma membrane and lead to increased SDF as well as affect concentration, motility, morphology, and capacitation [26, 32]. The term male oxidative stress infertility (MOSI) has been proposed to describe men with infertility and elevated OS who were previously classified as having idiopathic male infertility [33]. The WHO sixth identifies three examinations to measure oxidative stress: luminol, oxidation reduction potential, and total antioxidant capacity. However due to the lack of standardization and evidence from prospective trials, the EAU, AUA/ASRM, and EAA male infertility guidelines do not recommend ROS testing in the routine evaluation of male infertility [4, 18, 19]. Testing should be reserved for specific clinical scenarios and future studies may help shed more light on this.

The acrosome reaction occurs after capacitation and allows for spermatozoa to penetrate the oocyte zona pellucida and fuse with the oocyte plasma membrane. Calcium influx is believed to be an initiating event and can be stimulated by zona pellucida proteins and progesterone [34]. There are two tests detailed in the WHO sixth edition to assess acrosome functionality of sperm: assessment of acrosome status and induced acrosome reaction assay [5]. Further validation of these tests is necessary before they can be recommended in guidelines and be considered in the routine evaluation of male infertility.

Sperm chromatin structure is important for normal fertilization and normal embryo development. Abnormalities of chromatin structure are associated with increased SDF [35]. The aniline blue assessment and chromomycin A3 assessment are described in the WHO sixth edition to assess sperm chromatin structure [5]. Since abnormalities of sperm chromatin structure are closely associated with elevated SDF, they may be considered in scenarios of RPL, unexplained infertility, or previous ART failure. Future studies need to clarify if there is any benefit to performing these tests as opposed to measuring SDF directly, before they can be adopted by clinical guidelines.

Transmembrane ion flux and sperm transport are emerging research areas in male infertility. Several key functions of spermatozoa are activated by intracellular changes in pH, calcium concentration, or membrane voltage [5]. Abnormalities of sperm transmembrane ion flux can potentially impact motility, capacitation, and the acrosome reaction. CatSper gene abnormalities have been associated with male infertility due to altered sperm flagellum which ultimately affects motility and function [36]. Currently there are no clinically available tests under these categories but they remain an important target for future research and development.

Computer assisted semen analysis (CASA) technology uses electronic imaging to visualize spermatozoa and analyze several individual semen parameters including concentration, motility and sperm kinematics, and morphology. The main advantages of CASA over conventional semen analysis is that it ensures reliability, consistency, accuracy, and repeatability when processing several images from a semen sample. In addition, computer systems are being used to evaluate sperm hyperactivation [5]. However, clumping and pleiomorphic morphology of human spermatozoa, generally high viscosity of human semen, and background cellular debris have limited the use of CASA in clinical andrology labs [37]. Emerging technologies are also being developed in the realm of computational and technological advances to improve quality, visualization, and access to diagnostics related to male infertility. All of these diagnostics would need to undergo a rigorous validation process before being considered in male infertility guidelines.

Conclusions

The new edition of the WHO manual is technically sound, providing all the details needed to perform semen analysis. In the current edition of the WHO manual, it is stated that the semen analysis should be used to aid in

- the diagnosis of male reproductive disorders,
- identify lines of investigation,
- choose appropriate initial and follow-up therapy, and
- select appropriate Assisted Reproductive Technology (ART) procedures, if needed.

What is missing are the criteria for clinical use of these parameters especially due to the lack of reference values in the latest edition of the WHO guide. This move leaves the clinician confused about how to interpret the test result and what action to take. Thus, the objective of our book is to help resolve this uncertainty about test interpretation and significance so that the laboratory personnel and clinicians can utilize the WHO sixth edition correctly. This book is dedicated to a detailed presentation of all aspects of the new sixth edition of the WHO manual, discussing all its changes and analyzing both their advantages and limitations in fulfilling the multiple objectives of semen testing as proposed in the new manual. This book is intended to be a guide to the interpretation of the WHO manual. While the WHO manual seeks to evaluate the fertility of a male, our aim is to answer the questions that andrologists, embryologists and reproductive specialists will ask: What to expect from this or that sperm parameter? What are the physiology and causes of alteration of this parameter? What threshold should I use to make a clinical decision as to whether my patient needs treatment? Should I go further in the investigations? What tests should I associate with basic semen analysis? Which ART technique should I choose according to the results? In each chapter, each question will be answered through a systematic review of the literature, and through the development of decision trees and clinical scenarios. The aim is to give each chapter a global view by putting ourselves in the shoes of all readers (scientists, laboratory professionals, urologists, andrologists, reproductive medicine specialists…) and answering all the questions they may have. Thus, our book will bring a clinical perspective, with a "patient-centered" view to the WHO technical guide of semen analysis.

This book will thus be devoted to the clinical value of semen analysis and will make it possible to determine for each parameter, the indications of the test, the criteria of interpretation as well as the complementary examinations to be carried out, the treatments to be prescribed or the ART techniques to be chosen according to the altercations in a given parameter.

Take Home Messages
- When a couple presents with infertility it is important to evaluate both partners as a male factor is involved in 50% of cases.
- The basic male evaluation should include (at least) a history and the basic semen analysis.
- The need for further testing including advanced and extended semen tests, endocrine and genetic evaluation, and imaging should be based on the results of the initial basic evaluation.
- The WHO sixth edition does not provide reference ranges for laboratory examinations and it is up to the clinician to make a determination of the fertility potential based on the results.
- There are several extended and advanced semen tests that are described in the WHO sixth edition. Some of these have been validated in the literature and are being incorporated into male infertility guidelines but many need future studies to evaluate their clinical utility.

References

1. Agarwal A, Baskaran S, Parekh N, Cho CL, Henkel R, Vij S, et al. Male infertility. Lancet. 2021;397(10271):319–33.
2. Boitrelle F, Shah R, Saleh R, Henkel R, Kandil H, Chung E, et al. The sixth edition of the WHO manual for human semen analysis: a critical review and SWOT analysis. Life (Basel). 2021;11(12):1368.
3. Guzick DS, Overstreet JW, Factor-Litvak P, Brazil CK, Nakajima ST, Coutifaris C, et al. Sperm morphology, motility, and concentration in fertile and infertile men. N Engl J Med. 2001;345(19):1388–93.
4. Schlegel PN, Sigman M, Collura B, De Jonge CJ, Eisenberg ML, Lamb DJ, et al. Diagnosis and treatment of infertility in men: AUA/ASRM guideline part I. Fertil Steril. 2021;115(1):54–61.
5. World Health Organization. WHO laboratory manual for the examination and processing of human semen. 6th ed. Geneva: World Health Organization; 2021.
6. Barratt CLR, Björndahl L, De Jonge CJ, Lamb DJ, Osorio Martini F, McLachlan R, et al. The diagnosis of male infertility: an analysis of the evidence to support the development of global WHO guidance-challenges and future research opportunities. Hum Reprod Update. 2017;23(6):660–80.
7. Christman MS, Kraft KH, Tasian GE, Zderic SA, Kolon TF. Reproducibility and reliability of semen analysis in youths at risk for infertility. J Urol. 2013;190(2):683–8.
8. Francavilla F, Barbonetti A, Necozione S, Santucci R, Cordeschi G, Macerola B, et al. Within-subject variation of seminal parameters in men with infertile marriages. Int J Androl. 2007;30(3):174–81.
9. Leushuis E, van der Steeg JW, Steures P, Repping S, Bossuyt PMM, Blankenstein MA, et al. Reproducibility and reliability of repeated semen analyses in male partners of subfertile couples. Fertil Steril. 2010;94(7):2631–5.
10. Mishail A, Marshall S, Schulsinger D, Sheynkin Y. Impact of a second semen analysis on a treatment decision making in the infertile man with varicocele. Fertil Steril. 2009;91(5):1809–11.
11. Stokes-Riner A, Thurston SW, Brazil C, Guzick D, Liu F, Overstreet JW, et al. One semen sample or 2? Insights from a study of fertile men. J Androl. 2007;28(5):638–43.
12. Zhu QX, Gao ES, Pathak N, Wu JQ, Zhou WJ. Single or double semen samples: the dilemma in epidemiological studies on semen quality. Hum Reprod. 2016;31(3):511–7.
13. Berman NG, Wang C, Paulsen CA. Methodological issues in the analysis of human sperm concentration data. J Androl. 1996;17(1):68–73.
14. Carlsen E, Petersen JH, Andersson AM, Skakkebaek NE. Effects of ejaculatory frequency and season on variations in semen quality. Fertil Steril. 2004;82(2):358–66.
15. Castilla JA, Alvarez C, Aguilar J, González-Varea C, Gonzalvo MC, Martínez L. Influence of analytical and biological variation on the clinical interpretation of seminal parameters. Hum Reprod. 2006;21(4):847–51.
16. Keel BA. Within- and between-subject variation in semen parameters in infertile men and normal semen donors. Fertil Steril. 2006;85(1):128–34.
17. Poland ML, Moghissi KS, Giblin PT, Ager JW, Olson JM. Variation of semen measures within normal men. Fertil Steril. 1985;44(3):396–400.
18. Colpi GM, Francavilla S, Haidl G, Link K, Behre HM, Goulis DG, et al. European Academy of Andrology guideline management of oligo-astheno-teratozoospermia. Andrology. 2018;6(4):513–24.
19. Tharakan T, Bettocchi C, Carvalho J, Corona G, Jones TH, Kadioglu A, et al. European Association of Urology guidelines panel on male sexual and reproductive health: a clinical consultation guide on the indications for performing sperm DNA fragmentation testing in men with infertility and testicular sperm extraction in nonazoospermic men. Eur Urol Focus. 2022;8(1):339–50.
20. Gatimel N, Moreau J, Parinaud J, Léandri RD. Sperm morphology: assessment, pathophysiology, clinical relevance, and state of the art in 2017. Andrology. 2017;5(5):845–62.

21. Simon L, Emery B, Carrell DT. Sperm DNA fragmentation: consequences for reproduction. Adv Exp Med Biol. 2019;1166:87–105.
22. Tan J, Taskin O, Albert A, Bedaiwy MA. Association between sperm DNA fragmentation and idiopathic recurrent pregnancy loss: a systematic review and meta-analysis. Reprod Biomed Online. 2019;38(6):951–60.
23. Agarwal A, Majzoub A, Baskaran S, Panner Selvam MK, Cho CL, Henkel R, et al. Sperm DNA fragmentation: a new guideline for clinicians. World J Mens Health. 2020;38(4):412.
24. Rodrigo L, Meseguer M, Mateu E, Mercader A, Peinado V, Bori L, et al. Sperm chromosomal abnormalities and their contribution to human embryo aneuploidy. Biol Reprod. 2019;101(6):1091–101.
25. Agarwal A, Sharma RK, Nallella KP, Thomas AJ, Alvarez JG, Sikka SC. Reactive oxygen species as an independent marker of male factor infertility. Fertil Steril. 2006;86(4):878–85.
26. Agarwal A, Durairajanayagam D, Halabi J, Peng J, Vazquez-Levin M. Proteomics, oxidative stress and male infertility. Reprod Biomed Online. 2014;29(1):32–58.
27. Wagner H, Cheng JW, Ko EY. Role of reactive oxygen species in male infertility: an updated review of literature. Arab J Urol. 2018;16(1):35–43.
28. Aitken RJ, West K, Buckingham D. Leukocytic infiltration into the human ejaculate and its association with semen quality, oxidative stress, and sperm function. J Androl. 1994;15(4):343–52.
29. Cassina A, Silveira P, Cantu L, Montes JM, Radi R, Sapiro R. Defective human sperm cells are associated with mitochondrial dysfunction and oxidant production. Biol Reprod. 2015;93(5):119.
30. Sharma RK, Agarwal A. Role of reactive oxygen species in male infertility. Urology. 1996;48(6):835–50.
31. Walczak-Jedrzejowska R, Wolski JK, Slowikowska-Hilczer J. The role of oxidative stress and antioxidants in male fertility. Cent Eur J Urol. 2013;66(1):60–7.
32. Aitken RJ. Reactive oxygen species as mediators of sperm capacitation and pathological damage. Mol Reprod Dev. 2017;84(10):1039–52.
33. Agarwal A, Parekh N, Panner Selvam MK, Henkel R, Shah R, Homa ST, et al. Male oxidative stress infertility (MOSI): proposed terminology and clinical practice guidelines for management of idiopathic male infertility. World J Mens Health. 2019;37(3):296–312.
34. Beltrán C, Treviño CL, Mata-Martínez E, Chávez JC, Sánchez-Cárdenas C, Baker M, et al. Role of ion channels in the sperm acrosome reaction. Adv Anat Embryol Cell Biol. 2016;220:35–69.
35. Bungum M, Bungum L, Giwercman A. Sperm chromatin structure assay (SCSA): a tool in diagnosis and treatment of infertility. Asian J Androl. 2011;13(1):69–75.
36. Smith JF, Syritsyna O, Fellous M, Serres C, Mannowetz N, Kirichok Y, et al. Disruption of the principal, progesterone-activated sperm Ca^{2+} channel in a CatSper2-deficient infertile patient. Proc Natl Acad Sci USA. 2013;110(17):6823–8.
37. Mortimer ST, van der Horst G, Mortimer D. The future of computer-aided sperm analysis. Asian J Androl. 2015;17(4):545–53.

Macroscopic Semen Parameters

Raghavender Kosgi and Murat Gül

Introduction

Male subfertility and infertility impact numerous couples during their reproductive years. The prevalence of these conditions has been on the rise [1], leading to a substantial burden on healthcare systems [2]. This increase can be attributed to intentional postponement of childbearing by couples, particularly in developed nations, as well as environmental and lifestyle influences [3]. When a couple seeks medical guidance and support for achieving pregnancy, the assessment of female factors typically takes precedence, as it is commonly believed that female factors play a more significant role in determining the choice and success of assisted reproductive technology (ART) [4]. However, there has been a growing recognition of the importance of male factors, which directly or indirectly contribute to 20–70% of infertility cases in couples [4].

Semen analysis plays a pivotal role in evaluating infertile men since it provides a comprehensive assessment of sperm production by the testes, the patency of the reproductive tract, and the secretion activity of accessory glands [5]. This crucial information helps to establish accurate individual diagnoses and serves as the fundamental investigation for assessing male factors in couples suffering from infertility [6].

The process of semen analysis involves several sequential steps, including collection, macroscopic evaluation, and microscopic evaluation. In this particular chapter, we will focus extensively on the macroscopic evaluation of semen.

R. Kosgi (✉)
Department of Andrology and Men's Health, Apollo Hospitals, Jubileehills, Hyderabad, Telangana, India

M. Gül
Department of Urology, School of Medicine, Selcuk University, Konya, Turkey

A. Agarwal et al. (eds.), *Human Semen Analysis*, https://doi.org/10.1007/978-3-031-55337-0_3

Physiology of Human Ejaculate

Human ejaculate is a heterogenous mixture of secretions from male accessory glands and spermatozoa from the testis. Seminal plasma constitutes major portion of the semen. It consists of secretions from prostate, seminal vesicles, bulbourethral glands, epididymis, and small contributions from the litter and Tyson's glands. About 15–30% of semen volume comes from prostate, up to 85% from seminal vesicles and minor contributions from others [7]. Pathologies affecting these glands, alter the volume.

Seminal vesicle secretions contribute to alkaline nature of the semen. It helps in nourishment and transport of spermatozoa. Seminal vesicle secretions contain fructose, fibrinogen, and prostaglandins [7]. Fructose is the energy source for the ejaculated sperms. Fructose is absent/reduced in the ejaculate in cases of aplastic/hypoplastic seminal vesicles, respectively. Fibrinogen helps in the formation of semen coagulum. Prostaglandins are helpful in sperm transport by means of stimulating the contraction of smooth muscles in both male and female reproductive tract and make female cervical mucus receptive to sperms [8]. Bilateral absence or hypoplastic seminal vesicle will result in low volume acidic ejaculate due to available acidic prostatic secretions [9].

Prostate is a walnut-sized male gland located between the urogenital diaphragm and bladder neck surrounding the prostatic part of urethra and ejaculatory ducts, measuring about 18–20 cm^3 [9]. Prostatic fluid consists of acid phosphatases, prostatic specific antigen (PSA), prostate binding protein, citrate, zinc, and many proteins. It helps in sperm activation and sperm function along with seminal vesicle secretions. PSA helps in liquefaction of the semen. Zinc helps in the testes development and acts as an antioxidant, antibacterial agent [10]. Prostatic secretions are acidic in nature [11].

Pair of bulbourethral glands(Cowper's glands) are located below the prostatic gland in the urogenital diaphragm, posterior and lateral to the membranous urethra [12]. They secrete alkaline, mucus like substance known as pre-ejaculate or precum which enters the urethra during sexual arousal and may contain few sperms. It helps in lubrication and removal of residual urine from the urethra [9].

Epididymal secretions contain glycerol-phosphocholine, L-carnitine, myoinositol, and Alpha–glucosidase. Epididymal secretions help in maturation and acquiring motility for spermatozoa [13].

Macroscopic Parameters of Semen: Methodological Considerations

Ensuring a proper collection of the semen specimen and subsequent liquefaction are vital steps in semen assessment. These procedures aim to simulate the natural deposition of semen in the female reproductive tract as closely as possible. Inadequate liquefaction can have a negative impact on the physical and chemical properties of the sample [14]. Once liquefaction has occurred, the macroscopic analysis focuses on simple characteristics such as viscosity, appearance (colour), odour, pH, and volume. These factors are evaluated during the macroscopic analysis phase.

Collection of Semen Samples

Routinely semen sample is obtained near the laboratory in a private room with adequate privacy, to avoid time delay and temperature fluctuations. Sample container is labelled properly before handing it over to the patient. Proper written and verbal instructions are given about complete sample collection. Sample is collected into a clean, wide mouthed sterile container by means of masturbation with 3–5 days of abstinence from infertile male [14].

Liquefaction of Semen

Upon ejaculation, human semen rapidly forms a loose gel-like coagulum within a few seconds, primarily due to the crosslinking of seminal vesicle proteins, namely semenogelins and fibronectin [15]. This coagulum formation serves multiple purposes: it prevents sperm back-flow after deposition in the vagina, protects spermatozoa from the acidic vaginal environment, and helps to defend against immune attack. Subsequently, PSA gradually breaks down this clot, releasing the spermatozoa [16]. The liquefaction time, which can range from a few minutes in vivo to 15–30 min in vitro, depends on the enzymatic ability of PSA to digest the coagulum [14].

While liquefaction can occur at room temperature, it is generally recommended to maintain the specimen at 37 °C. Continuous gentle mixing or rotation of the sample container can aid in facilitating the liquefaction process. The semen sample is typically allowed to undergo liquefaction either at room temperature or in an incubator set at 37 °C for a duration of 15–20 min. The liquefaction process is considered complete when the sample achieves a homogeneous and watery consistency [17].

If liquefaction of the semen sample does not occur within 30 min, it is recommended to incubate the sample for an additional 30 min at either room temperature or in a 37 °C incubator [14]. An incomplete liquefaction of the sample is considered suboptimal for semen analysis [18]. If the semen sample fails to liquefy within 60 min, it is defined as delayed liquefaction [17], and additional mechanical or enzymatic methods may be necessary to break down the coagulum and increase fluidity.

Delayed liquefaction can have various clinical implications. It may suggest an incomplete collection of the ejaculate, potentially indicating the loss of the last portion of the ejaculate. If the collection of the specimen was complete and yet fails to liquefy, it may indicate impaired secretory activity of the male accessory glands, particularly the prostate [19]. Abnormal liquefaction may also indicate conditions such as ejaculatory duct obstruction (EDO), congenital bilateral absence of the seminal vesicles (CBASV), or genital tract infection [19, 20].

Viscosity of Semen

Following liquefaction, it is important to assess the viscosity of the semen sample. Liquefaction and viscosity are separate semen parameters with distinct clinical interpretations. Liquefaction refers to the transition of the sample from a semi-solid to a liquid state over time, whereas viscosity relates to the elastic properties of the sample after complete liquefaction.

To evaluate the viscosity of the semen, a disposable plastic pipette with an approximate diameter of 1.5 mm is used. A portion of the semen sample is aspirated into the pipette and then allowed to drop freely by applying gentle pressure. In normal cases, small dispersed drops are observed without the formation of any semen threads, indicating normal viscosity [14]. However, if a semen thread with a length exceeding 2 cm is formed, it indicates hyperviscosity [21]. The degree of hyperviscosity can be classified as slight, moderate, or high based on the length of the thread formed. Samples with a thread length of 2–4 cm are considered slightly hyperviscous, those with a thread length of 4–6 cm are categorized as moderately hyperviscous, and samples with a thread length greater than 6 cm are labelled as highly hyperviscous [21].

Semen hyperviscosity can be indicative of dysfunction in the accessory glands [21]. Abnormal viscosity has been linked to reduced function of the prostate or seminal vesicles, as these glands contribute the most to seminal plasma. Additionally, infections and inflammation of the accessory glands or other male fertility-related conditions can also cause semen hyperviscosity, even in individuals with normally functioning accessory glands [22].

Hyperviscosity hampers normal sperm motility, and the resistance created by the trapping effect can interfere with the energy required to achieve a certain velocity, thereby compromising sperm quality [21]. Although the exact mechanisms through which hyperviscosity affects male fertility require further investigation, it has been associated with lower fertilization rates in ART, disrupted embryo development, and increased rates of pregnancy failure [23].

Semen Colour

A normal liquefied Semen sample has a grey-opalescent appearance. It is less opaque if sperm count is too low. Sometimes, clear, colourless, viscous ejaculate may be from Cowper's gland secretion. Reddish-brown ejaculate may be because of presence of red blood cells (hemospermia) [14]. Appearance of semen in various conditions is given in Table 3.1.

Table 3.1 Appearance of semen

Colour of the semen	Cause
Grey-opalescent	Normal
Reddish-brown	Hemospermia
Slight yellowish	Prolonged abstinence
Clear yellow	Jaundice, vitamins or drugs
Brown	Spinal cord injury

Table 3.2 Causes of hemospermia

Infections/inflammatory	Cysts
Epididymitis	Seminal vesicle cyst
Epididymo-orchitis	Ejaculatory duct cyst
Prostatitis	Midline prostatic cysts
Seminal vesiculitis	Utricular cysts
Urethritis	Mullerian duct cyst
Calculi	**Obstruction**
Seminal vesicles	Ejaculatory duct obstruction
Ejaculatory duct	Seminal vesicular duct obstruction
Prostatic	Stricture urethra
Bladder/urethral	
Vascular malformations	**Miscellaneous**
Urethra	Prolonged abstinence
Prostatic varices	Anticoagulants/ antiplatelets
Seminal vehicles	Transrectal biopsy of prostate
	Radiotherapy

Hemospermia

Blood in the semen is known as hemospermia. It is also called as hematospermia or bloody ejaculate. It is commonly seen between 30 and 40 years of age but not uncommon in elderly. Various aetiologies such as infections, inflammations, cysts, tumours, obstructions, and vascular malformations of male reproductive tract are implicated [24] (Table. 3.2).

Duration of hemospermia, association with pain, clots, amount of bleeding, number of episodes, lower urinary tract symptoms should be noted. Persistent hemospermia is of clinical significance than the occasional episodic bleeding [25]. Thorough physical examination, focussing on the external genitalia and digital rectal examination is more important to find out any lumps in the testes, spermatic cord, prostatic nodules, and signs of infections/inflammation [26].

Laboratory investigations like, complete blood picture, routine urine analysis, prothrombin time with international normalized ratio, prostatic specific antigen, urine cytology, semen culture and urine culture, urine for AFB/Gene X pert culture, urethral swab and radiological studies like ultrasound of the abdomen, transrectal ultrasound are tailored to the patient presentation [27]. A computerized tomography (CT) scan of the abdomen and pelvis, magnetic resonance imaging (MRI) of abdomen and pelvis, urethra-cystoscopy and seminal vesiculoscopy are performed in persistent cases of hematospermia [26].

Though it is alarming to the patient, in majority of the cases it is of benign nature with self-limiting course [28]. Counselling and reassurance are the most important aspects to alleviate the patient anxiety. Infective/inflammatory causes can be dealt with antibiotics and anti-inflammatory agents. Hematospermia of prostatic origin may resolve the finasteride and alpha-blockers [29].

Regular follow-up is needed to monitor the patient. Most of the case resolve over a period of 2–3 months. In case of persistent hematospermia further evaluation and treatment according to the aetiological agent is needed. Seminal vesiculoscopy and cystourethroscopy are both diagnostic and therapeutic modalities with utilization of laser energy [25, 30]. Tumours of the male reproductive tract are dealt, based on the nature (benign/malignant), stage of the disease and considering various other parameters.

Semen Odour

Evaluation of seminal odour is added in sixth edition of WHO [14]. Smell of ejaculate may vary according to the individual perception. It is subjective in nature and difficult to standardize. But strong urinary odour or putrefaction has got clinical significance. It should be noted. In the era of new viral pandemics, it will jeopardize the safety of the lab personnel against respiratory illness [14].

Semen pH

pH measurement is a crucial aspect of semen analysis. It helps in assessing the acidity or alkalinity of the semen sample. Seminal vesicle secretions are primarily alkaline, while prostatic secretions are acidic. The overall pH of semen, under normal conditions, is mainly determined by the volume of seminal vesicle secretions, resulting in an alkaline pH [18].

An abnormal pH level in semen analysis can provide important insights into the functioning of the accessory glands, completeness of ejaculate collection, or the presence of an infection. If the pH exceeds 7.8, it may indicate accessory gland dysfunction or incomplete collection of the ejaculate, as well as the possibility of an infection [14].

On the other hand, if the semen sample has a pH level below 7.0, along with low volume and low sperm count/zero sperm count, potential diagnoses to consider are ejaculatory duct obstruction or congenital bilateral absent vas deference (CBAVD) [31]. These conditions should be considered as differential diagnoses when encountering semen samples with low pH, reduced volume, and decreased/zero sperm numbers.

Semen Volume

Accurate measurement of semen volume is most important, as it reflects the secretory function of the accessory glands [11]. Total number of spermatozoa, total number of non-sperm cells and the total amount of biochemical markers per ejaculate are calculated based on the semen volume [14]. Semen volume reliable estimation will give more accurate values of semen parameters.

Semen volume is measured by weighing the sample. Patient is given sterile, labelled, pre-weighed, wide mouthed container for sample collection. Volume is measured immediately within 5 min of collection. Container weight is subtracted to derive actual semen volume considering the Semen density as 1 g/mL [14].

Semen volume is also measured by completely aspirating the sample into a sterile graduated disposable serological pipette. Aspirating the entire sample into a pipette or syringe and decanting it into a measuring cylinder is not recommended, as it underestimates the volume. Unfortunately, majority of the labs still follow these methods [14].

Semen volume less than 1.5 mL is considered as hypovolemia [32]. Most common cause of low volume is spillage due to improper collection. Short abstinence, severe hypogonadism, partial retrograde ejaculation, partial/complete obstruction of ejaculatory ducts/seminal vesicular ducts, hypoplasia/agenesis of seminal of vesicles. Neurological causes such as multiple sclerosis, diabetic neuropathy, spinal cord injury and drugs like alpha blockers, antidepressants, bladder neck surgeries, transurethral resection of prostate, retroperitoneal lymph node dissection may cause low volume ejaculate due to ejaculatory dysfunction [33].

Semen volume more than 5–6 mL is considered as hypervolemia. It may be because of prolonged abstinence, seminal vesiculitis, or prostatitis. It may interfere with fertilization by diluting the sperms [32].

Summary

Macroscopic evaluation encompasses several crucial observations that may not be quantitatively measured or controlled by traditional numerical methods, but still hold significant clinical importance. These qualitative assessments include the evaluation of viscosity, pH, colour, odour, and volume of semen and provide valuable information that contributes to the overall interpretation of the semen analysis results, guides for further evaluation and management.

Take Home Messages

- Physiologic aspects of human ejaculate.
- Significance of semen volume in the assessment of functional status of the male accessory glands.
- The value of semen pH measurement in cases presented with low volume ejaculates.

- Diagnostic significance of semen colour in some cases of male infertility.
- Clinical implications and management of semen samples with delayed liquefaction and high viscosity.
- Laboratory and clinical implications of the finding of hematospermia.

References

1. Skakkebaek NE, et al. Male reproductive disorders and fertility trends: influences of environment and genetic susceptibility. Physiol Rev. 2016;96:55–97. https://doi.org/10.1152/physrev.00017.2015.
2. ESHRE Capri Workshop Group. Economic aspects of infertility care: a challenge for researchers and clinicians. Hum Reprod. 2015;30:2243–8. https://doi.org/10.1093/humrep/dev163.
3. Lalinde-Acevedo PC, et al. Physically active men show better semen parameters than their sedentary counterparts. Int J Fertil Steril. 2017;11:156–65. https://doi.org/10.22074/ijfs.2017.4881.
4. Agarwal A, Mulgund A, Hamada A, Chyatte MR. A unique view on male infertility around the globe. Reprod Biol Endocrinol. 2015;13:37. https://doi.org/10.1186/s12958-015-0032-1.
5. Centola GM. Semen assessment. Urol Clin North Am. 2014;41:163–7. https://doi.org/10.1016/j.ucl.2013.08.007.
6. Jequier AM. Clinical andrology—still a major problem in the treatment of infertility. Hum Reprod. 2004;19:1245–9. https://doi.org/10.1093/humrep/deh269.
7. Heath JW, Young B. Wheater's Functional Histology. 4th edi. Churchill Livingstone, London, 2000.
8. Hafez ESE. Techniques of human andrology, vol. 1. Amsterdam: North-Holland; 1977.
9. Risbridger GP, Taylor RA. Knobil and Neill's physiology of reproduction. Amsterdam: Elsevier; 2006. p. 1149–72.
10. Colagar AH, Marzony ET, Chaichi MJ. Zinc levels in seminal plasma are associated with sperm quality in fertile and infertile men. Nutr Res. 2009;29:82–8. https://doi.org/10.1016/j.nutres.2008.11.007.
11. Kandeel FR. Male reproductive dysfunction: pathophysiology and treatment. Boca Raton, FL: CRC Press; 2007.
12. Chughtai B, et al. A neglected gland: a review of Cowper's gland. Int J Androl. 2005;28:74–7.
13. Turner T. On the epididymis and its role in the development of the fertile ejaculate. J Androl. 1995;16:292–8.
14. Boitrelle et al. The sixth edition of The Who manual for human semen analysis: a critical review and swot analysis. Life. 2021.
15. De Lamirande E. Seminars in thrombosis and hemostasis. New York: Thieme Publishers, Inc.; 2007.
16. Rodríguez-Martínez H, Kvist U, Ernerudh J, Sanz L, Calvete JJ. Seminal plasma proteins: what role do they play? Am J Reprod Immunol. 2011;66(Suppl 1):11–22. https://doi.org/10.1111/j.1600-0897.2011.01033.x.
17. Cooper TG, et al. World Health Organization reference values for human semen characteristics. Hum Reprod Update. 2010;16:231–45. https://doi.org/10.1093/humupd/dmp048.
18. Sikka SC, Hellstrom WJ. Current updates on laboratory techniques for the diagnosis of male reproductive failure. Asian J Androl. 2016;18:392–401. https://doi.org/10.4103/1008-682x.179161.
19. Agarwal A, Bragais FM, Sabanegh E. Laboratory assessment of male infertility—a guide for the urologist. Eur Urol Rev. 2009;4:70–3.

20. Andrade-Rocha FT. Physical analysis of ejaculate to evaluate the secretory activity of the seminal vesicles and prostate. Clin Chem Lab Med. 2005;43:1203–10. https://doi.org/10.1515/cclm.2005.208.
21. Du Plessis SS, Gokul S, Agarwal A. Semen hyperviscosity: causes, consequences, and cures. Front Biosci (Elite Ed). 2013;5:224–31.
22. Elia J, et al. Human semen hyperviscosity: prevalence, pathogenesis and therapeutic aspects. Asian J Androl. 2009;11:609–15. https://doi.org/10.1038/aja.2009.46.
23. Esfandiari N, Burjaq H, Gotlieb L, Casper RF. Seminal hyperviscosity is associated with poor outcome of in vitro fertilization and embryo transfer: a prospective study. Fertil Steril. 2008;90:1739–43. https://doi.org/10.1016/j.fertnstert.2007.09.032.
24. Munkelwitz R, et al. Current perspectives on hematospermia: a review. J Androl. 1997;18:6–14.
25. Drury RH, King B, Herzog B, Hellstrom WJG. Hematospermia etiology, diagnosis, treatment, and sexual ramifications: a narrative review. Sex Med Rev. 2022;10:669–80. https://doi.org/10.1016/j.sxmr.2021.07.004.
26. Mulhall JP, Albertsen PC. Hemospermia: diagnosis and management. Urology. 1995;46:463–7. https://doi.org/10.1016/s0090-4295(99)80256-8.
27. Torigian DA, Ramchandani P. Hematospermia: imaging findings. Abdom Imaging. 2007;32:29–49. https://doi.org/10.1007/s00261-006-9013-3.
28. Furuya S, Masumori N, Takayanagi A. Natural history of hematospermia in 189 Japanese men. Int J Urol. 2016;23:934–40. https://doi.org/10.1111/iju.13176.
29. Badawy AA, Abdelhafez AA, Abuzeid AM. Finasteride for treatment of refractory hemospermia: prospective placebo-controlled study. Int Urol Nephrol. 2012;44:371–5. https://doi.org/10.1007/s11255-011-0057-0.
30. Byon S-K, Rha K-H, Yang S-C. Transutricular seminal-vesiculoscopy in the management of hematospermia. Korean J Urol. 2001;42:329–33.
31. Weiske WH, Sälzler N, Schroeder-Printzen I, Weidner W. Clinical findings in congenital absence of the vasa deferentia. Andrologia. 2000;32:13–8.
32. Poland ML, et al. Variation of semen measures within normal men. Fertil Steril. 1985;44:396–400.
33. Roberts M, Jarvi K. Steps in the investigation and management of low semen volume in the infertile man. Can Urol Assoc J. 2009;3:479.

Sperm Concentration and Total Sperm Count

4

Rafael Favero Ambar, Evangelos Maziotis,
and Mara Simopoulou (iD)

Introduction

Male factor infertility constitutes a major health issue induced by several factors such as testicular and hypothalamic-pituitary diseases, genetic conditions, cancer, systemic diseases, lifestyle-associated factors or oxidative stress [1–4]. Semen analysis constitutes a fundamental method for the evaluation of reproductive potential [5]. Furthermore, conventional semen parameters like total sperm count and semen concentration may provide insight into the testicular functionality of spermatozoa production (*WHO Laboratory Manual for the Examination and Processing of Human Semen*, n.d.). Hence, it is essential for the semen analysis protocol to be standardized, ascertaining uniformity and relevance to the test. In this context, over the past 40 years, the World Health Organization (WHO) Infertility Task Force have developed guidelines that represent global male population demographics noting the technological and scientific evolution in the field of reproduction [6].

It has been reported that conventional semen analysis may provide inadequate information regarding the etiology of infertility. To elaborate on that, semen analysis may identify azoospermia, but it may not provide data regarding the causative factor such as obstructive and non-obstructive azoospermia, hypogonadism or

R. F. Ambar
Urology Department of Centro Universitario em Saude do ABC/Andrology Group at Ideia Fertil Institute of Human Reproduction, Santo André, Brazil

Urology Department of Hospital do Servidor Público Estadual HSPE/IAMSPE, São Paulo, Brazil

E. Maziotis · M. Simopoulou (✉)
Department of Physiology, Medical School, National and Kapodistrian University of Athens, Athens, Greece

A. Agarwal et al. (eds.), *Human Semen Analysis*, https://doi.org/10.1007/978-3-031-55337-0_4

microdeletions of the Y chromosome (AZF) [7, 8]. Moreover, it cannot investigate sperm dysfunctions at cellular and molecular levels [9]. Thus, the accurate diagnosis of male infertility may require further investigation employing more advanced tests [7].

Hitherto, several invasive and non-invasive approaches have been developed for the management of male factor infertility. Techniques such as microsurgical epididymal sperm aspiration (MESA), testicular sperm extraction (TESE), testicular sperm aspiration (TESA), percutaneous epididymal sperm aspiration (PESA) have been employed for sperm retrieval surgically, in men with azoospermia [10, 11]. Additionally, intracytoplasmic sperm injection (ICSI) constitutes a fundamental method in cases of low sperm count, as only one spermatozoon is required to achieve oocyte fertilization [12].

The current chapter investigates:

- Methodology of sperm concentration and total sperm count testing.
- Sperm count and concentration diagnosing fertility and infertility.
- Sperm count and concentration and etiological diagnosis of male reproductive functions and dysfunctions.
- Further investigations of low sperm count and concentration.
- Sperm count and concentration and non-ART management—Treatment and treatment response monitoring.
- Sperm count and concentration and ART management.

Additionally, herein, two clinical scenarios as well as key points are included.

Physiology: Methodology of Sperm Concentration and Total Sperm Count Testing

Explaining the Test

Spermatogenesis is a series of complex processes occurring in the seminiferous tubules, leading to the production of the mature male gamete. This process includes the proliferation of spermatogonia and their differentiation into spermatocytes, which in turn divide meiotically producing spermatids. Round spermatids undergo maturation leading to the development of mature spermatozoa into the testicular tubule lumen [13]. It has been estimated that the spermatogenic process might vary between 42 and 76 days [14]. Furthermore, it has been reported that the daily sperm production per man ranges from 150 to 275 millions spermatozoa [13]. The total sperm count per ejaculate and the sperm concentration have been associated with both time to pregnancy [15] and pregnancy rates [16] and constitute predictors of conception [17].

Sperm concentration has been defined as the number of spermatozoa in millions per 1 mL of semen and is a function of the number of spermatozoa and the volume of fluid diluting them [18]. Total sperm count has been designated as the total number of sperm in the ejaculate and is obtained by multiplying the sperm concentration by the semen volume [18]. According to the WHO laboratory manual for the examination and processing of human semen, published in 2021, semen analysis includes the estimation of semen concentration and the total number of spermatozoa among several semen parameters [19].

Regarding the accurate assessment of the aforementioned parameters, a wet preparation and dilution of the ejaculate are required to immobilize spermatozoa and allow the separation of individual cells. The diluted samples are transferred into a hemocytometer, which consist of a thick glass microscope slide etched with a grid-like pattern. WHO recommends the employment of improve Neubauer hemocytometer for sperm count following the loading of the hemocytometer, sperm concentration is estimated from the number of spermatozoa observed in an entire high magnification microscopic field [19, 20].

Manual sperm count presents as the most robust method of sperm concentration evaluation. This method is based on the spermatozoa visualization employing especially designed chambers. Manual sperm count is a widely employed method in semen analysis, as it is relatively simple [20]. This method includes the employment of chambers in which cells may be counted within a known predefined area. While only modified Neubauer hemocytometers are recommended by WHO, a variety of chambers, namely the Makler chamber and disposable slide chambers either featuring a grid or not, are employed in clinical practice [20]. Additionally, spectrophotometers have been employed for the assessment of sperm concentration as an alternative to hemocytometers. This method does not include direct enumeration of sperm, nevertheless, precise and accurate outcomes may be obtained [20].

Computer-assisted semen analysis systems (CASAs) have been employed for automated analysis of sperm images. Employment of CASA provides fairly precise evaluation of sperm concentration [20]. Despite the fact that CASA may provide partial automation of routine semen analysis, CASA lacks wider employment due to its complicated operation [21] (for more information please read the chapter on this subject).

Significance of Sperm Count

The estimation of the total sperm count per ejaculate is of utmost importance in order to evaluate the testicular sperm production [22]. The sperm concentration and ejaculate volume are included in the estimation of the sperm count in the ejaculate. The sperm count is related to the sperm volume, in cases of unobstructed male tract with a short abstinence period [23, 24]. Hence, sperm count reveals the sperm production by the testes, the patency of the male tract and, the number of spermatozoa released to the female oviduct during intercourse [25].

Furthermore, sperm count demonstrates the active reveal of spermatozoa to the urethra through the contractions of smooth muscle in the epididymis and vasa deferentia. This process is affected by nerve signals to smooth muscle cells, like vas deferens, glands, and urinary bladder sphincter [10]. Moreover, smooth muscle cells control blood inflow of blood into and outflow from the erectile tissues of the penis, and the striated bulbocavernosus and perineal muscles affecting the erectile function and the transfer of sperm to the urethra [26].

Sperm concentration in the ejaculate depends on the volume of the secretions from the seminal vesicles and prostate. In contrast to sperm count, sperm concentration has not been related to testicular function, while it has been associated to fertilization and pregnancy rates [27].

Natural Variation

The sperm count may be affected by numerous variants, namely, environmental factors and lifestyle choices. To elaborate on this, smoking, alcohol consumption, obesity, diabetes, physical exercise, environment pollutants, and asymptomatic infections may constitute contributors of reactive oxygen species (ROS) production [28]. It has been reported that increased ROS levels in seminal plasma may reduce sperm count, leading to oligozoospermia [29]. Oligozoospermia has been associated with apoptosis within the developing germ cell population and increased DNA fragmentation index [28].

It has been observed that ejaculatory abstinence has an impact on semen parameters. Particularly, longer abstinence seems to enhance semen volume and sperm count [30]. According to WHO, semen analysis should be performed on sperm samples produced following a minimum of 2 days and a maximum of 7 days of abstinence [19]. Furthermore, sperm concentration seems to be affected by abstinence time as well as average sleep duration [31]. An additional contributing factor regarding sperm count and concentration seems to be age. Aging may impair sperm parameters, increasing oxidative stress, and ROS production [28, 31]. It has been reported that the complete collection of the ejaculate is required, in order to accurately evaluate the sperm count. Namely, the first ejaculated fraction constitutes the 15–45% of the whole ejaculate, being rich in sperm, epididymal, and prostatic secretions [32].

More Than One Test May Be Required

Spermatogenesis is a complex process that may be impeded by several etiologies. Lifestyle, health, and environmental conditions may affect spermatogenesis. Numerous animal studies have reported that heat stress and increased scrotum temperature may impede spermatogenesis lowering sperm concentration and motility [33, 34]. Moreover, recent infections even if not directly impacting the reproductive system, as recently demonstrated by COVID-19, may impact sperm quality [35]. Thus, it is necessary to repeat the test at least one more time prior to diagnosing oligozoospermia, cryptozoospermia, or azoospermia.

Special Measures If Count Is Very Low

It has been reported that in cases of low number of spermatozoa in the wet preparations, the semen sample may be centrifuged to determine the presence of spermatozoa [36]. This is essential for cases where no spermatozoa are detected in the semen sample. Following centrifugation if spermatozoa are detected and the whole process is repeated following an adequate interval assessing a new spermatogenesis cycle yielding similar results, the patient may be diagnosed with cryptozoospermia. In the case that no spermatozoa are observed in either case, then azoospermia diagnosis may be established. However, centrifugation is not recommended for the general population as it may impair sperm motility [37]. Besides centrifugation, sperm concentration may be evaluated by scanning wet preparations based on high-power field (HPF) observations [6]. Furthermore, the assessment of low sperm count may be performed in large-volume disposable chambers. The employment of fluorescent dye may facilitate the rapid detection of spermatozoa in large chambers scanning [38].

Sperm Count/Concentration and Diagnosis of Fertility and Infertility

Reference Ranges Employed by the WHO Manual

Infertility has been defined as the failure to establish spontaneous pregnancy within 1 year of regular unprotected sexual intercourse [18]. Semen analysis constitutes a fundamental method for the evaluation of reproductive potential and a significant diagnostic approach for the management of male factor infertility [5].

Therefore, the World Health Organization (WHO) has developed guidelines, establishing the methodology of semen analysis in order to achieve uniformity and relevance to this process [6]. The first edition was published in 1980 following four more editions of the WHO manual. Each edition focuses on the changes in global male population demographics, limitations from previous versions, and on the technological and scientific evolution noted in the field of reproduction [39].

In 2021, the sixth edition was published providing details regarding the basic examination and temporal manner, increasing the reproducibility of the protocol in any laboratory [39]. In spite of the simplifying of semen dilutions required for the assessment of sperm count, the estimation of 200 spermatozoa per replicate is still required. Albeit assesing a sample of low spermatozoa number may be more prone to error, it is essential to evaluate with accuracy the low sperm concentrations ($<2 \times 10^6$/mL) [40]. During the last decade, the reference values regarding sperm count, sperm concentration, and sperm volume have been revised based on the current data.

The lower limit value for semen volume has been estimated to be 1.4 mL with 95% confidence interval 1.3–1.5, for sperm concentration 16 million/mL (95% CI: 15–18) and for total sperm count 39 million per ejaculate (95% CI: 35–40), respectively (Table 4.1).

A significant improvement of the WHO manual concerns the adoption of decision limits which may distinguish normal from abnormal ejaculates [39]. The fifth percentile designates the lower reference limit, under which only the 5% of the reference population is estimated. The reference values may facilitate the interpretation of the results from an individual patient, but it is of utmost importance to pay attention regarding the over-interpretation of these limits. To elaborate on this, a degree of inconsistency has been observed with respect to the definition of the reference population [42]. The reference population includes men with infertility with a known time to pregnancy (TTP), in particular, the time to pregnancy should be at least 1 year of unprotected sexual intercourse without achieving a natural conception (TTP >12 months) [42]. However, a natural conception within a year despite problems in the ejaculate may occur. Additionally, men with normal ejaculates may be annotated as infertile due to female infertility factors. The aforementioned indicate the limitations regarding the employment of a dichotomous categorization to fertility. Furthermore, the essential overlap of the outcomes of semen analysis between fertile and infertile men is established knowledge [6]. Hence, the distinct employment of the lower fifth percentile does not constitute an adequate approach to define fertility or infertility, as infertility is a multivariable condition [39].

Hitherto, literature presents with conflicting results regarding the global trend in sperm count [43–45]. A significant reduction in sperm counts with respect to total sperm count and sperm concentration has been reported. Namely, a 50–60% decline among men from "Western" countries has been observed [44].

Table 4.1 In the WHO 2010 (fifth edition) and WHO 2021 (sixth edition), the fifth percentile and the 95% confidence interval of semen parameters were assessed in men from couples who successfully achieved pregnancy within a year of engaging in unprotected sexual intercourse

Semen parameters	WHO [41]	WHO [19, 41]
Semen volume (mL)	1.5; 1.4–1.7	1.4; 1.3–1.5
Sperm concentration (million/mL)	15; 12–16	16; 15–18
Sperm count (million/mL)	39; 33–46	39; 35–40

Additionally, it has been proposed that the decline of sperm counts may induce increased rates of male infertility [44]. Despite this hypothesis, an increase in male infertility rates has not been reported [46]. Male infertility constitutes a multifactorial condition that depends on numerous biological and environmental contributors [43]. Considering the above, it appears that the single metric of sperm count may fail to conclusively present as an adequate measure to determine infertility [47]. This has been verified by studies reporting that men with low sperm counts may achieve conception, in contrast to men featuring higher counts [48, 49].

Sperm Count/Concentration and Etiological Diagnosis of Male Reproductive Functions and Dysfunction

Causes Implied in Sperm Count/Concentration Decreasing

Male fertility may be impaired by abnormal sperm parameters and contributes to 50% of all cases of infertility. The main cause is low quality and quantity of sperm (Christin-Maitre and Young 2022). Sperm concentration can reflect the condition of male fertility and testicular function and it is positively associated with pregnancy rate [50].

Despite significant advances within the past few decades, an etiology for male factor infertility is not able to be identified in up to 50% of patients. The causal factors behind the most severe forms of impaired spermatogenesis are being studied and still need more explanations [51]. Although, a 9-year prospective clinical-epidemiological study showed semen impairment could be attributed to aspermia in 46/46 cases (100%), azoospermia in 321/388 cases (82.7%), and cryptozoospermia in 54/130 cases (41.5%). In contrast, 75% of oligozoospermia cases remained unexplained [52].

Decreased sperm concentration (oligozoospermia) may be considered if sperm count drops below 15 million cells/mL of ejaculate and a total sperm number below 39 million/mL [19, 53]. Yet, oligozoospermia can be classified as mild (10–15 million sperm/mL), moderate (5 and 10 million sperm/mL), or severe (<5 million sperm/mL) [50, 54, 55]. Differently, azoospermia refers to an ejaculate with no sperm detected during semen analysis [50, 54, 55].

A wide variety of conditions (Table 4.2) may result in oligozoospermia. Factors implied in decreasing sperm count include obesity, endocrine disturbances, intrinsic testicular defects, testicles trauma or surgery, anatomic alterations, medications, exposure to thermal or chemical environmental factors, or even idiopathic causes [55, 85]. There are various causes of low sperm count, which can be grouped into three main categories: medical, environmental, and lifestyle.

Table 4.2 Main etiology of human oligozoospermia

Predisposing factor	Description	References
Endocrine dysfunction	*Hypothalamic dysfunction* may be seen as a deficiency of GnRH secretion. Usually it is a congenital condition (e.g., Kallmann's syndrome). The diagnosis is based on lack of sexual maturation at puberty *Pituitary dysfunction* may occur because of several pathologies, including neoplasia and infiltrative disease. These situations may lead to deficiency of gonadotropins. On the other hand, pituitary activity can be affected by androgenic steroid use or abuse; glucocorticoid therapy *Adrenal dysfunction* such as adrenal hyperplasia, a congenital disease, leads to an enzymatic deficiency (21-hydroxylase) that impairs glucocorticoid production and increase the production of adrenal androgens due to a higher level of ACTH. This condition suppresses the hypothalamic–pituitary–gonadal axis that will affect normal spermatogenesis *Hyperthyroidism* may cause delayed spermatogenesis, reduced sperm motility, and decreased testis weight *Hypothyroidism* impairs seminal volume, arrest spermatogenesis, decrease the number of seminal tubules	[55–60]
Genetic abnormalities	*Constitutive chromosome abnormalities (e.g., Klinefelter's syndrome)* the extra X chromosome inherited leads to phenotypic abnormalities in Klinefelter patients such as gynecomastia, small form testes, hyalinization of seminiferous tubules, and hypergonadotropic hypogonadism and severe oligospermia/azoospermia *Y chromosome microdeletions* especially involved with azoospermia factor (AZF) locus on the q arm of the Y chromosome lead to male infertility. Depending on the AZF-altered region, the patient may present Sertoli cell only syndrome, maturation arrest, and hypospermatogenesis. Those alterations may be present in different regions of the testes leading to a variable histologic pattern *Cystic fibrosis* leads to a bilateral absence of the vas deferens which causes an obstructive azoospermia. The seminal vesicles atrophy and the epididymis malformation may be associated in in some patients	[57, 59, 61]

Anatomical disorders	*Varicocele* is presented as abnormally dilated and tortuous veins in the pampiniform plexus of the spermatic cord. The pathogenesis is complex and multifactorial and is not fully understood. It is believed that it may lead to scrotal hyperthermia, hypoxia, reflux of renal and adrenal metabolites, hormonal imbalances, and the formation of antisperm antibodies. The increased scrotal temperature impairs normal spermatogenesis affects semen quality, sperm function, testicular histology and reproductive hormones. Oxidative stress and lower levels of total antioxidant capacity leads to oxidation of fatty acids in sperm membrane causing impairment of sperm motility and function *Ejaculatory duct obstruction* may cause aspermia, azoospermia or oligoasthenospermia, among other symptoms. It may be caused by ejaculatory duct malformation, middle line prostatic cysts, fibrosis due to prostatitis or seminal vesiculitis, seminal vesicle stones or scarring after endoscopy *Cryptorchidism* can be an acquired or a congenital disorder. It is associated with reduced number of germ cells, reduced testicular size and germinal cells reduction. The loss of spermatogonial stem cells leads to azoospermia or oligozoospermia	[62–65]
Medications	*Antitumoral drugs* can be gonadotoxic. Combination treatment with radiotherapy and chemotherapy will induce more toxic effect than either modality alone. The gonadotoxic effect of radiotherapy depends on the gonadal dosage and the delivery method. Radiation doses begin to impair spermatogenesis at 0.1–1.2 Gy. Irreversible damage can occur at a 4 Gy dose. Several chemotherapeutic drugs cross the blood–testis barrier and affect germ cells directly or by hyalinization and fibrosis of testicular interstitial tissue *Opioids* at high doses decrease testosterone levels leading to hypogonadism. Morphine increases aromatase expression in testis decreasing its function *Glucocorticoids* may disrupt the hypothalamic–pituitary–gonadal axis, lowering testosterone levels *Sulfasalazine* when used at doses higher than 2 mg/day may cause azoospermia. Although this condition may be reversible *Cyclophosphamide* when used at doses higher than 7.5 mg/day may cause azoospermia. This condition may be irreversible	[59, 66–68]

(continued)

Table 4.2 (continued)

Predisposing factor	Description	References
Testicular injuries	*Infections* such as mumps may cause orchitis. Testicular damage is observed by scrotal swelling and pain. Consequences of mumps orchitis is the atrophy of germinal epithelium and spermatogenesis arrest *Vascular damage (torsion)* when unilateral may induce immunological damage to the opposite testis. Cryptorchidism has a tenfold increase in risk of testicular torsion. Patients with unilateral cryptorchidism show impaired spermatogenesis *Surgery (orchidectomy)* to treat testicular cancer, for example, may cause decrease in sperm count after unilateral orchidectomy. However the condition can be improved within 2–3 years	[59, 69, 70]
Environmental factors	*Pollutants agents* may affect sperm cells by altering plasma membrane fluidity and membrane potential. Also those chemical agents are able to activate the apoptotic cascade, alter mitochondrial function (upregulation of pro-apoptotic genes) and may act as endocrine disruptors *Heavy metals* such as Copper (Cu), Lead (Pb), and Cadmium (Cd) may alter reproductive hormone levels such as testosterone. Also heavy metals are able to induce oxidative stress and are considered endocrine disruptors which are harmful to testis. Cd is able to disrupt the blood–testis barrier, for example *Pesticides* are considered endocrine disrupters that are able to impair semen quality. Pesticides may affect spermatogenesis through a hormonal or genotoxic pathway. The organophosphorus compounds can affect sperm concentration by damaging the seminiferous epithelium through germ cell proliferation *Obesity* may lead to an increase in leptin and insulin resistance and consequently decreased the release of GnRH. Also, it has been observed an increase of aromatase expression leading to androgen deficiency (increase conversion of testosterone into estradiol)	[34, 71–80]

| Lifestyle factors | *Cigarette smoking* is associated with leukocytospermia (source of ROS) and has been negatively associated with sperm count, motility, and morphology
Alcohol consumption affects the hypothalamus–pituitary–gonadal axis interfering with GnRH, FSH, LH, and testosterone production and consequently impairing on spermatogenesis
Illicit drugs, such as cocaine, are associated with spermatogenesis disruption and testicular ultrastructure damage
Psychological stress activate the hypothalamic–pituitary–adrenal axis, increasing glucocorticoid that decrease (or inhibit) testosterone secretion, consequently impairing on spermatogenesis
Sleep disturbance may increase serotonin levels and it is negatively correlated to sperm concentration, motility, and morphology. The sleep duration is positively associated to sperm concentration | [2, 81–84] |

Sperm Count/Concentration Planning of Further Investigations

Diagnosis of oligozoospermia may lead to additional evaluations in order to investigate, and when possible, treat the causes of this diagnosis. This is especially true for cases of severe oligozoospermia defined as less than 5 million spermatozoa per mL [86]. Further evaluation of oligozoospermia may be also required for men presenting with sperm count and/or concentration lower than the 2.5th centile according to WHO manual, namely 29 million spermatozoa per ejaculate and 11 million spermatozoa per mL, respectively. Following routine clinical examination and recording of patient history, the practitioner may be required to suggest additional tests as recommended in Fig. 4.1. Patients below the fifth centile in sperm concentration/count should be referred for hormonal evaluation. The hormonal evaluation includes Follicle Stimulation Hormone (FSH), Luteinizing Hormone (LH), and Testosterone (T) mainly. It may also include evaluation of prolactin levels as well as iron saturation to exclude the possibility of hyperprolactinemia or hemochromatosis. According to the results of the hormonal evaluation, it may be necessary to further refer the patient for genetic testing and counseling. Judging by the physical

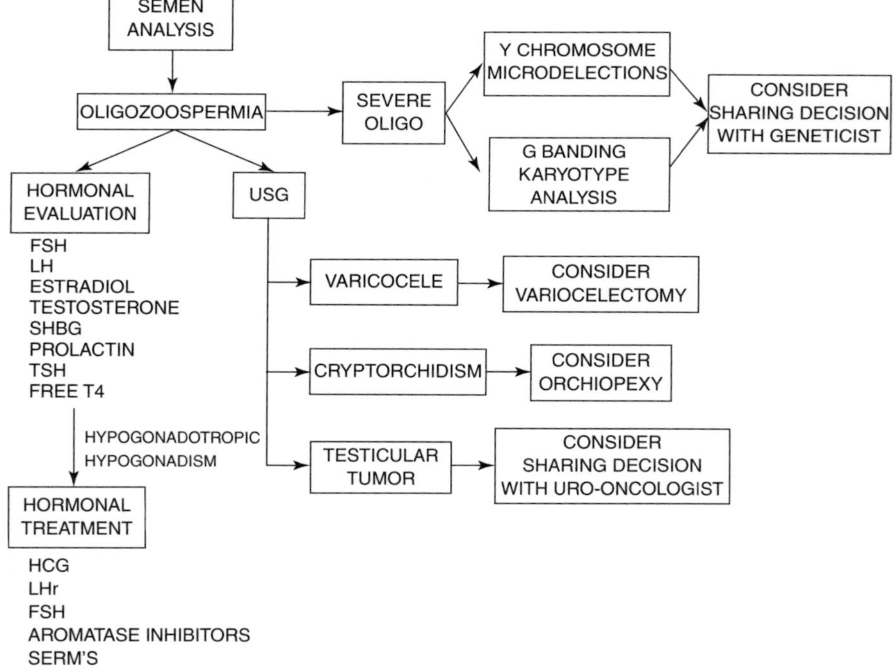

Fig. 4.1 Nomogram about oligozoospermia diagnosis and treatment. *USG* ultrasonography, *FSH* follicle-stimulating hormone, *LH* luteinizing hormone, *SHBG* sex hormone-binding globulin, *TSH* thyroid stimulating hormone, *T4* tetraiodothyronine, *HCG* human chorionic gonadotropin, *LHr* luteinizing hormone receptor, *SERM'S* selective estrogen receptor modulators

examination the practitioner may also suggest ultrasonography evaluation to determine the possibility of undiagnosed cryptorchidism.

It has been reported that oligozoospermia is associated with increased ROS levels and sperm DNA fragmentation. Thus, it may be beneficial for the patients to be referred for the aforementioned evaluations.

Sperm Count/Concentration and Non-ART Management: Treatment and Treatment Response Monitoring

Oligozoospermia is one of the most common causes of male infertility. Although most patients have no apparent cause for this condition, oligozoospermia can be caused by endocrine dysfunction, anatomical abnormalities, medications, or environmental exposures. When the urologist diagnoses a patient with irreversible oligozoospermia, employing assisted reproduction techniques can be suggested. However, it is possible to use clinical treatment for patients with reversible cases of this type of infertility [55].

Management of Oligozoospermic Patient Using Hormonal Treatment

For patients with oligozoospermia secondary to low concentrations of gonadotropins, treatment with gonadotropins can result in significant improvement in sperm production over time. The increase in sperm production can be noticed as early as 3–6 months after starting treatment. In most cases, the fertilizing potential of the sperm of these patients and the couple's ability to conceive are recovered after 1–2 years of therapy. As this human chorionic gonadotropin (hCG) treatment has a lower cost and longer half-life compared to recombinant LH, it is one of the preferred options for treating hypogonadotropic hypogonadism in men [55, 87].

In patients diagnosed with congenital idiopathic hypogonadotropic hypogonadism and/or testicular volume less than 4 mL, treatment with a combination of hCG and FSH is recommended. It is important for the physician to warn those patients who are about to start treatment with hormones for oligozoospermia, especially FSH, about the use of testosterone that inhibits the negative feedback on FSH secretion [55, 87, 88]. On the other hand, some researchers believe that reports of improved sperm parameter need confirmation and that are inadequate data to support gonadotropin therapy [89, 90].

Clomiphene citrate is a selective estrogen receptor modulator widely used to induce ovulation in infertile women. This medication has been used off-label to treat men with oligozoospermia from hypogonadotropic hypogonadism. However, several researchers have shown that the treatment of men with oligozoospermic infertility with clomiphene citrate are conflicting [91–93]. Importantly, aromatase inhibitors should not be given to patients with abnormally functioning or absent pituitary glands as this medication increases gonadotropin release from the reduced negative feedback of estrogen in the pituitary. Despite having been used as a possible treatment for patients with hypogonadotropic hypogonadism, it is not recommended to replace the treatment of hypogonadotropic hypogonadism using gonadotropins with the use of clomiphene citrate, as there is still no adequate scientific evidence for this type of treatment. In addition, antiestrogen therapy has been observed to impair both bone mineral density and male sexual function 94]. Therefore, aromatase inhibitors, when used to treat oligozoospermia, should not be used for periods longer than 12 months [95, 96].

Management of Oligozoospermic Patient Using Antioxidants

Reactive oxygen species (ROS) are essential for normal sperm function. ROS are widely known for their role as second messenger in crucial cellular events related to the fertilization process, such as capacitation, acrosome reaction, hyperactivation, and sperm-oocyte fusion [97]. High levels of ROS may induce oxidative stress leading to cellular damage such as lipid peroxidation of sperm membrane, loss of protein function and genomic and mitochondrial DNA fragmentation. Oxidative stress thereby negatively affects seminal parameters, fertilization rate, embryo development, and pregnancy rates. Increased concentration ROS can be caused among other factors by inflammation, cigarette smoking, caffeine, sleep disturbance, obesity, stress, alcohol intake, pollutant agents, drug abuse. The lifestyle factors correction is the first step of the treatment [98, 99].

Antioxidants have been used to treat patients diagnosed with infertility. Those substances are known to improve sperm motility and mitochondrial function [98]. Huang and co-workers conducted a double-blinded, randomized, controlled trial in oligozoospermic patients to evaluate the effects of folic acid on seminal parameters. They observed that folic acid supplementation has a beneficial effect on oligozoospermia and pregnancy outcome [99]. In accordance, Magdi et al. [100] suggested that antioxidative supplement in combination with modifying the lifestyle factors in a cumulative treatment period significantly improved the basic semen parameters. Bozhedomov and co-workers investigated the efficacy and safety of the L- and acetyl-L-carnitine complex, vitamins A, E, C, selenium, zinc, and other antioxidants to manage oligo, and/or astheno-and/or teratozoospermia. They found out that administration of L- and acetyl-L-carnitines and antioxidant complex (vitamins and minerals) provided some additional positive effect on the concentration of spermatozoa, but did not improve the morphology, progressive sperm motility, and pregnancy rates [101]. Amory et al. conducted a study for the evaluation of isotretinoin, an active form of vitamin A, in patients with oligozoospermia; despite promising results, these results need to be validated in a larger, randomized, blinded study before this treatment can be recommended for men with infertility from oligozoospermia [102]. A recent systematic review and meta-analysis [103] showed a significant improvement in some sperm parameters after supplementation with selenium (alone or in combination with N-acetylcysteine), a combination of zinc and folic acid, a combination of EPA and DHA, a combination of L-carnitine and LAC, and co-enzyme Q10. However, the authors point out that further studies with larger homogeneous cohorts are necessary to assess the effect of vitamins and minerals on the semen analysis, so that final recommendations concerning supplements in the treatment of male factor infertility can be provided.

Others believe that there are weak data about the benefits of antioxidants for improving fertility outcomes and properly controlled randomized controlled trials are needed [104]. A Cochrane review analyzed 61 RTCs that compared different types, doses, and combination of antioxidant therapy with placebo and no treatment groups of 6264 subfertile patients. The review showed that there is low-quality evidence about the benefit of antioxidant supplementation in subfertile patients to improve live-birth rates. Furthermore, it was observed that some adverse events such as mild gastrointestinal upsets during antioxidant therapy. In general, the authors found low-quality evidence in seven RCTs and concluded that benefits of antioxidant therapy to treat men infertility is inconclusive since there RTCs analyzed showed a high risk of bias due to poor reporting of methods of randomization and small overall sample size [59, 110].

Recently a systematic review and meta-analysis of RCTs including 4332 infertile patients conducted by Agarwal et al. (2023) showed that pregnancy rate was significantly higher in patients treated with antioxidants when compared to placebo or untreated groups. The antioxidant therapy was able to improve sperm concentration, sperm progressive motility, sperm total motility, and normal sperm morphology. The study also found that seminal levels of total antioxidant capacity in patients treated with antioxidant were improved when compared with controls. Yet, the seminal malondialdehyde acid was significantly lower in patients treated with antioxidant than control and placebo groups. The meta-analysis concluded that there is robust evidence to recommend antioxidant therapy to infertile patients to improve spontaneous pregnancy rates and sperm parameters (Agarwal; Cannarella; Saleh et al. 2023).

Management of Oligozoospermic Patient with Varicocelectomy

There are several surgical techniques to treat varicocele such as retroperitoneal, microsurgical inguinal and microsurgical subinguinal varicocelectomy. However, a microsurgical varicocelectomy can be considered a better approach since the technique has less post-operative complications [105]. After surgical correction of varicocele, semen parameters may be significantly improved [106–108].

A recent systematic review and metanalyses conducted by Majzoub and colleagues [105] showed that varicocelectomy is an efficient approach for treating severe oligozoospermic patients. Almekaty and co-workers (2019) evaluated the outcome of varicocelectomy in infertile men with severe oligozoospermia comparing internal spermatic artery preservation and artery ligation procedure. They showed that artery preservation varicocelectomy had better seminal parameters outcomes when compared with artery ligation technique. However, in a recent study

Addar et al. [109] observed that the improvement of seminal parameters after microsurgical varicocelectomy for severely oligozoospermic patients is less efficient than reported in mild male factor infertility.

Published scientific studies on the use of medical therapies for men with infertility secondary to oligozoospermia remain inconclusive. These studies are challenging because cases of spontaneous improvement in seminal parameters can be confounded and wrongly considered to be treatment effects. The fact is that there is currently no clear consensus on the clinical management of idiopathic oligozoospermia. Unproven medical practices to treat patients with oligozoospermia are unlikely to cause harm to health but involve costs for the patient. In addition, clinical (non-surgical) treatments make both the doctor and the patient feel that "something is being done" while waiting for a natural conception. However, before initiating hormone therapy or antioxidant supplementation for the management of oligozoospermia, a thorough and careful medical evaluation is essential to rule out any reversible causes [59, 110].

Sperm Count/Concentration and ART Management: Guide ART Choice

ART for Oligozoospermia

While during the past century diagnosis of oligozoospermia could lead to a childless couple, the introduction of in vitro fertilization (IVF) in 1978 and most importantly employment of Intracytoplasmic Sperm Injection (ICSI) practice in 1992 provided a solution for these couples. For couples diagnosed with oligozoospermia as the sole infertility factor, ART in the form of Intrauterine Insemination (IUI) as well as in vitro fertilization may be employed in order to achieve a pregnancy [55]. IUI may present as a cost-effective method, however, it may be less efficient than IVF, and this is especially true for more severe cases. ART in the form of conventional IVF and ICSI may assist in overcoming infertility for the majority of men diagnosed with oligozoospermia [111]. Further to this, additional treatments, namely sperm cryopreservation and testicular sperm extraction, have been proven beneficial for men with severe oligozoospermia.

IUI

Despite the advances in the field of ART, IUI remains a cost-effective method that may be employed as a first-line treatment for male infertility. The IUI procedure includes sperm preparation and may include employment of ovarian stimulation protocols. The techniques for sperm preparation are mainly based on migration, filtration, and centrifugation-based methods (Henkel et al. 2012). The techniques of sperm preparation are thoroughly discussed later herein (Chap. 17). Briefly the sperm preparation is commonly performed employing the swim-up technique, the density-gradient centrifugation (DGC), a combination of both or the novel magnetic-activated cell sorting (MACS) technique. Albeit IUI has been widely employed for decades, no consensus has been reached on the lower limit of sperm count to proceed for IUI, although a cut-off level of 5 million spermatozoa per mL has been proposed (Aribarg et al. 1995). It should be mentioned that according to the European Registry of ESHRE, IUI live-birth rates seem to be less than half when compared to IVF/ICSI (8.9% vs 23%) (Wyns et al. 2021).

IVF/ICSI

Conventional IVF and ICSI have been widely employed for the treatment of infertility. Since its inception in 1992, ICSI has become the gold standard when facing male infertility. Briefly, following oocyte retrieval, oocytes are denudated from the cumulus oophorous, employing enzymatic and mechanical denudation. This process is commonly called "stripping" allowing for oocyte maturity status identification. Following this, oocytes featuring an extruded first polar body indicating appropriate maturity are then injected with a single spermatozoon. When called to choose between IVF and ICSI, no consensus has been reached regarding the cut-off value of the sperm count. Most laboratories rely decision-making on the Total Motile Sperm Count (TMSC) of the sperm following preparation [112]. This identified inconsistency in decision-making on ICSI practice may be generating controversy in practice and has become a matter of debate inside and outside the laboratory. As a rule of thumb, ICSI should be mostly employed in cases of moderate and severe male infertility. Real world data originating from ESHRE and SART indicate similar results between IVF and ICSI (Wyns et al. 2021; SART National Summary 2020). However, it is a fact that ICSI practice irrespectively of indication is becoming more popular by year and according to the European Society for Human Reproduction and Embryology (ESHRE) fact sheer over 70% of the total number of cycles worldwide employ ICSI [113]. ICSI has been suggested for moderate and severe male factor infertility, which represents less than 50% of IVF cycles since the total cohort of male infertility represents 50%. This disproportionate employment of ICSI may not always be beneficial for the couples [114]. According to studies, ICSI employed for non-male factor infertility cases presents with similar fertilization rate, implantation rate, and live-birth rate when compared to IVF. Interestingly it was reported that ICSI presents with lower clinical pregnancy rate when compared to IVF [115]. Studies on epigenetics report that ICSI is associated with an increased risk of epigenetic disorders, congenital malformations, chromosomal alterations, and subfertility in babies born following ICSI compared to naturally conceived children [116], as well as differences in the methylation profile compared to IVF [117]. In light of the above, ICSI overuse should be avoided. Since publication of ASRM Recommendations on ICSI practice was published [118] decision-making on ICSI application should be straightforward. However, data shows that still, ICSI practice for non-male factor infertility persists [119]. This reinforces further the need to provide optimal sperm characterization [40, 120] (Palini et al. 2023).

Delving further into ICSI practices, novel ICSI variations have been proposed, and specifically the intracytoplasmic morphologically selected sperm injection (IMSI) employing ultra-high magnification and physiological ICSI (PICSI) employing hyaluronic acid for sperm slow and selection replacing the employment of PVP. Despite their high promise both these techniques have yet to cement their effectiveness and are still considered as add-ons [121–123].

Cryopreservation

Two methods are currently employed for sperm cryopreservation, namely, conventional rapid freezing and vitrification. Rapid freezing, which may be seen as an "update" of slow freezing, has been successfully employed for the cryopreservation of human sperm many times in the past [124]. The technique entails employment of a cryoprotectant and allowing sperm to freeze in vapors of liquid nitrogen or in a $-80\ ^{\circ}C$ freezer for 30 min to 2 h and then shifting to liquid nitrogen at $-196\ ^{\circ}C$ [125]. Vitrification is still considered to be a novel technique, slowly gaining ground as a growing alternative method of vapor freezing. Comparing the two methods, a meta-analysis reported that sperm cryopreservation employing vitrification resulted in better quality post-thaw samples [126].

Cryopreservation, employing the vitrification method, provides an effective approach to preserve human fertility in several possible disorders. Cryopreservation is usually suggested to patients undergoing chemotherapy or to patients that are administered medications that may impede future fertility. It has been suggested that for patients with declining sperm count that may become azoospermic, sperm cryopreservation could be an effective management. For these patients, sperm cryopreservation could be a supportive approach to preserve fertility. The vitrified sperm, following thawing may be employed for either IUI or IVF/ICSI.

The major drawback of the cryopreservation technique is the fact that cryopreservation has been reported to reduce both progressive motility and viability for approximately more than 35% in both fertile and infertile patients [127]. This reduction is suggested to be higher in subfertile and infertile patients due to the fact that spermatozoa may be more susceptible to osmotic and oxidative stress following cryopreservation. In order to compensate for this a very recent study has suggested that cryopreservation of prepared spermatozoa from oligozoospermic men with addition of seminal plasma from normozoospermic men may be of benefit [128]. However, novel approaches on that end remain to be validated.

For extremely low sperm counts and for patients with azoospermia who have undergone testicular sperm extraction the single sperm cryopreservation technique may be of benefit. The single sperm cryopreservation method is based on the principle of cryopreserving a low number of spermatozoa in an empty zona pellucida as first described by Walmsley and colleagues [129]. Despite its name this method entails cryopreservation of a small number of spermatozoa (usually less than 10) rather than a single spermatozoon. More than two decades later, numerous synthetic compounds have been developed in order to facilitate this technique. The synthetic compounds employed are cell sleeper, closed slice, Cryoleaf, Cryoloops, Cryopiece, Cryotop, culture dish with micro-droplets, and Sperm Vitrification Device [130].

Recently it has been reported that human spermatozoa, originating both from ejaculates and from testicular extraction may be cryopreserved for a short term in −80 °C freezers instead of liquid nitrogen. This method is suggested to present with similar or even enhanced results, regarding progressive motility and sperm DNA fragmentation, compared to liquid nitrogen vapors when evaluated for a maximum of 2 months [131]. This technique may be useful for severe oligozoospermic or azoospermic men, who are about to undergo an ICSI cycle in order to avoid cycle cancelation due to possible azoospermia (for more information, please read chapter on this subject).

Surgical Sperm Retrieval

Surgical sperm retrieval may present as the sole solution for men with azoospermia aiming to have children. The methods most usually employed are microsurgical epididymal sperm aspiration (MESA), testicular sperm aspiration (TESA), percutaneous sperm aspiration (PESA), testicular sperm extraction (TESE), and microdissection TESE (micro-TESE). A brief description of these methods is provided in Table 4.3.

Severe oligozoospermia has been associated with poor ICSI outcomes due to high ROS levels and sperm DNA fragmentation [7]. Higher clinical pregnancy and live-birth rates have been reported when employing testicular sperm in men with high sperm DNA fragmentation, however, the debate is still ongoing [132]. Testicular sperm has been reported to present with lower levels of DNA fragmentation and is associated with higher clinical pregnancy rates than with the use of ejaculated sperm in this specific population [133]. Both TESA and micro-TESE have been employed to evaluate this method. Data suggests that decision-making on employment of each method should be based on the ejaculate sperm concentration. More specifically for men presenting with less than 100,000 spermatozoa per mL, micro-TESE should be performed, whereas for men with more than the former

Table 4.3 Surgical sperm retrieval methods

	Anesthesia	Description	Indicated for NOA
TESA	Local or sedation	Aspiration of fluid and tissue from the testis	Yes
MESA	General	Surgical dissection of the epididymis and aspiration of the epididymal fluid	No
PESA	Local	Aspiration of epididymal fluid without surgery	No
TESE	Local or sedation	Surgical biopsy of the testis	Yes
Micro-TESE	General	Surgical retrieval of sperm from the seminiferous tubes	Yes

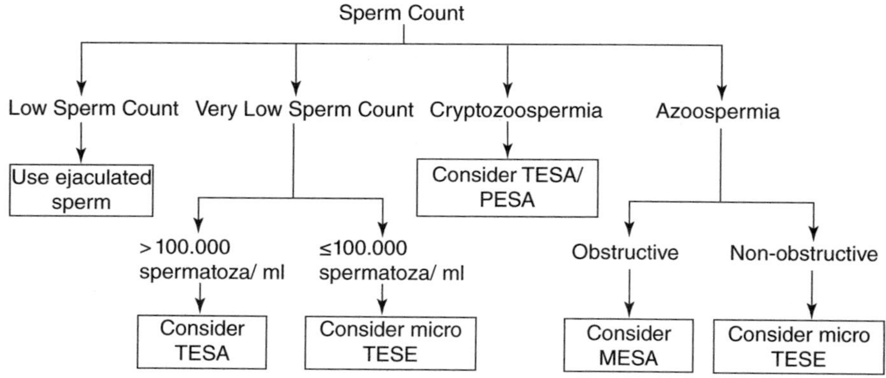

Fig. 4.2 Decision tree regarding the optimal method of sperm retrieval

cut-off value both techniques appear to perform equally, while for cryptozoospermia micro-TESE provides enhanced results compared to TESA [134]. In men with obstructive azoospermia, MESA presents with improved sperm retrieval rates in comparison to TESE [135, 136] while TESA performs marginally better than PESA [137]. For men presenting with NOA the optimal method seems to be micro-TESE, followed by conventional TESE and TESA [138]. A decision tree is presented in Fig. 4.2.

Two Clinical Scenarios

Case 1

A 34-year-old male, presented to the reproductive medicine center complaining of primary infertility for the last 2 years. He is physically fit and does not have a history of recent febrile illness or genitourinary infections. His past medical history was unremarkable. There is no family history of genetic issues. His is married to a 24-year-old woman who has a normal fertility evaluation. Physical examination revealed diminished testicular size, mainly on the left side, and bilateral grade III varicocele. A semen analysis provided by another laboratory demonstrated a volume of 2.8 mL, sperm concentration of 7 million/mL, total motility of 28% (progressive motility 18%) and normal morphology of 5%.

Repeat semen analysis with SDF testing was performed, using TUNEL, demonstrated a volume of 4.5 mL, sperm concentration 9 million/mL, total motility 20% (progressive motility 12%), normal morphology of 4%, and SDF of 49%. Hormonal profile was assessed and showed: testosterone 20.2 nmol/L (normal = 10.4–30.86 nmol/L), follicle-stimulating hormone (FSH) 3.6 IU/ L (normal = 1.5–12.4 IU/L), luteinizing hormone (LH) 5 IU/L (normal = 1.7–8.6 IU/L), estradiol 141 pmol/L (normal = 94.8–223 pmol/L), and prolactin 233 mIU/L (normal = 85–323 mIU/L).

Scrotal imaging was also requested and a Doppler ultrasound demonstrated bilateral varicocele with testicular vein reflux induced by Valsalva's maneuver. Right veins measure 3.2 mm and left measures 3.5 mm in maximum diameter. Testes were normal in shape and echotexture.

The patient was diagnosed with oligoasthenozoospermia and bilateral varicocele. He was submitted to a bilateral microsurgical subinguinal varicocelectomy, using microvascular Doppler, without any complications. Patient had a fast recover after the procedure and a new semen analysis was performed after 4 months in our center demonstrating a volume of 3.2 mL, sperm concentration of 22 million/mL, total motility of 52% (progressive motility 34%), and normal morphology of 6%. On the 6-month follow-up visit the patient reported that his wife was pregnant.

Case 2

E.M.A, male, 41 years old, presented to the male infertility unit reporting that he and his 29-year-old spouse have been trying unsuccessfully to conceive for the last 3.5 years. He is overweight (BMI 27.8 kg/m^2) with decreased libido. He did not smoke or consume alcohol. On genital examination, he had both testes of normal size and consistency, both epididymes were normal, vasa deferentia were palpable, and no varicocele was identified. The spouse reported regular menses, no gynecological problems, and a normal ovarian reserve (anti-mullerian hormone: 18.9 pmol/L, normal = 0.071–52.4 pmol/L).

Semen analysis demonstrated a volume of 2.5 mL, sperm concentration of 0.6 million/mL, total motility of 20% (13% progressive motility), and 5% normal morphology. At this point, SDF was also tested with other commercial Kit and it was high (75%). Hormone levels assessment showed testosterone 7.8 nmol/L (normal = 10.4–30.86 nmol/L), FSH 1.0 IU/L normal = 1.5–12.4 IU/L, LH 0.8 IU/L (normal = 1.7–8.6 IU/L), estradiol 95 pmol/L (normal = 94.8–223 pmol/L), and prolactin 1000 mIU/L (normal = 85–323 mIU/L). Scrotal ultrasound showed both testes with normal size, shape, and echotexture. Due to the hormonal discrepancies, a pituitary MRI was performed and a 16 × 14 × 21 mm lobulated pituitary mass was identified. Patient was started on cabergoline which successfully decreased his prolactin level to 100 pmol/L after 4 months. Despite this, the patient's testosterone level remained decreased, so it was decided to initiate hCG 1500 units SC three times per week.

After 16 weeks, the patient reported improvement of sexual activity and had a repeat semen analysis, which revealed a volume of 3.0 mL, sperm concentration of 15.3 million/mL, total motility of 42% (33% progressive motility), and 6% normal morphology. Despite the significant improvement, SDF was still high (60%) and the couple was unable to conceive. They underwent an IVF cycle in which sperm selection was performed using a microfluidics technique. They obtained three blastocysts and the couple achieved a pregnancy with the first embryo transfer.

Take Home Messages

- Since there is a natural variation of sperm count, semen analysis should be repeated at least once more prior to diagnosing oligozoospermia, cryptozoospermia, or azoospermia.
- If the sperm count is very low, special measures should be undertaken applying further techniques in order to determine the presence of spermatozoa.
- Oligozoospermia is a result of endocrine dysfunction, genetic abnormalities, anatomical disorders, testicular injuries, medications, environmental and lifestyle causes.
- Oligozoospermia can be managed by hormonal treatment, oral antioxidants or surgical techniques to treat varicocele, which may even enable natural conception prior to embarking on assisted reproductive techniques treatment.
- Sperm cryopreservation, surgical sperm retrieval and assisted reproductive techniques are options for oligozoospermic men to achieve pregnancy.

References

1. Agarwal A, Parekh N, Panner Selvam MK, Henkel R, Shah R, Homa ST, Ramasamy R, Ko E, Tremellen K, Esteves S, Majzoub A, Alvarez JG, Gardner DK, Jayasena CN, Ramsay JW, Cho CL, Saleh R, Sakkas D, Hotaling JM, et al. Male oxidative stress infertility (MOSI): proposed terminology and clinical practice guidelines for management of idiopathic male infertility. World J Mens Health. 2019;37(3):296–312. https://doi.org/10.5534/wjmh.190055.
2. Durairajanayagam D. Lifestyle causes of male infertility. Arab J Urol. 2018;16(1):10–20. https://doi.org/10.1016/j.aju.2017.12.004.
3. Fainberg J, Kashanian JA. Recent advances in understanding and managing male infertility. F1000Res. 2019;8:F1000 Faculty Rev-670. https://doi.org/10.12688/f1000research.17076.1.
4. Miyamoto T, Minase G, Shin T, Ueda H, Okada H, Sengoku K. Human male infertility and its genetic causes. Reprod Med Biol. 2017;16(2):81–8. https://doi.org/10.1002/rmb2.12017.
5. Zedan H, Ismail S, Gomaa A, Saleh R, Henkel R, Agarwal A. Evaluation of reference values of standard semen parameters in fertile Egyptian men. Andrologia. 2018;50(4):e12942. https://doi.org/10.1111/and.12942.
6. WHO laboratory manual for the examination and processing of human semen. https://www.who.int/publications-detail-redirect/9789240030787. Accessed 21 Jun 2022.
7. Barbăroşie C, Agarwal A, Henkel R. Diagnostic value of advanced semen analysis in evaluation of male infertility. Andrologia. 2021;53(2):e13625. https://doi.org/10.1111/and.13625.
8. Snow-Lisy D, Sabanegh E. What does the clinician need from an andrology laboratory? Front Biosci (Elite Ed). 2013;5(1):289–304. https://doi.org/10.2741/e616.
9. Agarwal A, Bui AD. Oxidation-reduction potential as a new marker for oxidative stress: correlation to male infertility. Invest Clin Urol. 2017;58(6):385–99. https://doi.org/10.4111/icu.2017.58.6.385.
10. Leaver RB. Male infertility: an overview of causes and treatment options. Br J Nurs. 2016;25(18):S35–40. https://doi.org/10.12968/bjon.2016.25.18.S35.
11. Shah R, Gupta C. Advances in sperm retrieval techniques in azoospermic men: a systematic review. Arab J Urol. 2018;16(1):125–31. https://doi.org/10.1016/j.aju.2017.11.010.
12. Esteves SC. Who cares about oligozoospermia when we have ICSI. Reprod Biomed Online. 2022;44(5):769–75. https://doi.org/10.1016/j.rbmo.2021.11.026.
13. Neto FTL, Bach PV, Najari BB, Li PS, Goldstein M. Spermatogenesis in humans and its affecting factors. Semin Cell Dev Biol. 2016;59:10–26. https://doi.org/10.1016/j.semcdb.2016.04.009.

14. Misell LM, Holochwost D, Boban D, Santi N, Shefi S, Hellerstein MK, Turek PJ. A stable isotope-mass spectrometric method for measuring human spermatogenesis kinetics in vivo. J Urol. 2006;175(1):242–6; discussion 246. https://doi.org/10.1016/S0022-5347(05)00053-4.

15. Slama R, Eustache F, Ducot B, Jensen TK, Jørgensen N, Horte A, Irvine S, Suominen J, Andersen AG, Auger J, Vierula M, Toppari J, Andersen AN, Keiding N, Skakkebaek NE, Spira A, Jouannet P. Time to pregnancy and semen parameters: a cross-sectional study among fertile couples from four European cities. Hum Reprod. 2002;17(2):503–15. https://doi.org/10.1093/humrep/17.2.503.

16. Zinaman MJ, Brown CC, Selevan SG, Clegg ED. Semen quality and human fertility: a prospective study with healthy couples. J Androl. 2000;21(1):145–53.

17. Borges E Jr, Setti AS, Braga DPAF, Figueira RCS, Iaconelli A Jr. Total motile sperm count has a superior predictive value over the WHO 2010 cut-off values for the outcomes of intra-cytoplasmic sperm injection cycles. Andrology. 2016;4(5):880–6. https://doi.org/10.1111/andr.12199.

18. International Committee for Monitoring Assisted Reproductive Technologies (ICMART). https://www.icmartivf.org. Accessed 21 Jun 2022.

19. World Health Organization. WHO laboratory manual for the examination and processing of human semen. 6th ed. Geneva: WHO Press; 2021. https://www.who.int/publications/i/item/9789240030787.

20. Brito LFC, Althouse GC, Aurich C, Chenoweth PJ, Eilts BE, Love CC, Luvoni GC, Mitchell JR, Peter AT, Pugh DG, Waberski D. Andrology laboratory review: evaluation of sperm concentration. Theriogenology. 2016;85(9):1507–27. https://doi.org/10.1016/j.theriogenology.2016.01.002.

21. Mortimer ST, van der Horst G, Mortimer D. The future of computer-aided sperm analysis. Asian J Androl. 2015;17(4):545–53. https://doi.org/10.4103/1008-682X.154312.

22. Patil PS, Humbarwadi RS, Patil AD, Gune AR. Immature germ cells in semen—correlation with total sperm count and sperm motility. J Cytol. 2013;30(3):185–9. https://doi.org/10.4103/0970-9371.117682.

23. Andersen AG, Jensen TK, Carlsen E, Jørgensen N, Andersson AM, Krarup T, Keiding N, Skakkebaek NE. High frequency of sub-optimal semen quality in an unselected population of young men. Hum Reprod. 2000;15(2):366–72. https://doi.org/10.1093/humrep/15.2.366.

24. Van BJP, Lawton E, Frazier JR, Zderic SA, Zaontz MR, Shukla AR, Srinivasan AK, Weiss DA, Long CJ, Canning DA, Kolon TF. Total motile sperm count in adolescent boys with varicocele is associated with hormone levels and total testicular volume. J Urol. 2021;205(3):888–94. https://doi.org/10.1097/JU.0000000000001405.

25. Mínguez-Alarcón L, Gaskins AJ, Chiu Y-H, Messerlian C, Williams PL, Ford JB, Souter I, Hauser R, Chavarro JE. Type of underwear worn and markers of testicular function among men attending a fertility center. Hum Reprod. 2018;33(9):1749–56. https://doi.org/10.1093/humrep/dey259.

26. Diaconu CC, Manea M, Marcu DR, Socea B, Spinu AD, Bratu OG. The erectile dysfunction as a marker of cardiovascular disease: a review. Acta Cardiol. 2020;75(4):286–92. https://doi.org/10.1080/00015385.2019.1590498.

27. Shabtaie SA, Gerkowicz SA, Kohn TP, Ramasamy R. Role of abnormal sperm morphology in predicting pregnancy outcomes. Curr Urol Rep. 2016;17(9):67. https://doi.org/10.1007/s11934-016-0623-1.

28. Sabeti P, Pourmasumi S, Rahiminia T, Akyash F, Talebi AR. Etiologies of sperm oxidative stress. Int J Reprod Biomed. 2016;14(4):231–40.

29. Agarwal A, Mulgund A, Sharma R, Sabanegh E. Mechanisms of oligozoospermia: an oxidative stress perspective. Syst Biol Reprod Med. 2014;60(4):206–16. https://doi.org/10.3109/19396368.2014.918675.

30. Hanson BM, Aston KI, Jenkins TG, Carrell DT, Hotaling JM. The impact of ejaculatory abstinence on semen analysis parameters: a systematic review. J Assist Reprod Genet. 2018;35(2):213–20. https://doi.org/10.1007/s10815-017-1086-0.

31. Shi X, Chan CPS, Waters T, Chi L, Chan DYL, Li T-C. Lifestyle and demographic factors associated with human semen quality and sperm function. Syst Biol Reprod Med. 2018;64(5):358–67. https://doi.org/10.1080/19396368.2018.1491074.

32. Hebles M, Dorado M, Gallardo M, González-Martínez M, Sánchez-Martín P. Seminal quality in the first fraction of ejaculate. Syst Biol Reprod Med. 2015;61(2):113–6. https://doi.org/10.3109/19396368.2014.999390.

33. Hansen PJ. Effects of heat stress on mammalian reproduction. Philos Trans R Soc B Biol Sci. 2009;364(1534):3341–50. https://doi.org/10.1098/rstb.2009.0131.

34. Sharpe RM. Environmental/lifestyle effects on spermatogenesis. Philos Trans R Soc B Biol Sci. 2010;365(1546):1697–712. https://doi.org/10.1098/rstb.2009.0206.

35. Donders GGG, Bosmans E, Reumers J, Donders F, Jonckheere J, Salembier G, Stern N, Jacquemyn Y, Ombelet W, Depuydt CE. Sperm quality and absence of SARS-CoV-2 RNA in semen after COVID-19 infection: a prospective, observational study and validation of the SpermCOVID test. Fertil Steril. 2022;117(2):287–96. https://doi.org/10.1016/j.fertnstert.2021.10.022.

36. Viswambharan N, Murugan M. Effect of wash and swim-up and density gradient sperm preparation on sperm DNA fragmentation. Mater Today Proc. 2021;45:2002–5. https://doi.org/10.1016/j.matpr.2020.09.423.

37. Lestari SW, Sari T, Pujianto DA. Sperm DNA fragmentation and apoptosis levels: a comparison of the swim up and the density gradient centrifugation methods for sperm preparation. Online J Biol Sci. 2016;16(4):152–8. https://doi.org/10.3844/ojbsci.2016.152.158.

38. Uribe P, Villegas JV, Boguen R, Treulen F, Sánchez R, Mallmann P, Isachenko V, Rahimi G, Isachenko E. Use of the fluorescent dye tetramethylrhodamine methyl ester perchlorate for mitochondrial membrane potential assessment in human spermatozoa. Andrologia. 2017;49(9):e12753. https://doi.org/10.1111/and.12753.

39. Kandil H, Agarwal A, Saleh R, Boitrelle F, Arafa M, Vogiatzi P, Henkel R, Zini A, Shah R. Editorial commentary on draft of World Health Organization sixth edition laboratory manual for the examination and processing of human semen. World J Mens Health. 2021;39(4):577–80. https://doi.org/10.5534/wjmh.210074.

40. Boitrelle F, Shah R, Saleh R, Henkel R, Kandil H, Chung E, Vogiatzi P, Zini A, Arafa M, Agarwal A. The sixth edition of the WHO manual for human semen analysis: a critical review and SWOT analysis. Life. 2021;11(12):1368. https://doi.org/10.3390/life11121368.

41. World Health Organization. WHO laboratory manual for the examination and processing of human semen. 5th ed. Geneva: WHO Press; 2010.

42. Campbell MJ, Lotti F, Baldi E, Schlatt S, Festin MPR, Björndahl L, Toskin I, Barratt CLR. Distribution of semen examination results 2020—a follow up of data collated for the WHO semen analysis manual 2010. Andrology. 2021;9(3):817–22. https://doi.org/10.1111/andr.12983.

43. Boulicault M, Perret M, Galka J, Borsa A, Gompers A, Reiches M, Richardson S. The future of sperm: a biovariability framework for understanding global sperm count trends. Hum Fertil. 2021;25(5):888–902. https://doi.org/10.1080/14647273.2021.1917778.

44. Levine H, Jørgensen N, Martino-Andrade A, Mendiola J, Weksler-Derri D, Mindlis I, Pinotti R, Swan SH. Temporal trends in sperm count: a systematic review and meta-regression analysis. Hum Reprod Update. 2017;23(6):646–59. https://doi.org/10.1093/humupd/dmx022.

45. Tong N, Witherspoon L, Dunne C, Flannigan R. Global decline of male fertility: fact or fiction? A broad summary of the published evidence on sperm-count and fertility trends. B C Med J. 2022;64(3):126–30.

46. Inhorn MC, Patrizio P. Infertility around the globe: new thinking on gender, reproductive technologies and global movements in the 21st century. Hum Reprod Update. 2015;21(4):411–26. https://doi.org/10.1093/humupd/dmv016.

47. Guzick DS, Overstreet JW, Factor-Litvak P, Brazil CK, Nakajima ST, Coutifaris C, Carson SA, Cisneros P, Steinkampf MP, Hill JA, Xu D, Vogel DL, National Cooperative Reproductive Medicine Network. Sperm morphology, motility, and concentration in fertile and infertile men. N Engl J Med. 2001;345(19):1388–93. https://doi.org/10.1056/NEJMoa003005.

48. Patel AS, Leong JY, Ramasamy R. Prediction of male infertility by the World Health Organization laboratory manual for assessment of semen analysis: a systematic review. Arab J Urol. 2018;16(1):96–102. https://doi.org/10.1016/j.aju.2017.10.005.
49. Wang C, Swerdloff RS. Limitations of semen analysis as a test of male fertility and anticipated needs from newer tests. Fertil Steril. 2014;102(6):1502–7. https://doi.org/10.1016/j.fertnstert.2014.10.021.
50. Ping P, Zheng Z, Ma Y, Zou SS, Chen XF. Comparison of intracytoplasmic sperm injection (ICSI) outcomes in infertile men with spermatogenic impairment of differing severity. Asian J Androl. 2022;24(3):299–304. https://doi.org/10.4103/aja202151.
51. Miller D, Vukina J. Recent advances in clinical diagnosis and treatment of male factor infertility. Postgrad Med. 2020;132(sup4):28–34. https://doi.org/10.1080/00325481.2020.1830589.
52. Punab M, Poolamets O, Paju P, Vihljajev V, Pomm K, Ladva R, Korrovits P, Laan M. Causes of male infertility: a 9-year prospective monocentre study on 1737 patients with reduced total sperm counts. Hum Reprod. 2017;32(1):18–31. https://doi.org/10.1093/humrep/dew284.
53. Pantos K, Sfakianoudis K, Maziotis E, Rapani A, Karantzali E, Gounari-Papaioannou A, Vaxevanoglou T, Koutsilieris M, Simopoulou M. Abnormal fertilization in ICSI and its association with abnormal semen parameters: a retrospective observational study on 1855 cases. Asian J Androl. 2021;23(4):376–85. https://doi.org/10.4103/aja.aja_84_20.
54. Castañeda JM, Miyata H, Ikawa M, Matzuk MM. Sperm defects. In: Skinner MK, editor. Encyclopedia of reproduction. 2nd ed. Oxford: Academic Press; 2018. p. 276–81.
55. Choy JT, Amory JK. Nonsurgical management of oligozoospermia. J Clin Endocrinol Metab. 2020;105(12):e4194–207. https://doi.org/10.1210/clinem/dgaa390.
56. Cangiano B, Swee DS, Quinton R, Bonomi M. Genetics of congenital hypogonadotropic hypogonadism: peculiarities and phenotype of an oligogenic disease. Hum Genet. 2021;140(1):77–111. https://doi.org/10.1007/s00439-020-02147-1.
57. Iammarrone E, Balet R, Lower AM, Gillott C, Grudzinskas JG. Male infertility. Best Pract Res Clin Obstet Gynaecol. 2003;17(2):211–29. https://doi.org/10.1016/s1521-6934(02)00147-5.
58. La Vignera S, Vita R. Thyroid dysfunction and semen quality. Int J Immunopathol Pharmacol. 2018;32:2058738418775241. https://doi.org/10.1177/2058738418775241.
59. McLachlan RI. Approach to the patient with oligozoospermia. J Clin Endocrinol Metab. 2013;98(3):873–80. https://doi.org/10.1210/jc.2012-3650.
60. Romano RM, Gomes SN, Cardoso NC, Schiessl L, Romano MA, Oliveira CA. New insights for male infertility revealed by alterations in spermatic function and differential testicular expression of thyroid-related genes. Endocrine. 2017;55(2):607–17. https://doi.org/10.1007/s12020-016-0952-3.
61. Krausz C, Casamonti E. Spermatogenic failure and the Y chromosome. Hum Genet. 2017;136(5):637–55. https://doi.org/10.1007/s00439-017-1793-8.
62. Fisch H, Lambert SM, Goluboff ET. Management of ejaculatory duct obstruction: etiology, diagnosis, and treatment. World J Urol. 2006;24(6):604–10. https://doi.org/10.1007/s00345-006-0129-4.
63. Gupta C, Chinchole A, Shah R, Pathak H, Talreja D, Kayal A. Microscopic varicocelectomy as a treatment option for patients with severe oligospermia. Investig Clin Urol. 2018;59(3):182–6. https://doi.org/10.4111/icu.2018.59.3.182.
64. Pallotti F, Paoli D, Carlini T, Vestri AR, Martino G, Lenzi A, Lombardo F. Varicocele and semen quality: a retrospective case-control study of 4230 patients from a single centre. J Endocrinol Invest. 2018;41(2):185–92. https://doi.org/10.1007/s40618-017-0713-z.
65. Ciongradi CI, Sarbu I, Iliescu Halitchi CO, Benchia D, Sarbu K. Fertility of cryptorchid testis—an unsolved mistery. Genes (Basel). 2021;12(12):1894. https://doi.org/10.3390/genes12121894.
66. Vakalopoulos I, Dimou P, Anagnostou I, Zeginiadou T. Impact of cancer and cancer treatment on male fertility. Hormones (Athens). 2015;14(4):579–89. https://doi.org/10.14310/horm.2002.1620.
67. Drobnis EZ, Nangia AK. Pain medications and male reproduction. Adv Exp Med Biol. 2017;1034:39–57. https://doi.org/10.1007/978-3-319-69535-8_6.

68. Bermas BL. Paternal safety of anti-rheumatic medications. Best Pract Res Clin Obstet Gynaecol. 2020;64:77–84. https://doi.org/10.1016/j.bpobgyn.2019.09.004.
69. Ternavasio-de la Vega HG, Boronat M, Ojeda A, Garcia-Delgado Y, Angel-Moreno A, Carranza-Rodriguez C, Bellini R, Frances A, Novoa FJ, Perez-Arellano JL. Mumps orchitis in the post-vaccine era (1967-2009): a single-center series of 67 patients and review of clinical outcome and trends. Medicine (Baltimore). 2010;89(2):96–116. https://doi.org/10.1097/MD.0b013e3181d63191.
70. Gacci M, Coppi M, Baldi E, Sebastianelli A, Zaccaro C, Morselli S, Pecoraro A, Manera A, Nicoletti R, Liaci A, Bisegna C, Gemma L, Giancane S, Pollini S, Antonelli A, Lagi F, Marchiani S, Dabizzi S, Degl'Innocenti S, Annunziato F, Maggi M, Vignozzi L, Bartoloni A, Rossolini GM, Serni S. Semen impairment and occurrence of SARS-CoV-2 virus in semen after recovery from COVID-19. Hum Reprod. 2021;36(6):1520–9. https://doi.org/10.1093/humrep/deab026.
71. Sermondade N, Faure C, Fezeu L, Levy R, Czernichow S, Obesity-Fertility Collaborative G. Obesity and increased risk for oligozoospermia and azoospermia. Arch Intern Med. 2012;172(5):440–2. https://doi.org/10.1001/archinternmed.2011.1382.
72. Sermondade N, Faure C, Fezeu L, Shayeb AG, Bonde JP, Jensen TK, Van Wely M, Cao J, Martini AC, Eskandar M, Chavarro JE, Koloszar S, Twigt JM, Ramlau-Hansen CH, Borges E Jr, Lotti F, Steegers-Theunissen RP, Zorn B, Polotsky AJ, La Vignera S, Eskenazi B, Tremellen K, Magnusdottir EV, Fejes I, Hercberg S, Levy R, Czernichow S. BMI in relation to sperm count: an updated systematic review and collaborative meta-analysis. Hum Reprod Update. 2013;19(3):221–31. https://doi.org/10.1093/humupd/dms050.
73. Mehrpour O, Karrari P, Zamani N, Tsatsakis AM, Abdollahi M. Occupational exposure to pesticides and consequences on male semen and fertility: a review. Toxicol Lett. 2014;230(2):146–56. https://doi.org/10.1016/j.toxlet.2014.01.029.
74. Vaiserman A. Early-life exposure to endocrine disrupting chemicals and later-life health outcomes: an epigenetic bridge? Aging Dis. 2014;5(6):419–29. https://doi.org/10.14336/AD.2014.0500419.
75. Fernandez CJ, Chacko EC, Pappachan JM. Male obesity-related secondary hypogonadism—pathophysiology, clinical implications and management. Eur Endocrinol. 2019;15(2):83–90. https://doi.org/10.17925/EE.2019.15.2.83.
76. Ma J, Wu L, Zhou Y, Zhang H, Xiong C, Peng Z, Bao W, Meng T, Liu Y. Association between BMI and semen quality: an observational study of 3966 sperm donors. Hum Reprod. 2019;34(1):155–62. https://doi.org/10.1093/humrep/dey328.
77. Kaminski P, Baszynski J, Jerzak I, Kavanagh BP, Nowacka-Chiari E, Polanin M, Szymanski M, Wozniak A, Kozera W. External and genetic conditions determining male infertility. Int J Mol Sci. 2020;21(15):5274. https://doi.org/10.3390/ijms21155274.
78. Calogero AE, Fiore M, Giacone F, Altomare M, Asero P, Ledda C, Romeo G, Mongioi LM, Copat C, Giuffrida M, Vicari E, Sciacca S, Ferrante M. Exposure to multiple metals/metalloids and human semen quality: a cross-sectional study. Ecotoxicol Environ Saf. 2021;215:112165. https://doi.org/10.1016/j.ecoenv.2021.112165.
79. Leisegang K, Sengupta P, Agarwal A, Henkel R. Obesity and male infertility: mechanisms and management. Andrologia. 2021;53(1):e13617. https://doi.org/10.1111/and.13617.
80. Pizzol D, Foresta C, Garolla A, Demurtas J, Trott M, Bertoldo A, Smith L. Pollutants and sperm quality: a systematic review and meta-analysis. Environ Sci Pollut Res Int. 2021;28(4):4095–103. https://doi.org/10.1007/s11356-020-11589-z.
81. Tang Q, Pan F, Wu X, Nichols CE, Wang X, Xia Y, London SJ, Wu W. Semen quality and cigarette smoking in a cohort of healthy fertile men. Environ Epidemiol. 2019;3(4):e055. https://doi.org/10.1097/EE9.0000000000000055.
82. Zou P, Sun L, Chen Q, Zhang G, Yang W, Zeng Y, Zhou N, Li Y, Liu J, Ao L, Cao J, Yang H. Social support modifies an association between work stress and semen quality: results from 384 Chinese male workers. J Psychosom Res. 2019;117:65–70. https://doi.org/10.1016/j.jpsychores.2018.10.013.

83. Bai S, Wan Y, Zong L, Li W, Xu X, Zhao Y, Hu X, Zuo Y, Xu B, Tong X, Guo T. Association of alcohol intake and semen parameters in men with primary and secondary infertility: a cross-sectional study. Front Physiol. 2020;11:566625. https://doi.org/10.3389/fphys.2020.566625.
84. Demirkol MK, Yildirim A, Gica S, Dogan NT, Resim S. Evaluation of the effect of shift working and sleep quality on semen parameters in men attending infertility clinic. Andrologia. 2021;53(8):e14116. https://doi.org/10.1111/and.14116.
85. Hussein A. Overview treatment and male reproductive medicine. In: Skinner MK, editor. Encyclopedia of reproduction. 2nd ed. Oxford: Academic Press; 2018. p. 307–13.
86. Padubidri V, Daftary SN. Shaw's textbook of gynecology e-book. New Delhi: Elsevier Health Sciences; 2014.
87. Young J, Xu C, Papadakis GE, Acierno JS, Maione L, Hietamaki J, Raivio T, Pitteloud N. Clinical management of congenital hypogonadotropic hypogonadism. Endocr Rev. 2019;40(2):669–710. https://doi.org/10.1210/er.2018-00116.
88. Prior M, Stewart J, McEleny K, Dwyer AA, Quinton R. Fertility induction in hypogonadotropic hypogonadal men. Clin Endocrinol (Oxf). 2018;89(6):712–8. https://doi.org/10.1111/cen.13850.
89. Attia AM, Abou-Setta AM, Al-Inany HG. Gonadotrophins for idiopathic male factor subfertility. Cochrane Database Syst Rev. 2013;(8):CD005071. https://doi.org/10.1002/14651858.CD005071.pub4.
90. Ferlin A, Vinanzi C, Selice R, Garolla A, Frigo AC, Foresta C. Toward a pharmacogenetic approach to male infertility: polymorphism of follicle-stimulating hormone beta-subunit promoter. Fertil Steril. 2011;96(6):1344–9.e1342. https://doi.org/10.1016/j.fertnstert.2011.09.034.
91. Awouters M, Vanderschueren D, Antonio L. Aromatase inhibitors and selective estrogen receptor modulators: unconventional therapies for functional hypogonadism? Andrology. 2020;8(6):1590–7. https://doi.org/10.1111/andr.12725.
92. Cannarella R, Condorelli RA, Mongioi LM, Barbagallo F, Calogero AE, La Vignera S. Effects of the selective estrogen receptor modulators for the treatment of male infertility: a systematic review and meta-analysis. Expert Opin Pharmacother. 2019;20(12):1517–25. https://doi.org/10.1080/14656566.2019.1615057.
93. Helo S, Wynia B, McCullough A. "Cherchez La Femme": modulation of estrogen receptor function with selective modulators: clinical implications in the field of urology. Sex Med Rev. 2017;5(3):365–86. https://doi.org/10.1016/j.sxmr.2017.03.003.
94. Del Giudice F, Busetto GM, De Berardinis E, Sperduti I, Ferro M, Maggi M, Gross MS, Sciarra A, Eisenberg ML. A systematic review and meta-analysis of clinical trials implementing aromatase inhibitors to treat male infertility. Asian J Androl. 2020;22(4):360–7. https://doi.org/10.4103/aja.aja_101_19.
95. Burnett-Bowie SA, McKay EA, Lee H, Leder BZ. Effects of aromatase inhibition on bone mineral density and bone turnover in older men with low testosterone levels. J Clin Endocrinol Metab. 2009;94(12):4785–92. https://doi.org/10.1210/jc.2009-0739.
96. Dias JP, Melvin D, Simonsick EM, Carlson O, Shardell MD, Ferrucci L, Chia CW, Basaria S, Egan JM. Effects of aromatase inhibition vs. testosterone in older men with low testosterone: randomized-controlled trial. Andrology. 2016;4(1):33–40. https://doi.org/10.1111/andr.12126.
97. Aitken RJ. Reactive oxygen species as mediators of sperm capacitation and pathological damage. Mol Reprod Dev. 2017;84(10):1039–52. https://doi.org/10.1002/mrd.22871.
98. Gambera L, Stendardi A, Ghelardi C, Fineschi B, Aini R. Effects of antioxidant treatment on seminal parameters in patients undergoing in vitro fertilization. Arch Ital Urol Androl. 2019;91(3) https://doi.org/10.4081/aiua.2019.3.187.
99. Huang WJ, Lu XL, Li JT, Zhang JM. Effects of folic acid on oligozoospermia with MTHFR polymorphisms in term of seminal parameters, DNA fragmentation, and live birth rate: a double-blind, randomized, placebo-controlled trial. Andrology. 2020;8(1):110–6. https://doi.org/10.1111/andr.12652.

100. Magdi Y, Darwish E, Elbashir S, Majzoub A, Agarwal A. Effect of modifiable lifestyle factors and antioxidant treatment on semen parameters of men with severe oligoasthenoteratozoospermia. Andrologia. 2017;49(7) https://doi.org/10.1111/and.12694.
101. Bozhedomov VA, Lipatova NA, Bozhedomova GE, Rokhlikov IM, Shcherbakova EV, Komarina RA. [Using L- and acetyl-L-carnintines in combination with clomiphene citrate and antioxidant complex for treating idiopathic male infertility: a prospective randomized trial]. Urologiia. 2017;(3):22–32. https://doi.org/10.18565/urol.2017.3.22-32.
102. Amory JK, Ostrowski KA, Gannon JR, Berkseth K, Stevison F, Isoherranen N, Muller CH, Walsh T. Isotretinoin administration improves sperm production in men with infertility from oligoasthenozoospermia: a pilot study. Andrology. 2017;5(6):1115–23. https://doi.org/10.1111/andr.12420.
103. Buhling K, Schumacher A, Eulenburg CZ, Laakmann E. Influence of oral vitamin and mineral supplementation on male infertility: a meta-analysis and systematic review. Reprod Biomed Online. 2019;39(2):269–79. https://doi.org/10.1016/j.rbmo.2019.03.099.
104. Showell MG, Mackenzie-Proctor R, Brown J, Yazdani A, Stankiewicz MT, Hart RJ. Antioxidants for male subfertility. Cochrane Database Syst Rev. 2014;(12):CD007411. https://doi.org/10.1002/14651858.CD007411.pub3.
105. Majzoub A, ElBardisi H, Covarrubias S, Mak N, Agarwal A, Henkel R, ElSaid S, Al-Malki AH, Arafa M. Effect of microsurgical varicocelectomy on fertility outcome and treatment plans of patients with severe oligozoospermia: an original report and meta-analysis. Andrologia. 2021;53(6):e14059. https://doi.org/10.1111/and.14059.
106. Agarwal A, Deepinder F, Cocuzza M, Agarwal R, Short RA, Sabanegh E, Marmar JL. Efficacy of varicocelectomy in improving semen parameters: new meta-analytical approach. Urology. 2007;70(3):532–8. https://doi.org/10.1016/j.urology.2007.04.011.
107. Agarwal A, Majzoub A, Parekh N, Henkel R. A schematic overview of the current status of male infertility practice. World J Mens Health. 2020;38(3):308–22. https://doi.org/10.5534/wjmh.190068.
108. Agarwal A, Sharma R, Harlev A, Esteves SC. Effect of varicocele on semen characteristics according to the new 2010 World Health Organization criteria: a systematic review and meta-analysis. Asian J Androl. 2016;18(2):163–70. https://doi.org/10.4103/1008-682X.172638.
109. Addar AM, Nazer A, Almardawi A, Al Hathal N, Kattan S. The yield of microscopic varicocelectomy in men with severe oligospermia. Urol Ann. 2021;13(3):268–71. https://doi.org/10.4103/UA.UA_53_20.
110. Khourdaji I, Lee H, Smith RP. Frontiers in hormone therapy for male infertility. Transl Androl Urol. 2018;7(Suppl 3):S353–66. https://doi.org/10.21037/tau.2018.04.03.
111. Reichman DE, Gunnala V, Meyer L, Spandorfer S, Schattman G, Davis OK, Rosenwaks Z. In vitro fertilization versus conversion to intrauterine insemination in the setting of three or fewer follicles: how should patients proceed when follicular response falls short of expectation? Fertil Steril. 2013;100(1):94–9. https://doi.org/10.1016/j.fertnstert.2013.02.049.
112. Moolenaar LM, Cissen M, de Bruin JP, Hompes PGA, Repping S, van der Veen F, Mol BWJ. Cost-effectiveness of assisted conception for male subfertility. Reprod Biomed Online. 2015;30(6):659–66. https://doi.org/10.1016/j.rbmo.2015.02.006.
113. ESHRE. Factsheets and infographics. 2022. https://www.eshre.eu/Europe/Factsheets-and-infographics.
114. Glenn TL, Kotlyar AM, Seifer DB. The impact of intracytoplasmic sperm injection in non-male factor infertility—a critical review. J Clin Med. 2021;10(12):2616. https://doi.org/10.3390/jcm10122616.
115. Abbas AM, Hussein RS, Elsenity MA, Samaha II, El Etriby KA, Abd El-Ghany MF, Khalifa MA, Abdelrheem SS, Ahmed AA, Khodry MM. Higher clinical pregnancy rate with in-vitro fertilization versus intracytoplasmic sperm injection in treatment of non-male factor infertility: systematic review and meta-analysis. J Gynecol Obstet Hum Reprod. 2020;49(6):101706. https://doi.org/10.1016/j.jogoh.2020.101706.
116. Sciorio R, Esteves SC. Contemporary use of ICSI and epigenetic risks to future generations. J Clin Med. 2022;11(8):2135. https://doi.org/10.3390/jcm11082135.

117. Yang H, Ma Z, Peng L, Kuhn C, Rahmeh M, Mahner S, Jeschke U, von Schönfeldt V. Comparison of histone H3K4me3 between IVF and ICSI technologies and between boy and girl offspring. Int J Mol Sci. 2021;22(16):8574. https://doi.org/10.3390/ijms22168574.

118. Practice Committees of the American Society for Reproductive Medicine and the Society for Assisted Reproductive Technology. Intracytoplasmic sperm injection (ICSI) for non-male factor indications: a committee opinion. Fertil Steril. 2020;114(2):239–45. https://doi.org/10.1016/j.fertnstert.2020.05.032.

119. Quaas AM. ICSI for non-male factor: do we practice what we preach? J Assist Reprod Genet. 2021;38(1):125–7. https://doi.org/10.1007/s10815-020-02016-w.

120. Sallam H, Boitrelle F, Palini S, Durairajanayagam D, Parmegiani L, Jindal S, Saleh R, Colpi G, Agarwal A. ICSI for non-male factor infertility: time to reappraise IVF? Panminerva Med. 2023;65(2):159–65. https://doi.org/10.23736/S0031-0808.23.04869-3.

121. Lepine S, McDowell S, Searle LM, Kroon B, Glujovsky D, Yazdani A. Advanced sperm selection techniques for assisted reproduction. Cochrane Database Syst Rev. 2019;7(7):CD010461. https://doi.org/10.1002/14651858.CD010461.pub3.

122. Stein J, Harper JC. Analysis of fertility clinic marketing of complementary therapy add-ons. Reprod Biomed Soc Online. 2021;13:24–36. https://doi.org/10.1016/j.rbms.2021.04.001.

123. Teixeira DM, Miyague AH, Barbosa MA, Navarro PA, Raine-Fenning N, Nastri CO, Martins WP. Regular (ICSI) versus ultra-high magnification (IMSI) sperm selection for assisted reproduction. Cochrane Database Syst Rev. 2020;2020(2):CD010167. https://doi.org/10.1002/14651858.CD010167.pub3.

124. Tao Y, Sanger E, Saewu A, Leveille M-C. Human sperm vitrification: the state of the art. Reprod Biol Endocrinol. 2020;18(1):17. https://doi.org/10.1186/s12958-020-00580-5.

125. Nagy ZP, Varghese AC, Agarwal A. Cryopreservation of mammalian gametes and embryos: methods and protocols. New York: Springer; 2017.

126. Li Y-X, Zhou L, Lv M-Q, Ge P, Liu Y-C, Zhou D-X. Vitrification and conventional freezing methods in sperm cryopreservation: a systematic review and meta-analysis. Eur J Obstet Gynecol Reprod Biol. 2019;233:84–92. https://doi.org/10.1016/j.ejogrb.2018.11.028.

127. Moody JA, Ahmed K, Yap T, Minhas S, Shabbir M. Fertility management in testicular cancer: the need to establish a standardized and evidence-based patient-centric pathway. BJU Int. 2019;123(1):160–72. https://doi.org/10.1111/bju.14455.

128. Eini F, Kutenaei MA, Shirzeyli MH, Dastjerdi ZS, Omidi M, Novin MG. Normal seminal plasma could preserve human spermatozoa against cryopreservation damages in oligozoospermic patients. BMC Mol Cell Biol. 2021;22(1):50. https://doi.org/10.1186/s12860-021-00390-6.

129. Walmsley R, Cohen J, Ferrara-Congedo T, Reing A, Garrisi J. The first births and ongoing pregnancies associated with sperm cryopreservation within evacuated egg zonae. Hum Reprod. 1998;13(Suppl 4):61–70. https://doi.org/10.1093/humrep/13.suppl_4.61.

130. Liu S, Li F. Cryopreservation of single-sperm: where are we today? Reprod Biol Endocrinol. 2020;18(1):41. https://doi.org/10.1186/s12958-020-00607-x.

131. Wang X, Lu F, Bai S, Wu L, Huang L, Zhou N, Xu B, Wan Y, Jin R, Jiang X, Tong X. A simple and efficient method to cryopreserve human ejaculated and testicular spermatozoa in −80°C freezer. Front Genet. 2022;12:815270. https://www.frontiersin.org/article/10.3389/fgene.2021.815270.

132. Mehta A, Esteves SC, Schlegel PN, Niederberger CI, Sigman M, Zini A, Brannigan RE. Use of testicular sperm in nonazoospermic males. Fertil Steril. 2018;109(6):981–7. https://doi.org/10.1016/j.fertnstert.2018.04.029.

133. Esteves SC, Sánchez-Martín F, Sánchez-Martín P, Schneider DT, Gosálvez J. Comparison of reproductive outcome in oligozoospermic men with high sperm DNA fragmentation undergoing intracytoplasmic sperm injection with ejaculated and testicular sperm. Fertil Steril. 2015;104(6):1398–405. https://doi.org/10.1016/j.fertnstert.2015.08.028.

134. Alkandari MH, Moryousef J, Phillips S, Zini A. Testicular sperm aspiration (TESA) or microdissection testicular sperm extraction (micro-TESE): which approach is better in men

with cryptozoospermia and severe oligozoospermia? Urology. 2021;154:164–9. https://doi.org/10.1016/j.urology.2021.04.037.

135. Hibi H, Sonohara M, Sugie M, Fukunaga N, Asada Y. Microscopic epididymal sperm aspiration (MESA) should be employed over testicular sperm extraction (TESE) sperm retrieval surgery for obstructive azoospermia (OA). Cureus. 2023;15(6):e40659. https://doi.org/10.7759/cureus.40659.

136. van Wely M, Barbey N, Meissner A, Repping S, Silber SJ. Live birth rates after MESA or TESE in men with obstructive azoospermia: is there a difference? Hum Reprod. 2015;30(4):761–6. https://doi.org/10.1093/humrep/dev032.

137. Shih K-W, Shen P-Y, Wu C-C, Kang Y-N. Testicular versus percutaneous epididymal sperm aspiration for patients with obstructive azoospermia: a systematic review and meta-analysis. Transl Androl Urol. 2019;8(6):631–40. https://doi.org/10.21037/tau.2019.11.20.

138. Bernie AM, Mata DA, Ramasamy R, Schlegel PN. Comparison of microdissection testicular sperm extraction, conventional testicular sperm extraction, and testicular sperm aspiration for nonobstructive azoospermia: a systematic review and meta-analysis. Fertil Steril. 2015;104(5):1099–103.e1–3. https://doi.org/10.1016/j.fertnstert.2015.07.1136.

Sperm Motility

5

Evangelini Evgeni and Priyank Kothari

Introduction

Sperm motility has long been recognized as one of the most important functional aspects of semen quality, incorporated in basic semen analysis as an integral constituent.

Human spermatozoa acquire their ability to move after their passage through the epididymis. During their existence in the testicular environment, spermatozoa exhibit no or feeble motion, due to the immature status of the plasmalemma. As soon as they proceed to the epididymis, occurring functional alterations lead to the development of motility characteristics. After ejaculation, spermatozoa are mixed with the accessory glands' secretions, hence undergoing motility activation.

The quantitative analysis of the motility types provides a useful tool for semen quality evaluation in the diagnosis of male fertility and infertility. During the past decades, additional indices beyond the plain categorization of motility types have been sought, aiming to depict more objectively specific aspects of sperm movement, in the context of sperm kinematics' evaluation via automated systems.

Following the new sixth WHO edition of the Manual, sperm motility is re-evaluated and methodologically scrutinized, in the scope of discovering its clinical importance in the investigation of male infertility. In this chapter, the role of sperm motility assessment and its clinical relevance is outlined under the new perspective of the WHO methodological recommendations.

E. Evgeni (✉)
Cryogonia Cryopreservation Bank, Athens, Greece
e-mail: lina.evgeni@cryogonia.gr

P. Kothari
B.Y.L Nair Ch Hospital, Mumbai, India

A. Agarwal et al. (eds.), *Human Semen Analysis*,
https://doi.org/10.1007/978-3-031-55337-0_5

Physiology: Methodology of Sperm Motility Testing

In order to reach the site of fertilization, spermatozoa must be able to swim actively and progress through a hostile environment from the site of deposition in the vagina via the cervix and uterus. The efficiency of sperm transport through the female genital tract is highly dependent on a strict natural selective process which eliminates spermatozoa of impaired motility. The first types of sperm that are withheld in the lower parts of the female body mainly present with tail defects (e.g., small flagellum and thin midpiece) that reduce the ability to exhibit linear progressive movement [1].

Spermatogenesis is a differentiation process through which immature spermatogonia are transformed to mature spermatozoa that are expelled into the proximal part of the epididymis. During their journey to the distal part of the epididymis, spermatozoa undergo functional alterations that provide them with motility, maturity, and fertilizing ability. After ejaculation, sperm enter the female reproductive tract, where they undergo capacitation with a series of modifications through which spermatozoa acquire a hyperactivated motility pattern, a prerequisite for sperm entrance through the oocyte zona [2].

Semen analysis constitutes the cornerstone laboratory tool for the evaluation of the functional competence of male testicular and accessory reproductive glands. The examined specimen consists of the comprehensive secretion of the epididymis and vas deferens, as well as the prostate and seminal vesicles. Normally, ejaculation is performed sequentially, with the first fraction containing the spermatozoa with prostatic fluid, whereas the following two thirds of the ejaculate mainly contain seminal vesicular fluid [3].

Sperm motility is a major parameter of semen analysis which may be considered as a fundamental aspect of sperm fertility potential. Progressive motility in particular has been recognized as a factor associated with pregnancy rates, in vivo and in vitro. Also, the total number of ejaculated progressively motile spermatozoa bears biological significance [4–6]. Clinical data from both manual assessment of sperm motility as well as automated sperm analysis demonstrate the importance of the identification of rapidly progressive spermatozoa [7–17]. Hence, the recent sixth edition of the WHO laboratory manual for the examination and processing of human semen (2021) has re-adopted the distinct assessment of the rapid and slow progressive motility pattern as part of a four-category grading system for motility evaluation.

According to the manual's recommendations, sperm motility must be evaluated in a completely liquefied semen sample, collected after 2–7 days of sexual abstinence, within 30 min post ejaculation. In case of incomplete liquefaction within the designated 30-min interval, another 30-min incubation is performed and counting begins afterwards. Any sign of delayed liquefaction is separately reported.

As temperature variations may interfere with sperm velocity, it is imperative that sperm motility is evaluated at a standardized temperature. Room temperature is difficult to control, therefore maintaining a standard of 37 °C is essential. This requires a fully equipped andrology laboratory setting including an incubator of 37 °C to warm the samples as well as the slides and coverslips used for the wet preparation and a heated microscope stage to preserve the same temperature throughout the counting process.

A minimum number of 200 spermatozoa counted in at least five fields, in two replicate separate wet preparations, is required to achieve a statistically accurate result.

The recommended categories for motility classification according to WHO 2021 are as follows:

1. Class a "rapid progressive"—including spermatozoa moving forward with a speed of at least 25 μm/s, covering a minimum distance of 25 μm (or ½ tail length) per second;
2. Class b "slow progressive"—including spermatozoa progressing with a speed of 5 to less than 25 μm/s (or at least one head length to less than ½ tail length) per second;
3. Class c "non-progressive"—including spermatozoa exhibiting all other patterns of active tail movement with an absence of progression, showing displacement of the head less than 5 μm (one head length) per second;
4. Class d "immotility"—completely immotile spermatozoa with no active tail movement.

The accurate measurement of sperm motility is heavily dependent on the capability of the observer to precisely discriminate the different types of progressively moving sperm. In a sample containing spermatozoa of low numbers or slow motility, the evaluation can be performed more easily. Contrastingly, the evaluation of samples of high concentration or increased progressive motility requires sophisticated skills acquired by specialized training and experience. This is partly a reason leading the editing committee of the previous WHO manual (2010) to the decision of merging the rapid and slow progressive motility categories in one, as a majority of technicians performing semen analysis were not adequately efficient in discriminating between motility categories a and b. The recent editing committee re-installed the four-category system (as in WHO 1999), based on the fact that rapid progressive movement has been associated with increased sperm fertility potential and optimal reproductive outcomes [18].

In a recent review by Boitrelle et al., the clinical utility of the distinction between rapid and slow progressive motility is further scrutinized, as the authors suggest that more recent data (after 2010) should be available to further support this decision [19]. In any case, the rationale on which the adoption of the categorization system should be based is clinical relevance and not the lack of adequate training of the laboratory scientists performing the assay. The access to educational seminars aiming to train laboratory andrologists, as well as the participation in External Quality Control Schemes can be of great value toward this direction [16].

In case an increased percentage of immotile spermatozoa is present in the ejaculate, namely more than 60%, it is important to identify the percentage of "live-immotile" against "dead-immotile" sperm. The confusion provoked by the WHO manual fifth edition, recommending sperm vitality evaluation in the presence of less than 40% progressive motility has been addressed in the recent sixth edition, stating that vitality assessment is very important in the presence of less than 40% total motility [20].

Motility evaluation should be performed in conjunction with sperm vitality in order to discriminate between dead and live immotile sperm. Furthermore, it can provide an additional counter-check for the accuracy of motility assessment, as the percentage of dead spermatozoa should not exceed that of immotile ones. This can aid the more efficient management of asthenozoospermia versus necrozoospermia, when properly distinguished.

The investigation of an extreme presence of asthenozoospermia exhibited by total immotility should incorporate sperm vitality assessment. The causes of necrozoospermia have been detailed described by Agarwal et al. to include mainly genital tract infections, testicular hyperthermia, pathological conditions such as varicocele, hyperthyroidism, polycystic kidney disease, antisperm antibodies or lifestyle factors, e.g., toxic substances, such as tobacco, cannabis and exposure to pesticides, advanced male age or idiopathic. Also, in the examination of sperm motility and vitality, one should not overlook the possibility of the ejaculate contamination with lubricants, antiseptic solutions, soap and water during collection [21].

Apart from the first line management of treatment and/or modifications of previously mentioned contributory factors, the ejaculatory frequency should also be considered. Prolonged storage in the epididymis may diminish sperm motility and vitality, which could be improved by repeated ejaculations at short intervals (e.g., within 60 min, 12 h or 24 h after the first ejaculate) [22–24].

In case a sample of extreme asthenozoospermia is to be used in assisted reproduction techniques (ART), namely intracytoplasmic sperm injection (ICSI), a vitality test is necessary to select live spermatozoa with functional membranes for insemination, i.e., hypoosmotic swelling (HOS) test, sperm tail flexibility test (STFT), laser assisted immotile sperm selection (LAISS), This could be further aided by the use of activating substances, e.g. pentoxifylline (PTX) or theophylline that can activate flagellar movement of immotile spermatozoa [25–29]. Absolute necrozoospermia, on the other hand, could be referred to testicular sperm extraction, as a means of retrieval of vital spermatozoa to be used in ICSI [30, 31]. As sperm death may be linked with a sequential degrading process triggered by excessive ROS generation causing lipid peroxidation and DNA damage, that lead to sperm membrane and nucleic acid deterioration, oxidative stress-related DNA fragmentation should also be considered in the diagnostic workup of these cases [32].

Abstinence time has been considered as a factor affecting the levels of conventional seminal parameters. The formal recommendation of the recent WHO manual for the designated abstinence time for semen analysis is an interval from 4 to 7 days [20]. The European Society of Human Reproduction and Embryology (ESHRE) and Nordic Association for Andrology (NAFA) guidelines limit abstinence time to a narrower interval, ranging from 3 to 4 days [33]. Although the correlation between abstinence time and sperm quality does not appear to be straightforward, it is generally recognized that sperm motility may improve with shorter abstinence time. A recent meta-analysis by Li et al. suggests that a shorter (less than 4 days) rather than a longer (from 4 to 7 days) abstinence period could provide better clinical outcomes in in vitro fertilization (IVF)/intracytoplasmic sperm injection (ICSI) [34]. Although data from distinct groups of fertile as well as infertile men may be conflicting, it seems that progressive motility in pooled data may improve when an abstinence period of 2–4 days is applied, with better clinical results in cases of IVF/ICSI. A potential explanation could be attributed to the shorter storage period of the spermatozoa in the male reproductive ducts, which potentially prevents oxidative stress-related detrimental effects on sperm quality [35]. Short storage in the epididymal tail (even with 1 day of abstinence) may prevent long time effect of ROS on sperm before their excretion to the ejaculate, therefore promoting better chances of success in ART in terms of both fertilization and implantation rates [36]. Also, short abstinence time could improve protein expression responsible for sperm functional aspects, e.g., motility, capacitation or acrosome reaction [37].

Semen hyperviscosity has been documented in 12–29% of ejaculates, a condition that can seriously impair the physical and chemical characteristics of seminal fluid, causing a reduction in sperm motility as well as lower success rates in ART. Several approaches have been suggested for reducing semen viscosity, such as overhydration and prostatic massage, gentle aspiration, and expulsion of the ejaculate through a 5-mL syringe (with no needle) as well as treatment with chymotrypsin and recently with DNase I. According to Nosi et al., as semen hyperviscosity is likely caused either by inflammation or by seminal gland dysfunction, it could be associated with genital tract viral infections that can be effectively addressed by DNase I treatment. Additional studies may be warranted to support the wide application of the latter approach [38].

Sperm agglutination is a phenomenon describing multiple motile sperm sticking in particular patterns, i.e., head-to-head, tail-to-tail or in a mixed way, exhibiting a frantic shaking motion or at times even limited motion, with an underlying cause of immunological response of the male body to the secreted spermatozoa. This should not be confused with plain sperm aggregations, where motile spermatozoa may be stuck to other cells or debris or immotile spermatozoa, often with mucus [20]. In the presence of >20% agglutinates, the major type of agglutination reflecting the degree and the site of attachment should be recorded. Sperm motility may be impaired due to this phenomenon, as a significant number of motile spermatozoa are withheld in the agglutinates. Sperm motility assessment should be performed in these cases in free spermatozoa (not bound in agglutinates) and further examination for antisperm antibodies (ASA) should be effectuated. As ASA are bound on spermatozoa post ejaculation, a laboratory technique to eliminate agglutination and provide more free motile spermatozoa for examination and use in ART, could incorporate the addition of a low volume of culture medium (approximately 1–2 mL) in the container before collection.

Sperm Motility and Diagnosis of Fertility and Infertility

During the last three decades, numerous manuals have been written, in order to provide guidance to the laboratory scientists on the methodological steps required for the proper and skillful performance of a reliable basic semen analysis [16, 33, 39]. In the scope of achieving universal standardization of a rather subjective analysis, the WHO has published five manuals for the examination of human semen from 1980 to 2010 [40–44]. The latest, most recent sixth edition of the WHO laboratory manual for the examination and processing of human semen aimed to improve the recommended methodology and update the global perception of the clinical utility of basic semen analysis, addressing many of the issues criticized in previous editions.

Considering the evolution of the reference values from the first WHO manual in 1980, based on a liberal consideration of "normality" to the WHO fifth edition where the concept of natural fertility was for the first time embodied in the interpretation of the results of the basic semen analysis, the additions in the recent WHO manual empower the statistical significance of the updated reference limits. The new reference values now include data from >3500 men from 11 countries and 5 continents, also adding China and Africa, accepted after scrutiny regarding methodological issues. All these men had achieved pregnancy within less than 12 months of unprotected intercourse, examined after 2–7 days of abstinence. Although still regionally restrictive, considering that South America is not represented and only one African country has been included, these values represent a more global distribution than the previous ones [45] (Table 5.1).

The lower fifth centile of the distribution of these values is adopted as the reference limit differentiating between "normal" and "abnormal" measurements of basic seminal parameters, however, with certain limitations: distribution values do not necessarily constitute limits of fertility. A time to pregnancy (TTP) less than 12 months may represent couples with a compromised sperm quality, but with enough luck to achieve natural pregnancy or contrastingly, a good quality sperm may be omitted from the distribution, if a female factor is present, preventing the pregnancy from happening in this designated time period [3, 45].

Since a significant overlap may be present between fertile and sub-fertile men, a wide consensus-based categorization of groups signifying "normal," "borderline," and "pathological" values has been suggested, representing a continuum rather than a dichotomic perception of semen quality [16, 47] (Table 5.2).

Considering the above, the recent WHO manual introduces (before retraction at the final step of publication) the concept of decision limits, a novel approach in the interpretation of semen analysis which may be more clinically relevant depending on the clinical perspective under which it is effectuated. For example, the assessment of male reproductive organ function revealing endocrine or genetic disorders, post-treatment evaluation, decision-making in the context of assisted reproduction technology (ART), epidemiological and environmental studies, or as a man's general health marker (male subfertility correlates with other dysfunctions, e.g., cardiovascular, metabolic) [18, 49].

Table 5.1 Reference values of major semen parameters as published in consecutive WHO manuals

Manual editions	WHO 1980 1st	WHO 1987 2nd	WHO 1992 3rd	WHO 1999 4th	WHO 2010 5th	WHO 2021 6th
Semen characteristics						
Volume(mL)	ND	≥2	≥2	≥2	1.5[a]	1.4[a]
Sperm count ($\times 10^6$/mL)	20–200	≥20	≥20	≥20	15[a]	16[a]
Total sperm count ($\times 10^6$)	ND	≥40	≥40	≥40	39[a]	39[a]
Total motility (% motile)	≥60	≥50	≥50	≥50	40[a]	42[a]
Progressive motility[b] (%)	≥2[c]	≥25	≥20 (Grade a)	≥25 (Grade a)	32 (Grade a + b)[a]	30 (Grade a + b)[a]
Vitality (% live)	ND	≥50	≥75	≥75	58[a]	54[a]
Morphology (% typical forms)	80.5	≥50	≥30[d]	14[e]	4[a,f]	4[a,f]
Leukocyte count ($\times 10^6$/mL)	<4.7	<1.0	<1.0	<1.0	<1.0	<1.0

[a] Lower reference limit obtained from fifth centile value, based on fertility criteria
[b] Grade a, rapid progressive motility (25%); Grade b, slow/sluggish progressive motility (5–25 μm/s); normal, 50% motility (Grade a + b) within 60 min of ejaculation
[c] Forward progression (scale 0–3)
[d] Arbitrary value
[e] Value not defined, but strict criterion suggested
[f] Strict (Tygerberg) criteria. *WHO* World Health Organization, *ND* not defined (adapted from Esteves [46])

Table 5.2 General (consensus-based) reference values for evaluation of main semen parameters

Characteristics	Units	Normal	Borderline	Pathological	Notes
Volume	mL	2.0–6.0	1.5–1.9	<1.5	a
Sperm concentration	10^6/mL	20–250	10–20	<10	a, b
Total sperm count	10^6/ejaculate	≥80	20–79	<20	a, b
Motility	% motile (total)	≥60	40–59	<40	c, d
	% progressive	≥50	35–49	<35	c, d
	% rapid progressive	≥25	–	–	c, d
	Progression rate	3 or 4	2	1 or 2	c, d, e
Morphology	% Typical forms	≥14	4–13	<4	f
Viability	Percent viable	>75	50–70	<50	g

[a] Evaluated after 2–4 days of abstinence
[b] For specimen with 2.0–6.0 mL volume
[c] Evaluated at 30 min post ejaculation
[d] Evaluated at 37 °C
[e] Based on a scale of 0–4, 0: no progression; 1: poor; 2: medium; 3: good; 4: very good/excellent
[f] Evaluated using Tygerberg Strict Criteria
[g] Evaluated by eosin dye exclusion at 30 min post ejaculation (adapted from Bjorndahl et al. [48])

Sperm motility, in particular, is a strong marker of male reproductive potential, mirroring detrimental effects of various conditions, e.g., varicocele [50]. Apart from the individual categorization of the four motility types, other indices of motility evaluation such as the total progressive sperm count (TPMSC) have been investigated in association with reproductive outcomes. In a large retrospective cohort study in couples diagnosed with varying infertility factors, undergoing intrauterine insemination (IUI), it was concluded that anovulatory patients benefitted most from IUI, irrespective of TPMSC and that in patients with unexplained infertility, TPMSC does not significantly affect the success rates of IUI [51]. According to another longitudinal cohort study, prewash total motile sperm count (TMSC) was better correlated with the natural conception ongoing pregnancy rate than the WHO 2010 classification [52].

Although no current consensus exists regarding the predictive value of individual parameters for IUI, post-wash motile sperm count of more than one million is generally considered as a predictive parameter [53, 54]. Lower pregnancy rates have been reported in cases of total motile sperm count in the ejaculate less than ten million, with a baseline limit ranging from three to five million motile spermatozoa inseminated. Even values of post-wash TMSC as low as 0.8 million have been reported to have prognostic value in couples who underwent IUI [55].

In general, IUI has been suggested as first-line therapy method of ART for unexplained male infertility, when a TMSC higher than five million is present [56]. In vitro fertilization (IVF) is the recommended method when two to five million motile sperm can be isolated from the ejaculate and intracytoplasmic sperm injection (ICSI) is recommended when less than two million motile spermatozoa can be yielded [57].

Sperm Motility and Etiological Diagnosis of Male Reproductive Functions and Dysfunctions

In recent years, many researchers have focused on possible factors leading to male infertility and revealed the existence of many cellular and molecular defects during sperm production and maturation. These defects finally affect the count and structure of spermatozoa and reduce their ability to reach and fertilize the egg. A decrease in sperm motility, called "asthenozoospermia (AZS)," is one of these important deficiencies, influenced by various cellular and molecular factors.

Based on the WHO 2010 guidelines, asthenozoospermia was defined as total motility <40% and progressive motility <32% in a semen sample [44]. Severe asthenozoospermia was also characterized by total sperm immotility or very low motile spermatozoa in the semen sample. It was elucidated that total sperm immotility may be related to genetic disorders [58]. Understating the cellular and molecular processes producing sperm motility is necessary to be able to segregate the causes that lead to asthenozoospermia. Sperm motility depends on a fully functional flagellum,

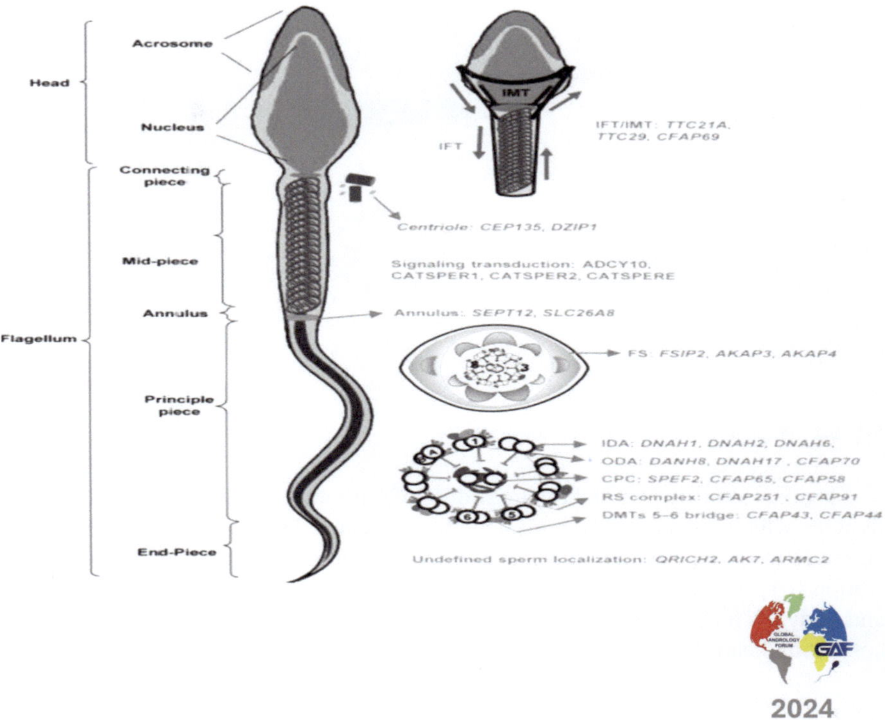

Fig. 5.1 Structure of spermatozoa with genes encoding various components

energy availability and efficient and coordinated signaling pathways that translate into external signals for motility.

Structural integrity of sperm flagella (Figs. 5.1 and 5.2), consisting of axonemal and periaxonemal parts, is a prerequisite for sperm motility [59]. The axoneme contains nine peripheral double microtubules (DMT) and a central pair (9 + 2). The nine microtubule doublets are connected to each other by the nexin—dynein regulatory complex (N-DRC) and to the central pair by projections and radial spokes (RSs). The periaxonemal structures contain the mitochondrial sheath (MS), fibrous sheath (FS) and outer dense fibers (ODFs), responsible for energy metabolism and signal transduction. The sperm flagellum can be divided into four regions: connecting piece, midpiece, principal piece, and end piece. The connecting piece contains the basal body which connects the tail and sperm head. The midpiece has a mitochondrial sheath and ODFs to ensure energy delivery for sperm motility and flagellar elasticity. The FS functions as a scaffolding for proteins in signaling pathways and enzymes in the glycolytic pathway [60]. The annulus connects the midpiece and principal piece and functions like a diffusion chamber (Fig. 5.1).

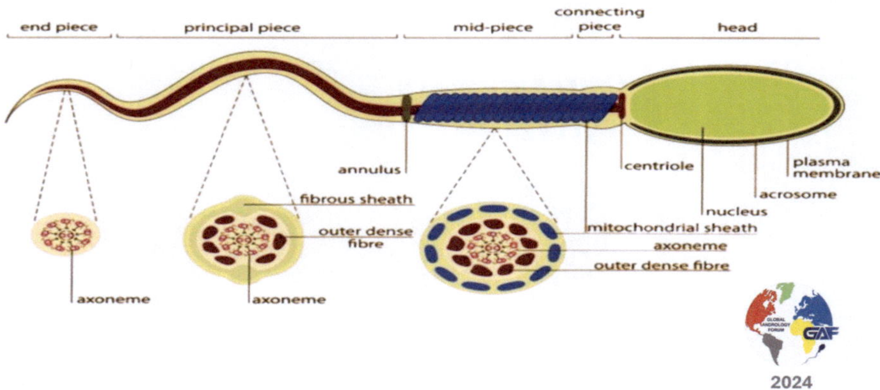

Fig. 5.2 Basic structure of the spermatozoon

Flagellar motility is based on the sliding of microtubule pairs through axonemal dyneins which mechanically reinforce the axonemes. Due to the main role of tail structure in sperm motility, flagellar defects may directly impair motility and fertilization [61]. Deficiencies in flagella structure may be related to other ciliopathies and body dysfunction, such as polycystic kidney disease, repeated chest infections, congenital heart disease, blindness, and obesity.

Flagellar/Ciliary Defects and Sperm Motility

AZS can be classified into two forms: isolated (without other ailments) and syndromic (characterized by additional symptoms with varied phenotypic expressivity), analyzed below:

- **Isolated**—Multiple morphological abnormalities of sperm flagella (MMAF) and AZS without oligo- and teratozoospermia. MMAF is characterized by aberrant flagellar types (short, angulated, irregular) and the origin seems to be genetic. It is the most frequent sperm defect observed in infertile men [62].
- **Syndromic**—Ciliopathy caused by ciliary dysfunction. The most characteristic abnormality is primary ciliary Dyskinesia (PCD), an autosomal recessive disease mainly characterized by chronic airway disease, rhinitis, bronchitis, and sinusitis due to dysfunction of cilia.

Genetic mutations in ciliary proteins of patients with Kartagener syndrome prompted the coining of the term Primary Ciliary Dyskinesia (PCD). It was found that dynein arms are absent in these patients contributing to defective epithelial cilia and sperm flagella. It was found that they had a common ultrastructural abnormality [63]. Patients suspected to have these disorders, although having high sperm concentrations, they exhibit 100% immotile sperm. In these cases, genetic testing of both partners is required, as this is an autosomal recessive disease with a possibility of transmission to the offspring of 25% (both alleles) from two carrier parents.

Ciliopathy has been used to refer to the general symptoms resulting from disorders of primary, motile, and sensory cilia. It is caused by many deficiencies, including male infertility due to similarity of sperm flagella and somatic cilia in axonemal structure and their formation mechanism [61]. Some defects apparent in cilia are not present in sperm flagella and vice versa, indicating differences between flagella and cilia. Ciliopathy occurs almost entirely due to genetic mutations, involving various organs associated with the flagella/cilia. Men with ciliopathy, such as PCD have totally immotile or very low motile spermatozoa in their semen sample (severe asthenozoospermia).

Energy-Driven Concept of Sperm Motility

Glycolysis and oxidative phosphorylation are two metabolic pathways responsible for ATP production in sperm cells. These processes occur in the flagellum's central piece, head, and in mitochondria. The head has no respiratory enzymes and ATP synthesis occurs through mitochondrial respiration and glycolysis in the flagellar sheath. Enzymes found in the fibrous sheath are phosphofructokinase, phosphoglucokinase isomerase, hexokinase, lactate dehydrogenase, glyceraldehyde-3-phosphate dehydrogenase (GAPD). When the chemical energy produced by ATP hydrolysis is converted by dynein into mechanical energy, a force is generated.

Sperm immotility is caused by impaired integrity of the mitochondrial membrane and sheath function [64]. It has also been implicated to malfunctions of sperm mitochondrial ultrastructure [65].

Changes in mitochondrial DNA (mtDNA) including deletions affecting cellular membrane integrity can lead to reduced sperm function and male infertility. Although few studies state that sperm motility may be affected by ETC inhibitors [66], other studies suggest that glycolysis plays a more important role and its suppression results in reduced sperm motility even when mitochondrial substrates are present [64]. Thus, glycolysis is the preferred source of energy for sperm motility, which is also supported by the fact that the glycolytic enzymes are present throughout the tail of the sperm. High levels of calcium affect sperm motility. A decrease in protein phosphorylation induced by calcium prevents substrate kinase interactions and hence translation of the ATP energy into mechanical energy [67, 68].

Sperm Motility and Lifestyle and Environmental Factors

Lifestyle habits, exposure to chemical pesticides and air pollution may disrupt sperm motility. There is a physiologic production of reactive oxygen species (ROS) during sperm maturation, ejaculation, and fertilization. Excessive production of ROS can lead to structural destruction and defective DNA methylation and damage. Pathological conditions such as leukocytospermia, varicocele, genitourinary tract infection, and chronic inflammation induce ROS and contribute to reduced sperm motility [69]. High levels of hydrogen peroxide impair the activity of G6PD, leading to decreased NADPH and thus increase in oxidative stress.

Tobacco inhalation is another common lifestyle factor known to contribute to compromised semen parameters. Inhalation of large number of toxins from tobacco smoking can affect spermatogenesis and semen quality, including motility. Even moderate smoking was shown to have significant adverse effects on progressive motility [69]. Tobacco smoke contains nicotine as the main hazardous chemical along with traces of tar, carbon monoxide, polycyclic aromatic hydrocarbons, and heavy metals. The decrease in motility could also be due to the epididymal dysfunction in smokers or elevated oxidative stress in the testicular environment. High malondialdehyde (MDA) and protein carbonyl levels and low levels of glutathione S-transferase (GST) and reduced glutathione (GSH) were reported in seminal plasma and spermatozoa of smokers. Other factors, such as high body mass index [70], intense physical activity, prolonged cell phone [71], laptop usage [72], and lack of sleep [73] are considered as potential risk factors for decrease in sperm motility. Therefore, lifestyle modification such as consuming nutritious diet, regular exercise and withdrawal from substance abuse, smoking, and alcohol consumption can improve semen parameters considerably.

The Role of Ion Channels in Sperm Motility

The main functions of channels located in the sperm tail membrane include controlling cell motility, mediating the transduction of ciliary signals, and sensing environmental cues [74]. The environmental cues are activated with the fluid in the genital tract penetrating the sperm membrane. A spermatozoon must adopt to the hostility in the female genital tract and acquire the required motility for successful fertilization.

Ion channels and transporters are essential for sperm survival and fertility as they regulate calcium concentration, membrane voltage, and intracellular pH of spermatozoa ($[Ca^{2+}]_i$) [75]. It may be possible to attribute many of idiopathic male infertility cases to impaired function of sperm ion channels and their effector molecules. Cation channels of sperm (CATSPER channels) are characterized among the main channels contributing to ion homeostasis, especially calcium ion, which is needed for physiological events like capacitation and hyperactivated motility [76].

In male patients with low sperm motility, the complete absence of CATSPER protein occurs due to nonsense mediated decay or severely truncated CATSPER1 protein without any transmembrane domain and channel pore. CATSPER channels have another important role as pH regulators in progressive motility. According to relative studies, defects in CATSPER channels resulted in less directed and sluggish spermatozoal movement. These defects may lead to asthenozoospermia. Sperm motility is pH sensitive, due to dynein protein ability to hydrolyze ATP and provide axonemal bending which is elevated with increase in intracellular pH. Intracellular protons are constantly generated by the motile flagellum and more acidic a flagellum becomes, the faster it moves [77].

Genetic Contribution to Sperm Motility

Most of the etiological factors leading to asthenozoospermia still remain unknown, leading to a lack of effective targeted therapy. Genetic factors are likely involved in a large proportion of isolated AZS with sperm flagellum defects. There are hundreds of proteins associated with sperm tail structure and function, thus many ultrastructural defects may be genetically originated [65]. The knowledge on monogenic causes of AZS is still very limited, however broadly divided into the following categories:

1. Structural defects of sperm flagella and related genes.
2. Genes related to energy supply and signaling pathways.
3. Annulus related genes.
4. Sperm mitochondria related genes.
5. Other genes.

Several studies have attempted to demonstrate the role of genes in poor sperm motility, finding that sperm motility is influenced by a variety of mutations which ultimately reduce spermatozoa movement, some of which also related to the sperm microenvironment. In Table 5.3, a review of the most common genes quoted in the literature is presented. A majority of these studies include findings from basic research in animals, which warrant further investigation before they can be generalized in humans. In a clinical setting, more studies need to be performed on human spermatozoa and models in order to elucidate the modes of treatment of these possible defects.

Deletions or mutations in mitochondrial DNA are correlated with elevated oxidative stress, sperm immotility, and male infertility. In addition, researchers have identified polymorphic mutations in genes encoding the oxidative phosphorylation

Table 5.3 List of genes with the defects they cause as quoted in various studies

Gene	Protein localisation (Figs. 5.1 and 5.2)	Defect	References
Isolated AZS			
DNAH1	IDA (inner dynein arms)	Lack IDA and disorganized FS	Wambergue et al. [78], Sha et al. [79]
DNAH 2	IDA	Lack IDA and disorganized axonemal structures	Li et al. [80]
DNAH 6	IDA	IDA and CPC	Tu et al. [81]
DNAH 8, 17	ODA	Lack ODA and CPC	Liu et al. [82]
CFAP 43,44	DMT	Misaligned CPC	Coutton et al. [83]
AKAP 3,4	FS	Disarranged axonemal structures (MMAF phenotype)	Xu et al. [60]
CEP 135	Next to proximal centriole	Short or absent tail	Sha et al. [84]
SLC26A8	Annulus	Atrophy of annulus	Dirami et al. [85]
EIF4G1	Sperm Head	Axonemal structure and MS defect	Sha et al. [86]
CATSPER 1, 2	FS calcium channels		Brown et al. [87]
Syndromic AZS			
DNAAF 1–4	Dynein assembly	Absence of ODA and IDA	Omran et al. [88], Mitchison et al. [89], Tarkar et al. [90], Horani et al. [91]
ZMYND10	Assembly of dynein complexes	Lack of ODA and IDA	(PCD) Paff et al. [92]
CCDC40	Assembly of N-DRC and radial spokes	IDA absent and MT disorganization	Antony et al. [93]
RSPH3, SPAG6	RS component	PCD	Wu et al. [94] (p. 3)
PKD 1	Sperm flagellum	Disarranged axonemal structures	Torra et al. [95]
Other genes			
CRISP2	Localized to acrosome and sperm tail for sperm egg fusion	Low sperm motility and abnormal morphology	Heidary et al. [96]
SEMG 1	Semenogelin 1	Associated with semen coagulation, hyperviscosity, and AZS	Yu et al. [97]
SPAG16L	Sperm associated antigen 16	Axonemal central apparatus—defective sperm motility	Zhang et al. [98]

DNAH dynein axonemal heavy chain, *IDA* inner dynein arms, *ODA* outer dynein arms, *CPC* central pair complex, *FS* fibrous sheath, *DMT* doublet microtubules, *CFAP* cilia and flagellar associated protein gene, *AKAP* a kinase anchoring protein, *PKD* polycystic kidney disease, *CRISP* cysteine rich secretory proteins complexes and transfer RNA of mitochondrial DNA associated with low sperm motility [99].

Role of Sexual Abstinence

The epididymis fails to provide a conducive environment to spermatozoa for a long time. Elevated oxidative content and poor antioxidant defense in the epididymal microenvironment may compromise sperm parameters under such circumstances. Shen et al. (2019) reported that ejaculates collected from men with short abstinence (1–3 h) period compared to 3–7 days of abstinence showed increased sperm concentration and higher percentage of motile spermatozoa [37]. Better sperm velocity, progressiveness, and hyperactivation were observed when the abstinence period was 2 h compared to 4–7 days [100]. This was true for oligozoospermic men as well. Dupesh et al. (2020) reported that <24 h abstinence in oligozoopermic men had the highest percentage of progressively motile spermatozoa [101].

Drugs Affecting Sperm Motility

In vitro studies have shown that psychotropic drugs (imipramine hydrochloride, desmethylimipramine, chlorpromazine, trifluoperazine, and nortriptyline hydrochloride) act as potent inhibitors of sperm motility [102]. Antiepileptic drugs (phenytoin, carbamazepine, and valproate) had adverse effects on motility both in vivo and in vitro [103]. Consumption of high amounts of acetaminophen, an antipyretic, has also shown to decrease sperm motility [104]. Lansoprazole, a proton pump inhibitor used to treat gastric illness, has shown to reduce the motility due to its calcium quenching effect or decreased Na^+-K^+-ATPase activity [105]. Moderate consumption of aspirin, a non-steroidal anti-inflammatory drug (NSAID), is known to demonstrate similar effects in young men [106]. In addition, regular consumption of recreational drugs, such as marijuana, is shown to affect spermatogenesis as well as sperm motility [107]. However, there are no clear reports in the literature to suggest whether the effects of these drugs on motility are reversible or irreversible.

Heat Exposure and Sperm Motility

Scrotal temperature is 2–5 °C lower than the core body temperature in mammals, which is essential for normal spermatogenesis to take place. It is suggested that high heat exposure may perturb regulation of intrascrotal temperature and increase intratesticular temperature, both of which have drastic effects on semen quality [108]. Heat stress decreases sperm motility by downregulating mitochondrial activity and decreasing ATP levels. Transient scrotal hyperthermia was shown to cause reversible reduction in proteins required for spermatogenesis, gamete interaction, and motility. Decreased antioxidant level, mitochondrial degeneration, and alterations in protein expression pattern have been associated with poor motility. Men exposed to higher temperatures due to their occupation (bakers, foundry workers, welders) and other factors which increase the intratesticular temperature, such as sedentary work habits, wearing tight under garments and frequent sauna use, may have an increased risk of defective sperm motility.

Psychological Stress Affecting Sperm Motility

Psychological stress is an "emotional experience" accompanied by several biochemical, physiological and behavioral changes or responses. During the events of stress, corticosterone elevation suppresses testosterone and inhibin levels [109]. Stress can affect male fertility through different mechanisms, mostly through altering testosterone secretion and through disruption of the blood–testis barrier. Inhibition of the hypothalamic–pituitary–gonadal axis via the inhibitory effect of gonadotropin-inhibitory hormone and activation of the hypothalamic–pituitary–adrenal axis by producing an inhibitory effect on hypothalamic-pituitary-gonadal and Leydig cells, consequently impairs spermatogenesis [110].

Infection and Sperm Motility

Experimental evidence suggests that bacteriospermia decreases sperm motility significantly due to bacterial infections, leucocyte accumulation (leukocytospermia), antibody buildup, inflammation, and oxidative stress [111]. Chlamydia trachomatis and Ureaplasma sp. infections affect sperm motility. Similarly, Burrello et al. reported that infections caused by Candida albicans, a pathogenic yeast, decreased sperm motility significantly by reducing mitochondrial membrane potential and increasing apoptosis of human spermatozoa in vitro [112]. Pathogens such as hepatitis B virus, human papillomaviruses [113], herpes simplex viruses, and adeno-associated virus were associated with significant reduction in sperm parameters, especially progressive motility. A recent report suggests that infection with SARS-Cov-2 coronavirus in men can lead to low sperm count and poor motility for 90 days following infection [114].

Sperm Motility and Planning Further Investigations

During a thorough investigation of male infertility, an in-depth evaluation of specialized parameters may be warranted to shed light in the etiology of sperm motility deterioration [115]. As previously described in detail, a variety of mechanisms may underlie sperm motility decrease, giving rise to the need for establishing etiological associations [73, 115–117]. In this view, a battery of additional examinations can be suggested (Fig. 5.3).

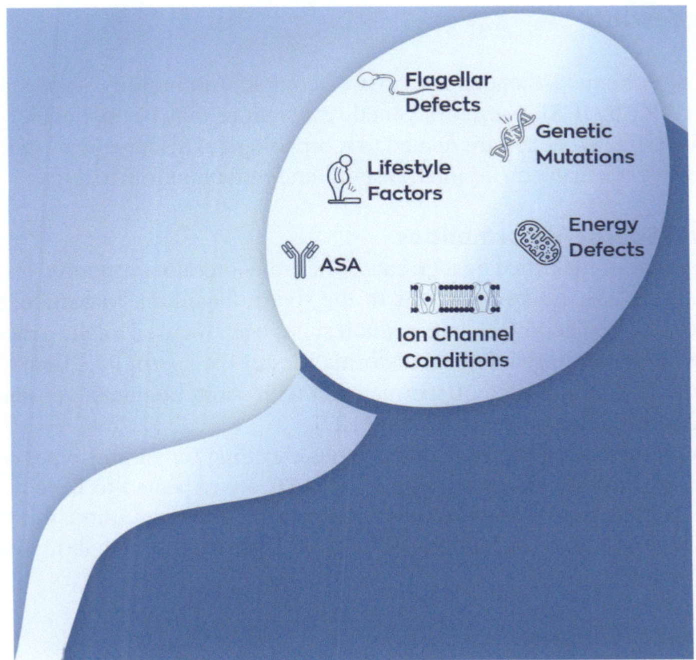

Fig. 5.3 Etiological mechanisms of sperm motility abberations, leading to additional investigations

With the advent of various advanced technologies in the methodology of semen quality evaluation, an exponential increase has been witnessed in research reports on the molecular defects involved in a variety of male reproductive deficiencies [49].

Oxidative Stress Evaluation

As in all cellular systems, a balance in the redox state exists at low physiological levels as reactive oxygen species (ROS) act in favor of optimal sperm functions such as motility, hyperactivation, capacitation, acrosome reaction, and sperm–oocyte fusion [118]. However, abnormally high levels of ROS produced by dysfunctional spermatozoa and leukocytes can adversely affect sperm function resulting in various defects among which sperm motility decrease [118–121].

In order to investigate the balance of oxidative and reductive agents and the possible etiological role of oxidative stress in cases of male asthenozoospermia, the MiOXSYS system can be applied for the reliable measurement of static oxidative–reductive potential (sORP) in semen and seminal plasma [116].

Genetic Testing

In cases of extreme asthenozoospermia or complete immotility, especially in the context of ART by ICSI, a series of genetic evaluations may be applicable. The main types of investigated genes are related to morphological discrepancies of the flagellum, defective mechanisms of ion transport, and mitochondrial activity.

Structural Sperm Abnormalities

A vast majority of identified genetic causes of asthenoteratozoospermia results from moderate or severe structural defects of the sperm flagellum. In particular, during the last decade, tremendous scientific interest has been focused on the genetic investigation of multiple morphological abnormalities of the sperm flagellum (MMAF), which present with a mosaic of spermatozoa with short, angulated, absent flagella or flagella of irregular shapes and sizes [122].

The examination of panels including genes encoding for various types of ciliopathies, e.g., primary ciliary dyskinesia or MMAF, are expected to have a powerful impact on the diagnostic improvement and possible treatment modalities of some types of male reproductive failure, and provide input on the probability of success in ICSI-IVF [49].

Ion Transport Channels

Genetic alterations affecting sperm ion transporters and channels have been related with asthenozoospermia. CATSPER is the first ion channel studied as a genetic cause of defects affecting sperm motility in humans, resulting in male sterility. Studies performed in various ethnic groups reveal the connection between genomic deletions of CATSPER2 and syndromic asthenozoospermia. A partial deletion was initially described in a French family presenting with a deafness-infertility syndrome (DIS) and asthenozoospermia. The identification of complete deletion of the gene was subsequently made in three unrelated Iranian families. Also, two consanguineous Iranian families with autosomal recessive non-syndromic male infertility, described with asthenozoospermia, low sperm count and abnormal sperm morphology were reported to harbor the CATSPER deletion. Intriguingly, a copy number variation leading to heterozygous CATSPER2 deletion was reported in a Chinese patient showing conventional analysis within the reference ranges, but with impaired sperm hyperactivation and zona pellucida penetration [122].

Genes encoding for the function of protein ion channel exchangers and transporters, such as CATSPER and Slo3 K$^+$ channels, are discussed in the sixth edition of the WHO Manual [49]. These novel tests are suggested as advanced tests for the sophisticated examination of human male infertility, although current techniques of assessment are too demanding to be implemented in routine laboratory practice [20].

Mitochondrial Gene Mutations

Mitochondrial DNA gene deletions or mutations have been associated with elevated oxidative stress-related male infertility exhibited with sperm immotility, e.g., a missense mutation (C119941) in the mitochondrial NADH dehydrogenase 4 gene.

Polymorphic mutations in genes encoding for oxidative phosphorylation complexes and transfer RNA of mitochondrial DNA have been identified as genetic causes associated with low sperm motility [57].

Antisperm Antibody (ASA) Testing

The effect of ASA on sperm motility has been debated in relative studies. Although some investigators report a negative effect, attributed to the engagement of moving spermatozoa in agglutinates that provoke their slowing down, others did not demonstrate any correlation between the presence of ASA and sperm motility. According to another group of studies, an immunological negative effect on motility has been associated with the severity of autoimmunization. This discrepancy may be explained by the different localization of the targeted antigen and the inclusion of patient groups with unmatched degrees of autoimmunity.

The current WHO guidelines recommend ASA determination directly on sperm surface by use of the mixed agglutination reaction (MAR) and immunobead tests (IBT), as they are widely available and easy-to-perform, or indirectly in serum or seminal plasma. The ELISA method has also been suggested for the detection of seminal ASA, to promote standardization, considering the significant correlation between seminal and sperm-bound ASA levels. Another advantage of the ELISA test is the possibility to perform the assay in one rum of collected stored samples, in contrast to IBT and MAR tests requiring fresh samples [123].

Microbiological Investigation

A comprehensive microbiological investigation may provide useful information in the context of asthenozoospermia. Bacteriospermia has been suggested as a cause of decreased sperm motility significantly due to infections, leukocytospermia, antibody generation, inflammation, and oxidative stress. Chlamydia trachomatis and Ureaplasma sp. infections have been linked to negative effects in sperm motility. Similarly, Candida albicans has been reported to significantly decrease sperm motility by reducing mitochondrial membrane potential and increasing apoptosis of human spermatozoa in vitro. The presence of viral pathogens such as hepatitis B virus, human papillomaviruses, herpes simplex viruses and adeno-associated virus has been correlated with significant deterioration of progressive motility [57].

Sperm Motility and Non-ART Management: Treatment and Treatment Response Monitoring

Effective treatment is not available for reversing the morphologic and/or motility defects in CATSPER related and genetically-linked asthenozoospermia. However, protecting the quality of spermatozoa and optimizing the existing motility is possible. Mainly oxidative stress-related factors can be avoided. Unhealthy lifestyle habits, toxic environmental and occupational exposure, physical inactivity, recreational use of tobacco, cigarettes, and alcohol can be avoided to reduce this oxidative stress. Although endocrine and cardiovascular disease cannot be completely reversed, it may be effectively managed by use of medications and lifestyle changes, so as to reduce oxidative stress.

Increasing the number of ejaculations and intercourse frequency may improve sperm motility, albeit not significantly as shown in a small study [124]. De Jonge et al. demonstrated that longer abstinence increased both sperm count and sample volume [125]. However, attributes such as pH, viability, morphology, motility, and DNA fragmentation were not affected. In a large scale relevant retrospective study, Levitas et al. reported on abstinence effects with general improvements in total motile count (TMC) with longer abstinence with optimized results in an abstinence from 3 to 6 days [126]. In a subgroup of men with low concentration at baseline ($<20 \times 10^6$ sperm/mL) declines in sample quality were noted after 2 days of abstinence. Hence, the evidence for the effect of frequent ejaculations and abstinence period on sperm motility is inconclusive to clearly support benefit for shorter abstinence or frequent ejaculations though it can be attempted as it might prove beneficial in certain cases.

Surgical management of varicocele, antibiotic treatment for infections of the genital tract and the use of corticosteroids for chronic inflammations can be used to reduce oxidative stress. Several antioxidants have been widely used for enhancing sperm motility. Antioxidant supplements are commonly recommended during 3–12 months and various clinical trials have studied their effect on sperm motility. These antioxidants can be used as a monotherapy or combination therapy.

Varicocele Repair for Isolated Asthenozoospermia

Surgical varicocele repair (varicocelectomy) is beneficial not only for alleviating oxidative stress-associated infertility, but also for preventing and protecting against the progressive character of varicocele and its consequent upregulations of systemic oxidative stress. A compromised testicular microenvironment due to elevated levels of highly reactive oxidants and reduced levels of antioxidant is commonly observed in this condition [127]. Plenty of evidence in the literature suggests that varicocele is associated with poor sperm motility [50, 127, 128]. A high percentage of inactive mitochondria, abnormal expression of mitochondrial proteins [129], decrease in ATP levels and altered calcium signaling cascade in spermatozoa of men with varicocele has been reported in the literature. There is a controversy regarding the indication for repair in individuals with isolated asthenozoospermia, but otherwise sperm counts above the fifth centile. In patients with oligoasthenozoospermia and clinical varicocele with reflux, varicocelectomy is proven to create oxidative stress and hence repair is beneficial with improvement in both count and motility [50, 130]. Few studies have shown no improvement in motility in patients with isolated asthenozoospermia post varicocelectomy [130], while others support treatment of isolated asthenozoospermia claiming improvement in spontaneous, IUI and ICSI pregnancy rates [131]. This discrepancy is unavoidable in studies using fifth centile as cut off for normal sperm concentration, which is used commonly. In our practice at B.Y.L Nair Charitable hospital, we proceed with correcting the varicocele in

Table 5.4 Depiction of various studies examining the effect of antioxidants on semen parameters in infertile men

Patient group and number (*n*)	Type of antioxidant and duration of consumption	Effect on semen parameters	References
Idiopathic OAT (228)	COQ 10 200 mg/day/28 weeks	Progressive motility improved significantly	Safarinejad et al. [132]
Idiopathic OAT (60)	200 mg CoQ/3 months	No difference in sperm parameters	Nadjarzadeh et al. [133]
Infertile men	Vit E 400 mg/day 6 months	Significant improvement in motility	Ghanem et al. [134]
Idiopathic OAT (90)	Vit E 400 mg 6 months	Mean total sperm motility improved in all patients	ElSheikh et al. [135]
Idiopathic asthenoteratozoospermia (114)	L carnitine 145 mg, fructose 250 mg, Se 50 µg, CoQ 20 mg, zinc 10 mg, ascorbic acid 90 mg, folic acid 200 µg (once a day × 4 months)	Progressive motility improved significantly	Busetto et al. [136]
Oligo, astheno, or terato- zoospermia (104)	L-carnitine and acetyl L carnitine	Progressive and total motility higher	Busetto et al. [137]
Infertile men	Docosahexenoic acid	No difference in sperm parameters	Martínez-Soto et al. [138]
Idiopathic asthenozoospermia (meta-analysis)	L carnitine/L-acetyl carnitine	Improvement in motility and morphology	Wei et al. [139]
Infertile men (metanalysis of RCTs for CoQ)	CoQ (200–300 mg)	Improvement in motility more than other parameters	Vishvkarma et al. [68]

OAT oligoasthenoteratozoospermia, *CoQ* Co enzyme Q

patients with isolated asthenozoospermia when medical therapy has failed and the ipsilateral testis is significantly smaller compared to the opposite testis with clinical varicocele and significant reflux on hand-held doppler study. As for the technique applied, microsurgical repair is associated with the best outcomes.

Large numbers of trials and meta-analyses with various antioxidants used individually or in combination have been effectuated, among which the most informative ones are listed Table 5.4.

Antioxidants such as vitamin E, coenzyme Q10, L-carnitine, vitamin C, and lycopene, alone or in combination with trace elements like selenium or zinc, have demonstrated improvement in sperm motility after oral administration. In a recent article, Tsounapi et al. reported significant improvement in sperm motility by using avanafil or combination of avanafil plus Profetil (mixture of micronutrients- L-carnitine, L-arginine, coenzyme Q10, vitamin E, zinc, folic acid, glutathione, and selenium) [140]. Pharmacological agents such as pentoxifylline and avanafil which are inhibitors of phosphodiesterase (PDE), and clomiphene citrate an antiestrogenic molecule that increases endogenous serum follicle-stimulating hormone (FSH), luteinizing hormone (LH) and testosterone, are proven to enhance sperm motility in vivo.

One large study has rightly concluded that even though the range of redox balance in human semen at normal physiological levels has been recently reported, the cut-off value is still unknown [141]. As such, the optimal combination of antioxidants needed to maintain the delicate redox balance in various conditions that impair fertility is still a matter of investigation. Furthermore, it is imperative to understand more clearly how antioxidants penetrate the blood–testis and blood–epididymis barriers, interact with the Sertoli, Leydig cells and the developing germ cells, as well as at which concentration and composition. This essential information needs be elucidated in order to develop effective treatments that address the physiological requirements of specific patient groups, such as those with asthenozoospermia, unexplained male factor infertility (UMI) or idiopathic male infertility (IMI).

Sperm Motility and ART Management: Guide to ART Choice

To decide upon effective treatment for correcting infertility, specialists depend upon semen parameters of the male partner. Motility is a parameter which plays an important role in deciding on the appropriate therapeutic insemination option for the infertile couple.

In general, to recommend intrauterine insemination (IUI), one should be able to extract at least five million motile sperm from the ejaculate; in vitro fertilization (IVF) is recommended when two to five million motile sperm can be extracted and intracytoplasmic sperm injection (ICSI) is recommended when samples yield less than two million motile spermatozoa. Kinematic parameters, such as straight line velocity (VSL) and curvilinear velocity (VCL), have prognostic value in predicting the fertilization potential of spermatozoa. If the spermatozoa have a VCL greater than 65 µm/s and VSL greater than 40 µm/s, IVF should be considered. If the velocities are lower than these values, ICSI is recommended to improve the fertilization rate, even if there is adequate percentage of motile spermatozoa to perform IVF [5].

Threshold for IUI in Male Factor Infertility

Infertile couples with male factor infertility or unexplained infertility may exhibit a wide range of semen parameter levels from normal to subnormal or extremely low count and/or motility. Clinical decisions regarding IUI vs IVF for men with oligospermia, asthenozoospermia, or oligoasthenozoospermia with normal female factor can be guided by two parameters commonly used: the initial sperm concentration and motility and post-wash total motile sperm count (TMSC). The thresholds have been reported with high variability in the literature. In a retrospective study of 526 IUI cycles in 294 couples, Madbouly et al. (2017) found post-wash TMSC to be an independent predictor of successful pregnancy after IUI with a TMSC of 5×10^6 sperm or more associated with a higher pregnancy rate [142]. Ok et al. (2013) in their study of 156 cycles in 141 couples reported that TMSC of 10×10^6 or more may be a useful threshold value of IUI success [143]. However, a meta-analysis of 16 studies by van Weert et al. (2004) demonstrated positive predictive values at lower cut-off levels, between 0.8 and 5×10^6 motile spermatozoa [55]. They concluded that post-wash TMSC provided a substantial discriminative performance for IUI outcomes. In a study by Akhil Muthigi et al. (2021), the analysis of 92,471 IUI cycles concluded that IUI pregnancy is optimized with a TMSC of 9×10^6, below which the rates gradually decline [144]. Although rare, pregnancies were achieved with TMSC of $<0.25 \times 10^6$. Since the decline in pregnancy was gradual and continuous, they did not recommend any specific threshold above which IUI could be applied. Dickey et al. (1999) in a study of 4056 cycles concluded that IUI is an effective therapy for male factor infertility when initial sperm motility is 30% and the total motile sperm count is $>5 \times 10^6$ [145]. Van Zyl et al. (1976) reported threshold values in fertile men of 10×10^6/mL and 30% motility [146]. Zukerman et al. (1977) also placed the threshold value for fertility at 10×10^6/mL [147]. Bostofte et al. (1982) placed the threshold at 5×10^6/mL and 20% motility [148]. Polansky and Lamb (1988) selected a threshold of 20×10^6/mL and 30% motility [149]. Another parameter commonly used is the number of inseminated progressively motile spermatozoa (NIPMS) which was considered a better predictive marker [150]. To achieve the best pregnancy rate in IUI, at least five million motile spermatozoa are thought to be essential. A systematic review conducted by Ombelet et al. [54] proposed that IUI can still be tried with an NIPMS of more than one million before directing the patient to IVF. They found that pregnancy probability significantly decreased when the NIPMS was less than one million.

In the case of insemination with cryopreserved semen samples, a total number of motile sperm less than 20 million significantly decreases pregnancy rate possibly due to the poor functional competence of frozen thawed spermatozoa.

To summarize, an absolute cut-off (threshold) cannot be set for IUI in cases of oligoasthenozoospermia, though there is a gradual decline in IUI success rates after a certain level as pointed out by these studies. Initial sperm motility of 30% with total motile sperm count of >5–10 million/mL can predict acceptable success rates with IUI. Similarly, a post-wash total motile sperm count (TMSC) of above 5–9×10^6 motile spermatozoa can predict acceptable success rate for IUI. Counts less than the above stated have lower success rates ranging from 1% to 12% per cycle as per various studies. With NIPMS less than 1 million/mL the probability decreases significantly and hence post-wash if NIPMS will be less than 1 million/mL then IUI can be avoided and IVF or ICSI might be a more appropriate choice. These values or a range can hence be used to provide personalized counseling and guide clinical decision-making.

Thresholds for IVF

It has been established in the past that spermatozoa having at least 30% motility and 15% progressive motility are required to perform IVF, with a sperm concentration of more than 2 million/mL. Sperm motility is known to have a strong correlation with IVF success and pregnancy outcome [151]. Superior sperm kinematic parameters are also considered to improve IVF outcome. The percentage of motile spermatozoa with an average path velocity (VAP) between 10 and 20 μm/s were known to significantly increase success rates during IVF. Donnelly et al. (1998) reported that values for VAP, VSL and VCL were significantly higher in samples that produced >50% fertilization, indicating a positive correlation between progressive motility and fertilization outcome [151]. Contrary to these reports, Moghadam et al. (2005) reported that motility did not enhance fertilization rate or improve pregnancy outcome through IVF [152].

If post-wash total sperm motility is poor, IVF with ICSI is the next option. Success with ICSI is not dependent on the presence of sperm with progressive motility as viable spermatozoa from the epididymis and testis have yielded similar fertilization rates. IVF outcome might depend on the presence of rapidly motile sperm, but in the current scenario, IVF and ICSI are considered in conjunction and use of conventional IVF alone has been drastically reduced. After evaluation of semen by the embryologist if the count and motility is low, ICSI is considered in the same setting in the laboratory to achieve higher rates of fertilization per cycle.

In Vitro Enhancement of Motility

Unlike other semen parameters, sperm motility is accessible to modulation under in vitro conditions, which serves as an advantage, especially for ART with agents like PDE (Phosphodiesterase) inhibitors. Compounds like 8-methoxy isobutyl methyl xanthine (8-MeOIBMX), rolipram, RS-25344, sildenafil, tadalafil, dipyridamole, isobutyl methyl xanthine (IBMX), ibudilast, tofisopam, etazolate hydrochloride, and papaverine were shown to increase sperm motility [153, 154]. Tardif et al. screened 43 commercially available compounds with reported PDE inhibitor activity, among which six compounds (dipyridamole, ibudilast, tofisopam, etazolate hydrochloride, papaverine, and 8-MeO-IBMX) were able to significantly increase the percentage of total and progressive motility in human spermatozoa [154]. Apart from PDE inhibitors, treatment of human sperm with cAMP analogues, such as dibutyryl cAMP, adenosine, 2-deoxyadenosine, or activator of adenylate cyclase enzyme, such as forskolin, have shown a significant increase in total motility for a short duration. Aitken et al. [155] reported that exposure of cryopreserved human spermatozoa to 2-deoxyadenosine resulted in significant increases in percentage of motility.

Absolute Asthenozoospermia Vs. Absolute Necrozoospermia

Sperm vitality testing is a basic semen examination that has been described in the World Health Organization (WHO) Laboratory Manual for the Examination and Processing of Human Semen. Several options can be used to test sperm vitality, such as the eosin–nigrosin (E–N) stain or the hypoosmotic swelling (HOS) test. In the 6th (2021) edition of the WHO Laboratory Manual, sperm vitality assessment is mainly recommended if the total motility is less than 40%. A motile spermatozoon is considered alive, however, in certain conditions an immotile spermatozoon can also be alive.

Necrozoospermia as per the WHO fifth edition is defined by the lower reference threshold of sperm vitality set at 58%. Normal sperm vitality is applied to samples with ≥58% (fifth centile; 95% confidence interval [CI], 55–63%) alive spermatozoa. The sixth edition of the WHO manual has argued that the boundaries between sperm from infertile and fertile men were not as clear.

Patients presenting with semen showing good counts, but 100% immotile sperm can be either absolute asthenozoospermic or necrozoospermic. Vitality testing can be the key to differentiating the two scenarios. Before proceeding with this evaluation, it should be confirmed that the collection of spermatozoa was done in a sterile container without any contaminants with an abstinence of 2–7 days. The terms "vitality" and "viability" are commonly used interchangeably as they both refer to sperm membrane function and therefore whether or not the sperm is dead or alive. If all the spermatozoa in the semen are immotile and >20–30% of these are viable (vital), then it can be deemed absolute asthenozoospermia. On the other hand, if all the immotile spermatozoa are dead, it is termed absolute necrozoospermia. Sometimes a few sperm are found to be viable in a fresh ejaculate, while the majority are dead, which can be considered almost absolute necrozoospermia. The viable sperm obtained in this scenario may have different characteristics and success rates with ICSI compared to those sperms used in case of absolute asthenozoospermia. Hence, the treatment options differ.

If the spermatozoa being tested are going to be further used for ICSI, HOS testing is preferred as Eosin–Nigrosin staining causes damage to the sperm. Spermatozoa that stain when Eosin and Nigrosin is used sequentially are considered dead, while those not being stained are live. The semipermeable membrane of dead sperm is defective and hence it takes up the staining easily. HOS testing evaluates the functional integrity of the sperm plasma membrane and also serves as a useful indicator of fertility potential [156]. Functional integrity can be demonstrated by allowing sperm to react in a hypoosmotic medium. The membrane is semipermeable in live cells, therefore cells with intact membranes (live) will swell in hypotonic solutions and their tails will get curled. The embryologist should aspirate the selected spermatozoon head first with the injecting needle and immerse the flagellum in a hypoosmotic solution for less than 5 min (WHO Manual). As soon as the tail swelling is visualized, the spermatozoon is considered viable, is removed from the hypoosmotic solution and rinsed in culture medium.

Activating substances such as pentoxifylline (PTX) have a role in activating flagellar movement of immotile spermatozoa. PTX is a 3′5′ nucleotidase phosphodiesterase inhibitor that improves sperm motility by increasing intracellular cyclic adenosine monophosphate. Thus, PTX can induce sperm motility in immotile but alive spermatozoa [29]. Their safety has been demonstrated in studies [27, 29]. However, given their potential toxicity, it is necessary to rinse the spermatozoon before injecting it into the oocyte.

If absolute necrozoospermia in the ejaculate is confirmed, then testicular sperm extraction should be considered since it allows the extraction of live spermatozoa. Necrozoospermia has been shown to be correlated with sperm DNA fragmentation (SDF). Samplaski et al. (2015) reported a strong direct correlation between sperm vitality and normal DNA integrity [157]. SDF was significantly higher in sperm with necrozoospermia [158] as well as in cases of leukocytospermia. The loss of viability could be due to a progressive oxidative process due to excessive ROS (reactive oxygen species), leading to peroxidation of membrane lipids and DNA damage, ending in sperm DNA fragmentation and ultimately death. Even if some immotile spermatozoa are alive, there can be DNA damage due to the oxidative nuclear DNA damage. Thus, testing for DNA fragmentation can be useful in deciding whether to use live ejaculated sperm in ICSI or to use testicular sperm extraction. The most frequently used tests are the TUNEL assay (terminal deoxynucleotidyl transferase-mediated deoxyuridine triphosphate nick end labeling) [32], Sperm Chromatin Dispersion Assay (SCD), Sperm Chromatin structure Assay (SCSA) [158], and COMET. Values higher than 30% are considered to be raised for the TUNEL assay while SCSA values above 20% are considered abnormal. Use of testicular sperm should be considered in cases of Increased SDF especially in cases of previous failed ICSI.

Flagellar Dyskinesia and Primary Ciliary Dyskinesia (PCD)

The presence of a large proportion of live but immotile spermatozoa may indeed be indicative of structural defects in the flagellum. There is no definition in the latest edition of the WHO manual of this "large proportion of immotile living spermatozoa", but it is considered that "if more than 25–30% of all spermatozoa are alive and immotile, a genetic ciliary problem may be the cause" (WHO manual sixth edition). If flagellar dyskinesia is suspected, it can be corroborated by considering other sperm characteristics and clinical phenotype. For example, the observation of short, bent or coiled flagella may be suggestive of such flagellar/ciliary problems [141]. Other commonly associated sperm anomalies are oligoasthenozoospermia and asthenoteratozoospermia. Flagellar dysfunction can be isolated (isolated asthenozoospermia) or as a part of complex of ciliary disorders (primary ciliary dyskinesia) as described in previous sections. Isolated asthenozoospermia is primarily due to axonemal and sperm motility machinery defects which may be due to known or unknown genetic mutations. Commonly patients with primary ciliary dyskinesia are diagnosed in childhood due to recurrent respiratory complaints and during treatment of bronchitis episodes and are diagnosed as having ciliary defects. In adulthood these patients are in need of counselling and assessment for fertility.

Primary ciliary dyskinesia is a genetic condition affecting approximately 1:10,000–40,000 individuals worldwide [159] It is an autosomal recessive disorder transmitted from one generation to another, which goes undetected as it is asymptomatic in traits. Evaluation and genetic counseling of patients and their siblings should be performed in view of this pattern of inheritance and if genetic testing is found to be positive, then semen analysis should be done. Confirmatory diagnosis of PCD is based on genetic testing for mutation and nasal epithelium ciliary biopsy. Symptoms frequently start in the neonatal period and include a chronic nasal discharge and wet cough, progressing in childhood to recurrent ear, nose, and chest infections and eventual scarring of the lungs in the form of bronchiectasis. The cause of the symptoms is the malfunction of airway motile cilia, which are responsible for mucus clearance in the airways. Motile cilia are also present in the brain, oviduct, Eustachian tube and middle ear, where they function in fluid movement and in the embryonic node during development. PCD is a lifelong condition, the impact of symptoms changing as the patient reaches adulthood. Ear symptoms often attenuate, but bronchiectasis usually progresses and many patients seek counseling and treatment for fertility problems when they reach adulthood.

Seventy-five to eighty percent of men with Primary Ciliary Dyskinesia are expected to be infertile. Currently, due to preserved sperm function in some cases of PCD, the fertility phenotype should be assessed by laboratory confirmation alongside or ideally prior to counseling of patients. Male infertility is caused by severe or total asthenozoospermia and is currently treated with IVF or ICSI. However, spontaneous fatherhood of PCD patients has been reported. Due to poor motility, success is more likely with ICSI than with IUI or IVF, although rare pregnancies with either method have been reported. Successful ICSI outcomes of PCD sperm have been reported for 28% of cases with live births [160], although the fertilization rate was much higher, at 80%. The low live birth rate compared to fertilization rate may imply developmental problems during embryogenesis. This may be due to poor embryo quality, which could result from functional failure of the sperm-derived centrosome. ICSI is thus the treatment of choice for infertile males with ciliary dyskinesia. Outcomes of ICSI are reported to be improved through testicular sperm extraction and with the addition of pentoxifylline treatment [161]. ICSI outcome for MMAF patients, sperm from *DNAH1* mutation carriers shows good prognosis, possibly due to these mutations primarily affecting the structure of the sperm axonemal inner dynein arms [78].

Clinical Scenarios

In the following section, two case scenarios for ART and Non-ART management of asthenozoospermia are described:

Case Scenario 1

Subjects: 27-year-old male and 26-year-old female, married since 5 years, experiencing primary infertility.

History-clinical evaluation: The evaluation of the female factor was normal.

The male partner has been diagnosed with varicocele (left subclinical with mild reflux). Right testis—20 cc; Left Testis—20 cc, Epididymis, vas deferens, cord found normal.

Semen analysis:

Semen volume: 2 mL
Fructose +
Sperm Concentration: 15 million/mL
Sperm Motility: 10% rapidly progressive motility; 10% sluggishly progressive motility; 10% non-progressive; 70% immotile
Sperm Morphology: 36% normal forms according to Strict Criteria

Management: IUI was attempted once– failed (post-wash semen quality: 3 mill/mL—60% motile).

Male patient started on lifestyle changes, smoking cessation, weight loss, and dietary modifications along with CoQ 100 mg in combination with lycopene and carnitine, once a day for 3 months.

Repeat semen analysis:

Semen volume: 2.5 mL
Sperm Concentration: 20 mill/mL
Sperm Motility: 30% rapidly progressive motility; 20% sluggishly progressive; 10% non-progressive motility; 40% immotile

Medications continued for 3 more months and by the end of 6 months the female partner conceived with singleton pregnancy.

Case Scenario 2

Subjects: 35-year-old male painter by profession; 34-year-old female trying to conceive for 6 years.

History—clinical evaluation: Normal female factor. Patient does not have history of chronic bronchitis, on examination no varicocele.

Semen analysis:

Sperm concentration: 5 million/mL
Sperm motility: 100% immotile sperms

Previously ICSI was tried with a few viable sperms found in the ejaculate but failed twice. Three semen analysis have yielded a few viable immotile sperms confirmed by HOS and vitality testing.

Management: Patient underwent Testis-ICSI with few viable sperms obtained twice. On the second attempt the couple conceived but had a pregnancy loss at 18 weeks. DNA fragmentation was performed, evaluated at a level of 35% with TUNEL assay. The patient was started on antioxidants and had a change in profession.

Few motile sperm appeared in the ejaculate after 1 year and ICSI was done with successful outcome.

Clinical Decision Tree

ART Management of Male Factor Infertility (Oligoasthenospermia): After Non-ART management has failed (A and B)

A. Considerations for IUI for Oligoasthenospermia

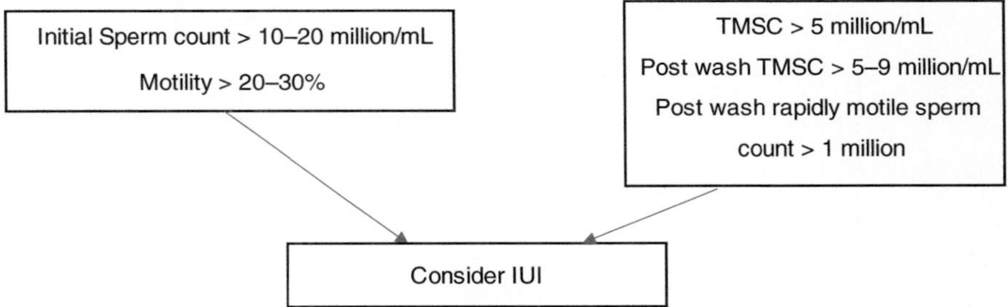

For values less than the above-mentioned thresholds the success rate with IUI declines progressively and the success rate per cycle varies from 4% to 12%. Counseling needs to be done as per these values and a sound clinical decision needs to be taken.

There is no absolute cut off for the parameters and the success rate for the above-mentioned ranges varies as per the couple and the studies have found success rates from 10% to 16% per cycle and are widely accepted as acceptable rates for proceeding with IUI.

B. ART Considerations for Severe Oligoasthenospermia

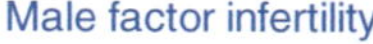

ART Considerations for Absolute Necrozoospermia

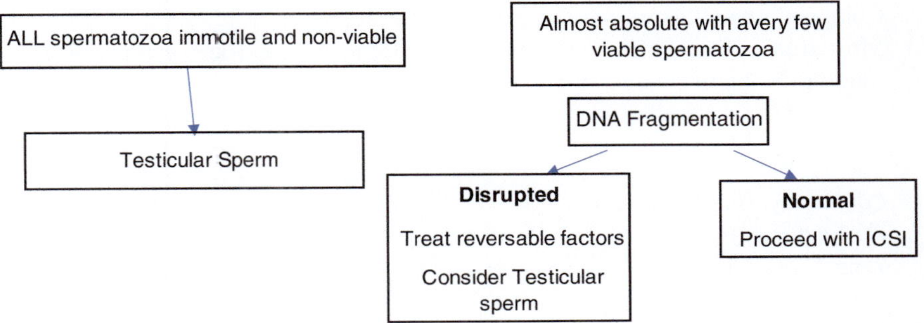

ART Considerations for Absolute Asthenozoospermia

100% immotile spermatozoawith > 20–30% viable

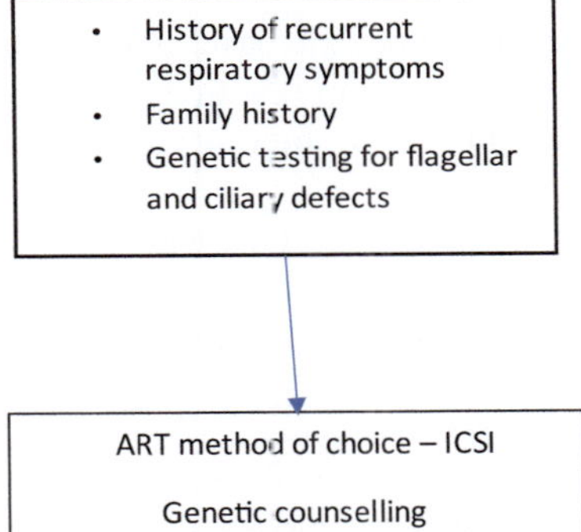

Non-ART Management of Asthenospermia

Look for concomitant oligo and teratozoospermia.
Look for lifestyle factors and correct them—smoking, obesity, sedentary lifestyle, occupational factors, varicocele, genital infection.

Oral treatment with Antioxidants.

Composition and duration of treatment is not defined.

Most studies suggest 3–6 months treatment, but no specific combination is found to be more beneficial than others.

Commonly Used Antioxidants
Co Enzyme Q
Zinc, Vit C, Vit E
Lycopene
Carnitine
Selenium
Glutathione
B complex vitamins

Take Home Messages
- Sperm motility is a long-standing integral constituent of the basic semen analysis, with important significance in the evaluation of sperm function, provided it is evaluated under strict conditions involving laboratory equipment, methodology, and training.
- Various factors affecting sperm motility may include environmental conditions, i.e., abstinence, lifestyle, exposure to toxicants, smoking, stress, as well as pathologies linked to molecular and cellular mechanisms, i.e., oxidative stress, membrane dysfunction, infections, autoimmunity, pathways of energy production, varicocele, and genetic causes.
- The etiological diagnosis of sperm motility disorders may include a thorough clinical and laboratory investigation, comprising detailed history taking, andrological workup, vitality testing, antisperm antibody investigation, DNA fragmentation, and oxidative stress evaluation, as well as genetic testing focused on genes associated with certain deficiencies in cilial, flagellar, and mitochondrial defects.
- The management of sperm motility dysfunction may involve antioxidant, antibiotic treatment, lifestyle alterations, varicocele repair and the application of ART methods, involving in vitro enhancement of motility, in cases where all conventional treatments have failed to produce a significant improvement.
- The determination of exact thresholds for the prediction of a successful treatment of sperm motility defects remains to be elucidated. In general, IUI has been recommended in cases of unexplained male infertility, when a TMSC higher than five million is present, while IVF is applied when two to five million motile sperm can be isolated from the ejaculate, while ICSI is the method of choice when less than two million motile spermatozoa can be yielded.

References

1. García-Vázquez FA, Gadea J, Matás C, Holt WV. Importance of sperm morphology during sperm transport and fertilization in mammals. Asian J Androl. 2016;18(6):844–50. https://doi.org/10.4103/1008-682X.186880.
2. Khatun A, Rahman MS, Pang MG. Clinical assessment of the male fertility. Obstet Gynecol Sci. 2018;61(2):179–91. https://doi.org/10.5468/ogs.2018.61.2.179.
3. Sikka SC, Hellstrom WJ. Current updates on laboratory techniques for the diagnosis of male reproductive failure. Asian J Androl. 2016;18(3):392–401. https://doi.org/10.4103/1008-682X.179161.
4. Jouannet P, Ducot B, Feneux D, Spira A. Male factors and the likelihood of pregnancy in infertile couples. I. Study of sperm characteristics. Int J Androl. 1988;11(5):379–94. https://doi.org/10.1111/j.1365-2605.1988.tb01011.x.
5. Larsen L, Scheike T, Jensen TK, et al. Computer-assisted semen analysis parameters as predictors for fertility of men from the general population. The Danish First Pregnancy Planner Study Team. Hum Reprod. 2000;15(7):1562–7. https://doi.org/10.1093/humrep/15.7.1562.
6. Zinaman MJ, Brown CC, Selevan SG, Clegg ED. Semen quality and human fertility: a prospective study with healthy couples. J Androl. 2000;21(1):145–53.
7. Aitken RJ, Sutton M, Warner P, Richardson DW. Relationship between the movement characteristics of human spermatozoa and their ability to penetrate cervical mucus and zona-free hamster oocytes. J Reprod Fertil. 1985;73(2):441–9. https://doi.org/10.1530/jrf.0.0730441.
8. Irvine DS, Aitken RJ. Predictive value of in-vitro sperm function tests in the context of an AID service. Hum Reprod. 1986;1(8):539–45. https://doi.org/10.1093/oxfordjournals.humrep.a136470.
9. Mortimer D, Pandya IJ, Sawers RS. Relationship between human sperm motility characteristics and sperm penetration into human cervical mucus in vitro. J Reprod Fertil. 1986;78(1):93–102. https://doi.org/10.1530/jrf.0.0780093.
10. Comhaire FH, Vermeulen L, Hinting A, Schoonjans F. Accuracy of sperm characteristics in predicting the in vitro fertilizing capacity of semen. J Vitro Fertil Embryo Transf IVF. 1988;5(6):326–31. https://doi.org/10.1007/BF01129567.
11. Barratt CL, McLeod ID, Dunphy BC, Cooke ID. Prognostic value of two putative sperm function tests: hypo-osmotic swelling and bovine sperm mucus penetration test (Penetrak). Hum Reprod. 1992;7(9):1240–4. https://doi.org/10.1093/oxfordjournals.humrep.a137834.
12. Barratt CLR, Björndahl L, Menkveld R, Mortimer D. ESHRE special interest group for andrology basic semen analysis course: a continued focus on accuracy, quality, efficiency and clinical relevance. Hum Reprod. 2011;26(12):3207–12. https://doi.org/10.1093/humrep/der312.
13. Bollendorf A, Check JH, Lurie D. Evaluation of the effect of the absence of sperm with rapid and linear progressive motility on subsequent pregnancy rates following intrauterine insemination or in vitro fertilization. J Androl. 1996;17(5):550–7.
14. Van den Bergh M, Emiliani S, Biramane J, Vannin AS, Englert Y. A first prospective study of the individual straight line velocity of the spermatozoon and its influences on the fertilization rate after intracytoplasmic sperm injection. Hum Reprod. 1998;13(11):3103–7. https://doi.org/10.1093/humrep/13.11.3103.
15. Sifer C, Sasportes T, Barraud V, et al. World Health Organization grade 'a' motility and zona-binding test accurately predict IVF outcome for mild male factor and unexplained infertilities. Hum Reprod. 2005;20(10):2769–75. https://doi.org/10.1093/humrep/dei118.
16. Björndahl L. The usefulness and significance of assessing rapidly progressive spermatozoa. Asian J Androl. 2010;12(1):33–5. https://doi.org/10.1038/aja.2008.50.
17. Eliasson R. Semen analysis with regard to sperm number, sperm morphology and functional aspects. Asian J Androl. 2010;12(1):26–32. https://doi.org/10.1038/aja.2008.58.

18. Björndahl L, Brown JK. The sixth edition of the WHO laboratory manual for the examination and processing of human semen: ensuring quality and standardization in basic examination of human ejaculates. Fertil Steril. 2022;117(2):246–51.

19. Boitrelle F, Shah R, Saleh R, et al. The sixth edition of the WHO manual for human semen analysis: a critical review and SWOT analysis. Life. 2021;11(12):1368. https://doi.org/10.3390/life11121368.

20. World Health Organization. WHO laboratory manual for the examination and processing of human semen. 6th ed. Cambridge: Cambridge University Press; 2021.

21. Agarwal A, Sharma RK, Gupta S, et al. Sperm vitality and necrozoospermia: diagnosis, management, and results of a global survey of clinical practice. World J Mens Health. 2022;40(2):228–42. https://doi.org/10.5534/wjmh.210149.

22. Wilton LJ, Temple-Smith PD, Baker HW, de Kretser DM. Human male infertility caused by degeneration and death of sperm in the epididymis. Fertil Steril. 1988;49(6):1052–8. https://doi.org/10.1016/s0015-0282(16)59960-9.

23. Ron-El R, Strassburger D, Friedler S, Komarovsky D, Bern O, Raziel A. Repetitive ejaculation before intracytoplasmic sperm injection in patients with absolute immotile spermatozoa. Hum Reprod. 1998;13(3):630–3. https://doi.org/10.1093/humrep/13.3.630.

24. Hanson BM, Aston KI, Jenkins TG, Carrell DT, Hotaling JM. The impact of ejaculatory abstinence on semen analysis parameters: a systematic review. J Assist Reprod Genet. 2018;35(2):213–20. https://doi.org/10.1007/s10815-017-1086-0.

25. Soares JB, Glina S, Antunes N, Wonchockier R, Galuppo AG, Mizrahi FE. Sperm tail flexibility test: a simple test for selecting viable spermatozoa for intracytoplasmic sperm injection from semen samples without motile spermatozoa. Rev Hosp Clin. 2003;58(5):250–3. https://doi.org/10.1590/s0041-87812003000500003.

26. Aktan TM, Montag M, Duman S, Gorkemli H, Rink K, Yurdakul T. Use of a laser to detect viable but immotile spermatozoa. Andrologia. 2004;36(6):366–9. https://doi.org/10.1111/j.1439-0272.2004.00636.x.

27. Ortega C, Verheyen G, Raick D, Camus M, Devroey P, Tournaye H. Absolute asthenozoospermia and ICSI: what are the options? Hum Reprod Update. 2011;17(5):684–92. https://doi.org/10.1093/humupd/dmr018.

28. Nordhoff V. How to select immotile but viable spermatozoa on the day of intracytoplasmic sperm injection? An embryologist's view. Andrology. 2015;3(2):156–62. https://doi.org/10.1111/andr.286.

29. Aydos K, Aydos OS. Sperm selection procedures for optimizing the outcome of ICSI in patients with NOA. J Clin Med. 2021;10(12):2687. https://doi.org/10.3390/jcm10122687.

30. Tournaye H, Liu J, Nagy Z, Verheyen G, Van Steirteghem A, Devroey P. The use of testicular sperm for intracytoplasmic sperm injection in patients with necrozoospermia. Fertil Steril. 1996;66(2):331–4. https://doi.org/10.1016/s0015-0282(16)58462-3.

31. Negri L, Patrizio P, Albani E, et al. ICSI outcome is significantly better with testicular spermatozoa in patients with necrozoospermia: a retrospective study. Gynecol Endocrinol. 2014;30(1):48–52. https://doi.org/10.3109/09513590.2013.848427.

32. Aitken RJ, De Iuliis GN. On the possible origins of DNA damage in human spermatozoa. Mol Hum Reprod. 2010;16(1):3–13. https://doi.org/10.1093/molehr/gap059.

33. Kvist U, Björndahl L. Manual on basic semen analysis: 2002. Rev. Published in Association with ESHRE by Oxford University Press; 2002.

34. Li J, Shi Q, Li X, et al. The effect of male sexual abstinence periods on the clinical outcomes of fresh embryo transfer cycles following assisted reproductive technology: a meta-analysis. Am J Mens Health. 2020;14(4):1557988320933758. https://doi.org/10.1177/1557988320933758.

35. Sokol P, Drakopoulos P, Polyzos NP. The effect of ejaculatory abstinence interval on sperm parameters and clinical outcome of ART. A systematic review of the literature. J Clin Med. 2021;10(15):3213. https://doi.org/10.3390/jcm10153213.

36. Okada FK, Andretta RR, Spaine DM. One day is better than four days of ejaculatory abstinence for sperm function. Reprod Fertil. 2020;1(1):1–10. https://doi.org/10.1530/RAF-20-0018.

37. Shen ZQ, Shi B, Wang TR, et al. Characterization of the sperm proteome and reproductive outcomes with *in vitro*, fertilization after a reduction in male ejaculatory abstinence period. Mol Cell Proteomics. 2019;18(Suppl 1):S109–17. https://doi.org/10.1074/mcp.ra117.000541.
38. Nosi E, Gritzapis AD, Makarounis K, et al. Improvement of sperm quality in hyperviscous semen following DNase I treatment. Int J Endocrinol. 2019;2019:6325169. https://doi.org/10.1155/2019/6325169.
39. Mortimer D. Laboratory standards in routine clinical andrology. Reprod Med Rev. 1994;3(2):97–111.
40. World Health Organization. WHO laboratory manual for the examination of human semen and sperm-cervical mucus interaction. 1st ed. Press Concern; 1980.
41. World Health Organization. WHO laboratory manual for the examination of human semen and sperm-cervical mucus interaction. 2nd ed. Cambridge: Cambridge University Press; 1987.
42. World Health Organization. WHO laboratory manual for the examination of human semen and sperm-cervical mucus interaction. 3rd ed. Cambridge: Cambridge University Press; 1992.
43. World Health Organization. WHO laboratory manual for the examination of human semen and sperm-cervical mucus interaction. 4th ed. Cambridge: Cambridge University Press; 1999.
44. World Health Organization, editor. WHO laboratory manual for the examination and processing of human semen. 5th ed. Geneva: World Health Organization; 2010.
45. Campbell MJ, Lotti F, Baldi E, et al. Distribution of semen examination results 2020—a follow up of data collated for the WHO semen analysis manual 2010. Andrology. 2021;9(3):817–22. https://doi.org/10.1111/andr.12983.
46. Esteves SC. Clinical relevance of routine semen analysis and controversies surrounding the 2010 World Health Organization criteria for semen examination. Int Braz J Urol. 2014;40:443–53.
47. Chung E, Arafa M, Boitrelle F, et al. The new 6th edition of the WHO laboratory manual for the examination and processing of human semen: is it a step toward better standard operating procedure? Asian J Androl. 2022;24(2):123.
48. Bjorndahl L, Mortimer D, Barratt CLR, Castilla HA, Menkveld R, Kvist U, Alvarez JG, Kaugen TB. A practical guide to basic laboratory andrology. Cambridge: Cambridge University Press; 2012. p. 264. ISBN: 978-0-521-73590-2
49. Barratt CLR, Wang C, Baldi E, et al. What advances may the future bring to the diagnosis, treatment, and care of male sexual and reproductive health? Fertil Steril. 2022;117(2):258–67. https://doi.org/10.1016/j.fertnstert.2021.12.013.
50. Agarwal A, Sharma R, Harlev A, Esteves SC. Effect of varicocele on semen characteristics according to the new 2010 World Health Organization criteria: a systematic review and meta-analysis. Asian J Androl. 2016;18(2):163–70. https://doi.org/10.4103/1008-682X.172638.
51. Lin H, Li Y, Ou S, et al. Role of the total progressive motile sperm count (TPMSC) in different infertility factors in IUI: a retrospective cohort study. BMJ Open. 2021;11(2):e040563. https://doi.org/10.1136/bmjopen-2020-040563.
52. Hamilton JAM, Cissen M, Brandes M, et al. Total motile sperm count: a better indicator for the severity of male factor infertility than the WHO sperm classification system. Hum Reprod. 2015;30(5):1110–21. https://doi.org/10.1093/humrep/dev058.
53. Merviel P, Heraud MH, Grenier N, Lourdel E, Sanguinet P, Copin H. Predictive factors for pregnancy after intrauterine insemination (IUI): an analysis of 1038 cycles and a review of the literature. Fertil Steril. 2010;93(1):79–88. https://doi.org/10.1016/j.fertnstert.2008.09.058.
54. Ombelet W, Dhont N, Thijssen A, Bosmans E, Kruger T. Semen quality and prediction of IUI success in male subfertility: a systematic review. Reprod Biomed Online. 2014;28(3):300–9. https://doi.org/10.1016/j.rbmo.2013.10.023.
55. van Weert JM, Repping S, Van Voorhis BJ, van der Veen F, Bossuyt PMM, Mol BWJ. Performance of the postwash total motile sperm count as a predictor of pregnancy at the time of intrauterine insemination: a meta-analysis. Fertil Steril. 2004;82(3):612–20. https://doi.org/10.1016/j.fertnstert.2004.01.042.

56. Hajder M, Hajder E, Husic A. The effects of total motile sperm count on spontaneous pregnancy rate and pregnancy after IUI treatment in couples with male factor and unexplained infertility. Med Arch Sarajevo Bosnia Herzeg. 2016;70(1):39–43. https://doi.org/10.5455/medarh.2016.70.39-43.

57. Dcunha R, Hussein RS, Ananda H, et al. Current insights and latest updates in sperm motility and associated applications in assisted reproduction. Reprod Sci. 2022;29(1):7–25. https://doi.org/10.1007/s43032-020-00408-y.

58. Blouin JL, Meeks M, Radhakrishna U, et al. Primary ciliary dyskinesia: a genome-wide linkage analysis reveals extensive locus heterogeneity. Eur J Hum Genet. 2000;8(2):109–18. https://doi.org/10.1038/sj.ejhg.5200429.

59. Inaba K. Sperm flagella: comparative and phylogenetic perspectives of protein components. Mol Hum Reprod. 2011;17(8):524–38. https://doi.org/10.1093/molehr/gar034.

60. Xu K, Yang L, Zhang L, Qi H. Lack of AKAP3 disrupts integrity of the subcellular structure and proteome of mouse sperm and causes male sterility. Development. 2020;147(2):dev181057. https://doi.org/10.1242/dev.181057.

61. Inaba K, Mizuno K. Sperm dysfunction and ciliopathy. Reprod Med Biol. 2016;15(2):77–94. https://doi.org/10.1007/s12522-015-0225-5.

62. Curi SM, Ariagno JI, Chenlo PH, et al. Asthenozoospermia: analysis of a large population. Arch Androl. 2003;49(5):343–9. https://doi.org/10.1080/01485010390219656.

63. Queiroz RM, Filho FB. Kartagener's syndrome. Pan Afr Med J. 2018;29:160. https://doi.org/10.11604/pamj.2018.29.160.14927.

64. du Plessis SS, Agarwal A, Mohanty G, van der Linde M. Oxidative phosphorylation versus glycolysis: what fuel do spermatozoa use? Asian J Androl. 2015;17(2):230–5. https://doi.org/10.4103/1008-682X.135123.

65. Amaral A, Castillo J, Estanyol JM, Ballescà JL, Ramalho-Santos J, Oliva R. Human sperm tail proteome suggests new endogenous metabolic pathways. Mol Cell Proteomics MCP. 2013;12(2):330–42. https://doi.org/10.1074/mcp.M112.020552.

66. Ferramosca A, Provenzano SP, Coppola L, Zara V. Mitochondrial respiratory efficiency is positively correlated with human sperm motility. Urology. 2012;79(4):809–14. https://doi.org/10.1016/j.urology.2011.12.042.

67. Mukai C, Okuno M. Glycolysis plays a major role for adenosine triphosphate supplementation in mouse sperm flagellar movement. Biol Reprod. 2004;71(2):540–7. https://doi.org/10.1095/biolreprod.103.026054.

68. Vishvkarma R, Alahmar AT, Gupta G, Rajender S. Coenzyme Q10 effect on semen parameters: profound or meagre? Andrologia. 2020;52(6):e13570. https://doi.org/10.1111/and.13570.

69. Mostafa RM, Nasrallah YS, Hassan MM, Farrag AF, Majzoub A, Agarwal A. The effect of cigarette smoking on human seminal parameters, sperm chromatin structure and condensation. Andrologia. 2018;50(3):e12910. https://doi.org/10.1111/and.12910.

70. Belloc S, Cohen-Bacrie M, Amar E, et al. High body mass index has a deleterious effect on semen parameters except morphology: results from a large cohort study. Fertil Steril. 2014;102(5):1268–73. https://doi.org/10.1016/j.fertnstert.2014.07.1212.

71. Gorpinchenko I, Nikitin O, Banyra O, Shulyak A. The influence of direct mobile phone radiation on sperm quality. Cent Eur J Urol. 2014;67(1):65–71. https://doi.org/10.5173/ceju.2014.01.art14.

72. Avendaño C, Mata A, Sanchez Sarmiento CA, Doncel GF. Use of laptop computers connected to internet through Wi-Fi decreases human sperm motility and increases sperm DNA fragmentation. Fertil Steril. 2012;97(1):39–45.e2. https://doi.org/10.1016/j.fertnstert.2011.10.012.

73. Liu MM, Liu L, Chen L, et al. Sleep deprivation and late bedtime impair sperm health through increasing antisperm antibody production: a prospective study of 981 healthy men. Med Sci Monit Int Med J Exp Clin Res. 2017;23:1842–8. https://doi.org/10.12659/MSM.900101.

74. Miller MR, Mansell SA, Meyers SA, Lishko PV. Flagellar ion channels of sperm: similarities and differences between species. Cell Calcium. 2015;58(1):105–13. https://doi.org/10.1016/j.ceca.2014.10.009.

75. Beltrán C, Treviño CL, Mata-Martínez E, et al. Role of ion channels in the sperm acrosome reaction. Adv Anat Embryol Cell Biol. 2016;220:35–69. https://doi.org/10.1007/978-3-319-30567-7_3.
76. Singh AP, Rajender S. CatSper channel, sperm function and male fertility. Reprod Biomed Online. 2015;30(1):28–38. https://doi.org/10.1016/j.rbmo.2014.09.014.
77. Mishra AK, Kumar A, Swain DK, Yadav S, Nigam R. Insights into pH regulatory mechanisms in mediating spermatozoa functions. Vet World. 2018;11(6):852–8. https://doi.org/10.14202/vetworld.2018.852-858.
78. Wambergue C, Zouari R, Fourati Ben Mustapha S, et al. Patients with multiple morphological abnormalities of the sperm flagella due to DNAH1 mutations have a good prognosis following intracytoplasmic sperm injection. Hum Reprod. 2016;31(6):1164–72.
79. Sha Y, Yang X, Mei L, et al. DNAH1 gene mutations and their potential association with dysplasia of the sperm fibrous sheath and infertility in the Han Chinese population. Fertil Steril. 2017;107(6):1312–8.e2. https://doi.org/10.1016/j.fertnstert.2017.04.007.
80. Li Y, Sha Y, Wang X, et al. DNAH2 is a novel candidate gene associated with multiple morphological abnormalities of the sperm flagella. Clin Genet. 2019;95(5):590–600. https://doi.org/10.1111/cge.13525.
81. Tu C, Nie H, Meng L, et al. Identification of DNAH6 mutations in infertile men with multiple morphological abnormalities of the sperm flagella. Sci Rep. 2019;9(1):15864. https://doi.org/10.1038/s41598-019-52436-7.
82. Liu C, Miyata H, Gao Y, et al. Bi-allelic DNAH8 variants lead to multiple morphological abnormalities of the sperm flagella and primary male infertility. Am J Hum Genet. 2020;107(2):330–41. https://doi.org/10.1016/j.ajhg.2020.06.004.
83. Coutton C, Vargas AS, Amiri-Yekta A, et al. Mutations in CFAP43 and CFAP44 cause male infertility and flagellum defects in Trypanosoma and human. Nat Commun. 2018;9(1):686. https://doi.org/10.1038/s41467-017-02792-7.
84. Sha YW, Xu X, Mei LB, et al. A homozygous CEP135 mutation is associated with multiple morphological abnormalities of the sperm flagella (MMAF). Gene. 2017;633:48–53. https://doi.org/10.1016/j.gene.2017.08.033.
85. Dirami T, Rode B, Jollivet M, et al. Missense mutations in SLC26A8, encoding a sperm-specific activator of CFTR, are associated with human asthenozoospermia. Am J Hum Genet. 2013;92(5):760–5. https://doi.org/10.1016/j.ajhg.2013.03.016.
86. Sha Y, Liu W, Huang X, et al. EIF4G1 is a novel candidate gene associated with severe asthenozoospermia. Mol Genet Genomic Med. 2019;7(8):e807. https://doi.org/10.1002/mgg3.807.
87. Brown SG, Miller MR, Lishko PV, et al. Homozygous in-frame deletion in CATSPERE in a man producing spermatozoa with loss of CatSper function and compromised fertilizing capacity. Hum Reprod. 2018;33(10):1812–6. https://doi.org/10.1093/humrep/dey278.
88. Omran H, Kobayashi D, Olbrich H, et al. Ktu/PF13 is required for cytoplasmic pre-assembly of axonemal dyneins. Nature. 2008;456(7222):611–6. https://doi.org/10.1038/nature07471.
89. Mitchison HM, Schmidts M, Loges NT, et al. Mutations in axonemal dynein assembly factor DNAAF3 cause primary ciliary dyskinesia. Nat Genet. 2012;44(4):381–9, S1–2. https://doi.org/10.1038/ng.1106.
90. Tarkar A, Loges NT, Slagle CE, et al. DYX1C1 is required for axonemal dynein assembly and ciliary motility. Nat Genet. 2013;45(9):995–1003. https://doi.org/10.1038/ng.2707.
91. Horani A, Ustione A, Huang T, et al. Establishment of the early cilia preassembly protein complex during motile ciliogenesis. Proc Natl Acad Sci. 2018;115(6):E1221–8. https://doi.org/10.1073/pnas.1715915115.
92. Paff T, Loges NT, Aprea I, et al. Mutations in PIH1D3 cause X-linked primary ciliary dyskinesia with outer and inner dynein arm defects. Am J Hum Genet. 2017;100(1):160–8. https://doi.org/10.1016/j.ajhg.2016.11.019.
93. Antony D, Becker-Heck A, Zariwala MA, et al. Mutations in CCDC39 and CCDC40 are the major cause of primary ciliary dyskinesia with axonemal disorganization and absent inner dynein arms. Hum Mutat. 2013;34(3):462–72. https://doi.org/10.1002/humu.22261.

94. Wu H, Wang J, Cheng H, et al. Patients with severe asthenoteratospermia carrying SPAG6 or RSPH3 mutations have a positive pregnancy outcome following intracytoplasmic sperm injection. J Assist Reprod Genet. 2020;37(4):829–40. https://doi.org/10.1007/s10815-020-01721-w.

95. Torra R, Sarquella J, Calabia J, et al. Prevalence of cysts in seminal tract and abnormal semen parameters in patients with autosomal dominant polycystic kidney disease. Clin J Am Soc Nephrol CJASN. 2008;3(3):790–3. https://doi.org/10.2215/CJN.05311107.

96. Heidary Z, Zaki-Dizaji M, Saliminejad K, Khorramkhorshid HR. Expression analysis of the CRISP2, CATSPER1, PATE1 and SEMG1 in the sperm of men with idiopathic asthenozoospermia. J Reprod Infertil. 2019;20(2):70–5. https://www.ncbi.nlm.nih.gov/pmc/articles/PMC6486568/. Accessed 7 Sept 2022.

97. Yu Q, Zhou Q, Wei Q, Li J, Feng C, Mao X. SEMG1 may be the candidate gene for idiopathic asthenozoospermia. Andrologia. 2014;46(2):158–66. https://doi.org/10.1111/and.12064.

98. Zhang L, Liu Y, Li W, et al. Transcriptional regulation of human sperm-associated antigen 16 gene by S-SOX5. BMC Mol Biol. 2017;18(1):2. https://doi.org/10.1186/s12867-017-0082-3.

99. Ruiz-Pesini E, Lapeña AC, Díez-Sánchez C, et al. Human mtDNA haplogroups associated with high or reduced spermatozoa motility. Am J Hum Genet. 2000;67(3):682–96. https://doi.org/10.1086/303040.

100. Alipour H, Van Der Horst G, Christiansen OB, et al. Improved sperm kinematics in semen samples collected after 2 h versus 4-7 days of ejaculation abstinence. Hum Reprod. 2017;32(7):1364–72. https://doi.org/10.1093/humrep/dex101.

101. Dupesh S, Pandiyan N, Pandiyan R, Kartheeswaran J, Prakash B. Ejaculatory abstinence in semen analysis: does it make any sense? Ther Adv Reprod Health. 2020;14:2633494120906882. https://doi.org/10.1177/2633494120906882.

102. Levin RM, Amsterdam JD, Winokur A, Wein AJ. Effects of psychotropic drugs on human sperm motility. Fertil Steril. 1981;36(4):503–6.

103. Chen SS, Shen MR, Chen TJ, Lai SL. Effects of antiepileptic drugs on sperm motility of normal controls and epileptic patients with long-term therapy. Epilepsia. 1992;33(1):149–53. https://doi.org/10.1111/j.1528-1157.1992.tb02298.x.

104. Banihani SA. Effect of paracetamol on semen quality. Andrologia. 2018;50(1):e12874.

105. Banihani SA, Khasawneh FH. Effect of lansoprazole on human sperm motility, sperm viability, seminal nitric oxide production, and seminal calcium chelation. Res Pharm Sci. 2018;13(5):460–8. https://doi.org/10.4103/1735-5362.236839.

106. Stutz G, Zamudio J, Santillán ME, Vincenti L, de Cuneo MF, Ruiz RD. The effect of alcohol, tobacco, and aspirin consumption on seminal quality among healthy young men. Arch Environ Health. 2004;59(11):548–52. https://doi.org/10.1080/00039890409603432.

107. du Plessis SS, Agarwal A, Syriac A. Marijuana, phytocannabinoids, the endocannabinoid system, and male fertility. J Assist Reprod Genet. 2015;32(11):1575–88. https://doi.org/10.1007/s10815-015-0553-8.

108. Thonneau P, Bujan L, Multigner L, Mieusset R. Occupational heat exposure and male fertility: a review. Hum Reprod. 1998;13(8):2122–5. https://doi.org/10.1093/humrep/13.8.2122.

109. Durairajanayagam D. Lifestyle causes of male infertility. Arab J Urol. 2018;16(1):10–20. https://doi.org/10.1016/j.aju.2017.12.004.

110. Kirby ED, Geraghty AC, Ubuka T, Bentley GE, Kaufer D. Stress increases putative gonadotropin inhibitory hormone and decreases luteinizing hormone in male rats. Proc Natl Acad Sci USA. 2009;106(27):11324–9. https://doi.org/10.1073/pnas.0901176106.

111. Shang Y, Liu C, Cui D, Han G, Yi S. The effect of chronic bacterial prostatitis on semen quality in adult men: a meta-analysis of case-control studies. Sci Rep. 2014;4:7233. https://doi.org/10.1038/srep07233.

112. Burrello N, Salmeri M, Perdichizzi A, et al. Candida albicans experimental infection: effects on human sperm motility, mitochondrial membrane potential and apoptosis. Reprod Biomed Online. 2009;18(4):496–501. https://doi.org/10.1016/s1472-6483(10)60125-3.

113. Foresta C, Garolla A, Zuccarello D, et al. Human papillomavirus found in sperm head of young adult males affects the progressive motility. Fertil Steril. 2010;93(3):802–6. https://doi.org/10.1016/j.fertnstert.2008.10.050.

114. Segars J, Katler Q, McQueen DB, et al. Prior and novel coronaviruses, coronavirus disease 2019 (COVID-19), and human reproduction: what is known? Fertil Steril. 2020;113(6):1140–9. https://doi.org/10.1016/j.fertnstert.2020.04.025.

115. Turner KA, Rambhatla A, Schon S, et al. Male infertility is a women's health issue-research and clinical evaluation of male infertility is needed. Cells. 2020;9(4):E990. https://doi.org/10.3390/cells9040990.

116. Agarwal A, Sharma R, Roychoudhury S, Du Plessis S, Sabanegh E. MiOXSYS: a novel method of measuring oxidation reduction potential in semen and seminal plasma. Fertil Steril. 2016;106(3):566–573.e10. https://doi.org/10.1016/j.fertnstert.2016.05.013.

117. Balawender K, Orkisz S. The impact of selected modifiable lifestyle factors on male fertility in the modern world. Cent Eur J Urol. 2020;73(4):563–8. https://doi.org/10.5173/ceju.2020.1975.

118. Agarwal A, Virk G, Ong C, du Plessis SS. Effect of oxidative stress on male reproduction. World J Mens Health. 2014;32(1):1–17. https://doi.org/10.5534/wjmh.2014.32.1.1.

119. Agarwal A, Durairajanayagam D, Halabi J, Peng J, Vazquez-Levin M. Proteomics, oxidative stress and male infertility. Reprod Biomed Online. 2014;29(1):32–58. https://doi.org/10.1016/j.rbmo.2014.02.013.

120. Agarwal A, Mulgund A, Sharma R, Sabanegh E. Mechanisms of oligozoospermia: an oxidative stress perspective. Syst Biol Reprod Med. 2014;60(4):206–16. https://doi.org/10.3109/19396368.2014.918675.

121. Agarwal A, Arafa M, Chandrakumar R, Majzoub A, AlSaid S, Elbardisi H. A multicenter study to evaluate oxidative stress by oxidation-reduction potential, a reliable and reproducible method. Andrology. 2017;5(5):939–45. https://doi.org/10.1111/andr.12395.

122. Cavarocchi E, Whitfield M, Saez F, Touré A. Sperm ion transporters and channels in human asthenozoospermia: genetic etiology, lessons from animal models, and clinical perspectives. Int J Mol Sci. 2022;23(7):3926. https://doi.org/10.3390/ijms23073926.

123. El-Sherbiny AF, Ali TA, Hassan EA, Mehaney AB, Elshemy HA. The prognostic value of seminal anti-sperm antibodies screening in men prepared for ICSI: a call to change the current antibody-directed viewpoint of sperm autoimmunity testing. Ther Adv Urol. 2021;13:1756287220981488. https://doi.org/10.1177/1756287220981488.

124. Welliver C, Benson AD, Frederick L, et al. Analysis of semen parameters during 2 weeks of daily ejaculation: a first in humans study. Transl Androl Urol. 2016;5(5):749–55. https://doi.org/10.21037/tau.2016.08.20.

125. De Jonge C, LaFromboise M, Bosmans E, Ombelet W, Cox A, Nijs M. Influence of the abstinence period on human sperm quality. Fertil Steril. 2004;82(1):57–65. https://doi.org/10.1016/j.fertnstert.2004.03.014.

126. Levitas E, Lunenfeld E, Weiss N, et al. Relationship between the duration of sexual abstinence and semen quality: analysis of 9,489 semen samples. Fertil Steril. 2005;83(6):1680–6. https://doi.org/10.1016/j.fertnstert.2004.12.045.

127. Abd-Elmoaty MA, Saleh R, Sharma R, Agarwal A. Increased levels of oxidants and reduced antioxidants in semen of infertile men with varicocele. Fertil Steril. 2010;94(4):1531–4. https://doi.org/10.1016/j.fertnstert.2009.12.039.

128. Zargooshi J. Sperm count and sperm motility in incidental high-grade varicocele. Fertil Steril. 2007;88(5):1470–3. https://doi.org/10.1016/j.fertnstert.2007.01.016.

129. Samanta L, Agarwal A, Swain N, et al. Proteomic signatures of sperm mitochondria in varicocele: clinical use as biomarkers of varicocele associated infertility. J Urol. 2018;200(2):414–22. https://doi.org/10.1016/j.juro.2018.03.009.

130. Okeke L, Ikuerowo O, Chiekwe I, Etukakpan B, Shittu O, Olapade-Olaopa O. Is varicocelectomy indicated in subfertile men with clinical varicoceles who have asthenospermia or teratospermia and normal sperm density? Int J Urol. 2007;14(8):729–32. https://doi.org/10.1111/j.1442-2042.2007.01786.x.

131. Boman JM, Libman J, Zini A. Microsurgical varicocelectomy for isolated asthenospermia. J Urol. 2008;180(5):2129–32. https://doi.org/10.1016/j.juro.2008.07.046.

132. Safarinejad MR, Safarinejad S, Shafiei N, Safarinejad S. Effects of the reduced form of coenzyme Q10 (ubiquinol) on semen parameters in men with idiopathic infertility: a double-blind, placebo controlled, randomized study. J Urol. 2012;188(2):526–31. https://doi.org/10.1016/j.juro.2012.03.131.

133. Nadjarzadeh A, Sadeghi MR, Amirjannati N, et al. Coenzyme Q10 improves seminal oxidative defense but does not affect on semen parameters in idiopathic oligoasthenoteratozoospermia: a randomized double-blind, placebo controlled trial. J Endocrinol Investig. 2011;34(8):e224–8. https://doi.org/10.3275/7572.

134. Ghanem H, Shaeer O, El-Segini A. Combination clomiphene citrate and antioxidant therapy for idiopathic male infertility: a randomized controlled trial. Fertil Steril. 2010;93(7):2232–5. https://doi.org/10.1016/j.fertnstert.2009.01.117.

135. ElSheikh MG, Hosny MB, Elshenoufy A, Elghamrawi H, Fayad A, Abdelrahman S. Combination of vitamin E and clomiphene citrate in treating patients with idiopathic oligoasthenozoospermia: a prospective, randomized trial. Andrology. 2015;3(5):864–7. https://doi.org/10.1111/andr.12086.

136. Busetto GM, Koverech A, Messano M, Antonini G, De Berardinis E, Gentile V. Prospective open-label study on the efficacy and tolerability of a combination of nutritional supplements in primary infertile patients with idiopathic astenoteratozoospermia. Arch Ital Urol Androl. 2012;84(3):137–40.

137. Busetto GM, Agarwal A, Virmani A, et al. Effect of metabolic and antioxidant supplementation on sperm parameters in oligo-astheno-teratozoospermia, with and without varicocele: a double-blind placebo-controlled study. Andrologia. 2018;50(3):e12927. https://doi.org/10.1111/and.12927.

138. Martínez-Soto JC, Domingo JC, Cordobilla B, et al. Dietary supplementation with docosahexaenoic acid (DHA) improves seminal antioxidant status and decreases sperm DNA fragmentation. Syst Biol Reprod Med. 2016;62(6):387–95. https://doi.org/10.1080/19396368.2016.1246623.

139. Wei G, Zhou Z, Cui Y, et al. A meta-analysis of the efficacy of L-carnitine/L-acetyl-carnitine or N-acetyl-cysteine in men with idiopathic asthenozoospermia. Am J Mens Health. 2021;15(2):15579883211011372. https://doi.org/10.1177/15579883211011371.

140. Tsounapi P, Honda M, Dimitriadis F, et al. Effects of a micronutrient supplementation combined with a phosphodiesterase type 5 inhibitor on sperm quantitative and qualitative parameters, percentage of mature spermatozoa and sperm capacity to undergo hyperactivation: a randomised controlled trial. Andrologia. 2018;50(8):e13071. https://doi.org/10.1111/and.13071.

141. Agarwal A, Selvam MKP, Baskaran S, et al. Highly cited articles in the field of male infertility and antioxidants: a scientometric analysis. World J Mens Health. 2021;39(4):760–75. https://doi.org/10.5534/wjmh.200181.

142. Madbouly K, Isa A, Habous M, Almannie R, Abu-Rafea B, Binsaleh S. Postwash total motile sperm count: should it be included as a standard male infertility work up. Can J Urol. 2017;24(3):8847–52.

143. Ok EK, Doğan ÖE, Okyay RE, Gülekli B. The effect of post-wash total progressive motile sperm count and semen volume on pregnancy outcomes in intrauterine insemination cycles: a retrospective study. J Turk Ger Gynecol Assoc. 2013;14(3):142–5. https://doi.org/10.5152/jtgga.2013.52280.

144. Muthigi A, Jahandideh S, Bishop LA, et al. Clarifying the relationship between total motile sperm counts and intrauterine insemination pregnancy rates. Fertil Steril. 2021;115(6):1454–60. https://doi.org/10.1016/j.fertnstert.2021.01.014.

145. Dickey RP, Pyrzak R, Lu PY, Taylor SN, Rye PH. Comparison of the sperm quality necessary for successful intrauterine insemination with World Health Organization threshold values for normal sperm. Fertil Steril. 1999;71(4):684–9. https://doi.org/10.1016/S0015-0282(98)00519-6.

146. Van Zyl J, Menkveld R, Kotze T, Van Niekerk W. The importance of spermiograms that meet the requirements of international standards and the most important factors that influence semen parameters, vol. 2. Paris: Diffusion Doin Editeurs; 1976. p. 263–71.
147. Zukerman Z, Rodriguez-Rigau LJ, Smith KD, Steinberger E. Frequency distribution of sperm counts in fertile and infertile males. Fertil Steril. 1977;28(12):1310–3. https://doi.org/10.1016/s0015-0282(16)42975-4.
148. Bostofte E, Serup J, Rebbe H. Relation between sperm count and semen volume, and pregnancies obtained during a twenty-year follow-up period. Int J Androl. 1982;5(3):267–75. https://doi.org/10.1111/j.1365-2605.1982.tb00255.x.
149. Polansky FF, Lamb EJ. Do the results of semen analysis predict future fertility? A survival analysis study. Fertil Steril. 1988;49(6):1059–65. https://doi.org/10.1016/s0015-0282(16)59961-0.
150. Tomlinson M, Lewis S, Morroll D, British Fertility Society. Sperm quality and its relationship to natural and assisted conception: British Fertility Society guidelines for practice. Hum Fertil. 2013;16(3):175–93. https://doi.org/10.3109/14647273.2013.807522.
151. Donnelly ET, Lewis SE, McNally JA, Thompson W. In vitro fertilization and pregnancy rates: the influence of sperm motility and morphology on IVF outcome. Fertil Steril. 1998;70(2):305–14. https://doi.org/10.1016/s0015-0282(98)00146-0.
152. Moghadam KK, Nett R, Robins JC, et al. The motility of epididymal or testicular spermatozoa does not directly affect IVF/ICSI pregnancy outcomes. J Androl. 2005;26(5):619–23.
153. Leclerc P, de Lamirande E, Gagnon C. Cyclic adenosine 3′,5′monophosphate-dependent regulation of protein tyrosine phosphorylation in relation to human sperm capacitation and motility. Biol Reprod. 1996;55(3):684–92. https://doi.org/10.1095/biolreprod55.3.684.
154. Tardif S, Madamidola OA, Brown SG, et al. Clinically relevant enhancement of human sperm motility using compounds with reported phosphodiesterase inhibitor activity. Hum Reprod. 2014;29(10):2123–35. https://doi.org/10.1093/humrep/deu196.
155. Aitken R, Mattei A, Irvine S. Paradoxical stimulation of human sperm motility by 2-deoxyadenosine. Reproduction. 1986;78(2):515–27.
156. Jeyendran RS, Van der Ven HH, Perez-Pelaez M, Crabo BG, Zaneveld LJ. Development of an assay to assess the functional integrity of the human sperm membrane and its relationship to other semen characteristics. J Reprod Fertil. 1984;70(1):219–28. https://doi.org/10.1530/jrf.0.0700219.
157. Samplaski MK, Dimitromanolakis A, Lo KC, et al. The relationship between sperm viability and DNA fragmentation rates. Reprod Biol Endocrinol RBE. 2015;13:42. https://doi.org/10.1186/s12958-015-0035-y.
158. Derbel R, Sellami H, Sakka R, et al. Relationship between nuclear DNA fragmentation, mitochondrial DNA damage and standard sperm parameters in spermatozoa of infertile patients with leukocytospermia. J Gynecol Obstet Hum Reprod. 2021;50(5):102101. https://doi.org/10.1016/j.jogoh.2021.102101.
159. Praveen K, Davis EE, Katsanis N. Unique among ciliopathies: primary ciliary dyskinesia, a motile cilia disorder. F1000Prime Rep. 2015;7:36. https://doi.org/10.12703/P7-36.
160. Kawasaki A, Okamoto H, Wada A, et al. A case of primary ciliary dyskinesia treated with ICSI using testicular spermatozoa: case report and a review of the literature. Reprod Med Biol. 2015;14(4):195–200. https://doi.org/10.1007/s12522-015-0210-z.
161. Yildirim G, Ficicioglu C, Akcin O, Attar R, Tecellioglu N, Yencilek F. Can pentoxifylline improve the sperm motion and ICSI success in the primary ciliary dyskinesia? Arch Gynecol Obstet. 2009;279(2):213–5. https://doi.org/10.1007/s00404-008-0671-y.

Sperm Vitality

6

Gianmaria Salvio and Cătălina Zenoaga-Barbăroșie

Introduction

The recent introduction of the new edition of *World Health Organization (WHO) laboratory manual for the examination and processing of human semen* has brought several changes in the interpretation of seminal parameters, the most important of which remains the progressive abandonment of reference values. Despite these changes, the assessment of sperm viability has maintained its fundamental role in the diagnosis of male infertility, and the new manual states that it may be determined routinely on all ejaculates, especially if less than 40% of spermatozoa are motile to discriminate between immotile dead sperms and immotile live sperms [1]. This represents a fundamental distinction, because the two conditions are determined by different causes and differ both diagnostically and therapeutically. For this reason, this chapter aims to provide a detailed overview of the pathophysiological mechanisms underlying reduced sperm viability, a description of the technical details of the examination, and a narrative review of the causes of reduced viability that can be sought in the medical history of the infertile patient. A description of possible interventions aimed at overcoming this condition (with regard to both spontaneous and medically assisted reproduction) is also provided, along with a discussion of some typical clinical scenarios.

G. Salvio (✉)
Department of Endocrinology, Polytechnic University of Marche, Ancona, Italy

C. Zenoaga-Barbăroșie
Department of Genetics, Faculty of Biology, University of Bucharest, Bucharest, Romania

© The Author(s), under exclusive license to Springer Nature Switzerland AG 2024

A. Agarwal et al. (eds.), *Human Semen Analysis*,
https://doi.org/10.1007/978-3-031-55337-0_6

103

Physiology: Methodology of Sperm Vitality Testing

Cell vitality represents the proportion of living sperm in the ejaculate. It is an important parameter when analysing human sperm and it is determined by the cellular and/or membrane integrity. The old definition for necrozoospermia states that it is the condition in which the percentage of alive spermatozoa is less than 58% [2]. The incidence of necrozoospermia is considered to be around 0.2–0.4% [3]. All samples which exceeded the threshold of 58% were considered having normal sperm vitality. However, the newly updated WHO laboratory manual for the examination and processing of human semen (sixth edition) mentions no reference threshold should be taken into consideration because there are no clear borderlines between sperm samples from fertile and infertile men [1, 4].

Tests assessing sperm vitality are recommended to be performed together with motility testing. The vitality test done for sperm samples with low sperm motility allow the differentiation between live or death immotile spermatozoa [2]. Moreover, motility and vitality tests allow to differentiate between asthenozoospermia and necrozoospermia, conditions that have different approaches and management. Also, assessing sperm vitality helps clinicians elucidating the cause of fertility problems and differentiating between sperm structural defects (live immotile sperm) [5], epididymal pathology (dead immotile sperm) [6] or immunological reaction as a result of an infection [2].

Deoxyribonucleic acid (DNA) is highly condensed in sperm cells because of the presence of protamines and formation of high number of disulphide bonds. The specific conformation of sperm DNA makes it possible to resist both physical and chemical denaturation and ensures cell viability during sperm transport [3]. However, due to several reasons, the function of sperm may deteriorate even starting from spermatogenesis. Moreover, it has also been shown that the viability of the sperm rapidly decreases after ejaculation [7].

There is a strong correlation between necrozoospermia and the degree of sperm DNA fragmentation, the latter being considered the last step before death of spermatozoa [3]. Viability of the sperm decreases until is totally lost as a result of a cascade of events. The excessive generation of reactive oxygen species (ROS) affects the membrane lipids and sperm DNA, which in turn, results in DNA fragmentation and death of the cell. Apart from stress, abortive apoptosis and chromatin condensation defects could also generate sperm DNA fragmentation [4, 8].

Tests for Sperm Vitality Assessment

According to the last edition (sixth edition) of WHO manual vitality testing can be performed routinely in all samples, but it is not mandatory if sperm motility is at least 40% [2].

Sperm vitality should be evaluated as soon as possible after semen liquefaction and no later than 1 h after collection, as dehydration and changes in temperatures negatively affect the sample [9]. The most common laboratory methods which assess sperm vitality are the eosin/eosin-nigrosin (E-N) staining and the hypo-osmotic swelling test (HOST) [2].

E-N staining assesses the integrity and permeability of the cell membrane. This technique is based on the fact that intact sperm cells have the ability to exclude the dye and appear with white heads (or only neck region stained), while non-viable cells with a damaged membrane will be stained in light-to-dark pink [10, 11]. Eosin is used to colour the dead cells, while nigrosin is used as a contrast dye to colour the background and make easier to discern between dead and alive sperm cells [9]. There is the option of using only eosin for vitality testing, but even if it is an easy and rapid test, no quality control cannot be done and there is need of a phase contrast optics for reliable results. As nigrosin is not used, there will be no contrast dye. E-N staining is the recommended diagnostic test for vitality by WHO [1]. However, spermatozoa assessed by this assay can no longer be used in assisted reproductive technology (ART). When the objective is to use the tested spermatozoa for therapeutic procedures (e.g., intracytoplasmic sperm injection—ICSI), staining methods are not an option, and other vitality tests should be used, such as hypo-osmotic swelling test.

HOST assess the structural and functional plasma membrane integrity [12]. The cell membrane of a viable cell sperm, in normal conditions, is semi-permeable. Therefore, it has the ability to transport fluid across membrane in a hypo-osmotic medium, resulting in swelling of the cell and change its tail's shape. On the other hand, a dead cell has a damaged and leaky membrane and the cell does not swell or curl its tail [13, 14]. When sperm is placed in a hypo-osmotic media, the water will enter into the cell and will take approximately 5 min while the flagellum of a live sperm changes its morphology. By around 30 min, all flagellar shapes of viable spermatozoa will be stablished [15]. After the identification of viable spermatozoa, they are retrieved and placed in a normo-osmotic fluid to reach the normal form before ICSI. This technique is also validated by WHO guidelines and can be used both as a diagnostic of therapeutic technique [2].

There are five additional tests to assess sperm viability which are based on physical properties of live sperm. They are more difficult to include in current practices as there are not sufficient studies to prove the advantages over the conventional methods. They also require expensive equipment and experienced laboratory personnel [9], which made them difficult to be applied in ART laboratories.

The sperm tail flexibility test (STFT) is one of them and it requires an optical microscope to verify the sperm tail flexibility before ICSI. If the tail moves up and down independently of the movement of the head, the tail is flexible. On the other head, if the movement of the tail occur together with the head's movement, the tails is considered inflexible [16].

Another technique uses a laser to detect viable but immotile spermatozoa and its name is **laser assisted immotile sperm selection** (LAISS). It has been observed that when a direct laser shot touches the far end of the tail sperm responds by curling it. The sperm that reacts to the laser shot are considered viable and used for ICSI. Presumably dead sperm do not react to the laser system [17].

Sperm head's birefringence. The use of polarized light has been used to analyse the human motile sperm head birefringence to check for structural normality of sperm. This technique is based on the fact that alive sperm cells are birefringent, while dead cells are not. Therefore, the microscope light is double refracted when it passes through the sperm structure [18, 19].

For the purpose of sperm selection, chemical substances that induce the movement of the tail can be used. For example, **pentoxifylline (PTX) and theophylline** are methylxanthine derivatives which can induce flagellar movement of immotile spermatozoa by inhibiting the phosphodiesterase activity, which, in consequence, increases intracellular cyclic adenosine monophosphate (cAMP) levels. Papaverine is another chemical substance with positive effects on sperm motility. It showed similar effects on motility but without decreasing the vitality or affecting DNA integrity [20]. Although studies have demonstrated these chemical substances are safe, they are still considered potential toxic and the spermatozoon should be rinsed before being used in ICSI procedure [4].

A few years ago, it was proposed to use **adenosine triphosphate/magnesium sulphate** (ATP/MgSO$_4$) in samples with no motile sperm in order to identify viable spermatozoa. ATP/MgSO$_4$ stimulates the kinetic machinery and thus can be differentiated viable from dead spermatozoa [21, 22].

Sperm Vitality and Diagnosis of Fertility and Infertility

According with the previous edition of the WHO manual, the lower reference limit for vitality test (using E-N, eosin alone, or HOST) was set at 58%. This threshold corresponded to the fifth centile (95% CI 55–63) of the reference population of the fifth edition of the WHO manual [2], but there was no direct evidence that this value could distinguish between fertile and infertile subjects. In the new edition of the manual, the use of the E-N staining is recommended, while eosin alone and HOST are considered as "alternative vitality tests". Although the technical aspects of the test have not changed, the novelty of the sixth edition of the WHO manual lies in the interpretation of the results and the abandonment of the reference value. In fact, the goal of the viability test becomes that of distinguishing between immobile dead spermatozoa and immobile live spermatozoa. The presence of an adequate proportion of live spermatozoa (for which there is no exact limit, but 25–30% can be used as a reference) suggests the presence of ciliary pathology of possible genetic origin, which makes the success of medical therapy unlikely [1]. In other cases, i.e., when the percentage of dead spermatozoa is high, proper etiological investigation and correction of risk factors can lead to improvement of this condition and should be considered mandatory.

Sperm Vitality and Etiological Diagnosis of Male Reproductive Functions and Dysfunctions

Ageing

Semen parameters change with age and it has been shown that semen viability decreases with the patients' age [23], especially starting from the age of 35 [24, 25]. It is considered that age-related changes that occur at testicular level lead to decrease of sperm parameters, such as vitality [26]. The exact pathogenic mechanism by which advancing age does negatively affect sperm vitality is unknown, but it may be due to sperm death regulation by the seminal plasma enzymes [25], secretory alteration of accessory glands, increase in oxidative stress (OS), and decrease of DNA quality [25, 27].

Studies present similar results when comparing men's age and sperm vitality. A study published in 2011 has shown that sperm vitality decreases with the increase of men's age ($r = -0.219$; $P = 0.01$) [23]. Another study concluded that sperm vitality is negatively correlated with age in patients with less or equal to 35 years old, aged between 36 and 45 years old and in those with more than 45 years old (66.7% ± 14.6, 64% ± 15.3, and 60.1% ± 18.3, respectively) [28]. Similarly, a comparative study has showed that sperm vitality ($r = -0.253$, $P = 0.020$) significantly decreases with age ranging from 60.1% in men with less than 30 years old, 42.9% in men aged between 30 and 40, and finally 28.5% in men with more than 40 years old [29]. Recently, similar results were reported by several authors, who found a negative correlation between age and sperm vitality [24, 27, 30]. Nazari et al. reported a decrease in sperm vitality from 63.70 ± 41.18 to 53.94 ± 23.47 with a cut-off of 35 years [31]. The same cut-off was proposed by Demirkol et al., who observed a decrease in sperm vitality from 65.14 ± 6.28% to 61.25 ± 11.07% for patients 30–34 to 35–39 years old, respectively [32]. Conversely, a study by Kaarouch et al. showed no significant differences in conventional semen parameters, including sperm vitality, in men with advanced age (>40 years) from couples undergoing ART. By the way, paternal age significantly affected unconventional semen parameters, including sperm DNA fragmentation (SDF), chromatin condensation, and aneuploidy, resulting in significant impairment of ART outcomes [33].

Tobacco

The smoke of tobacco contains more than 4000 types of substances with negative effects on male fertility [34]. It has been suggested that tobacco negatively influences sperm parameters, including vitality, due to increased leukocytospermia [34], OS [35], sperm DNA damage, DNA methylation [36], secretory alteration of accessory glands [37], dysregulation of sperm mitochondrial respiratory activity [34].

Despite a general consensus regarding the negative influence of smoking on male fertility, the results of the studies regarding the effects on sperm vitality are controversial. This may depend on many factors, including heterogeneous study populations, other unhealthy lifestyle habits (such as alcohol consumption) involved in the decrease of sperm parameters apart from tobacco exposure, the number of smoked cigarettes per day and the time of exposure to tobacco. While two studies have reported that cigarette smoking negatively affects sperm vitality in fertile men [38], infertile men [39], and in men with oligoasthenoteratozoospermia and varicocele [40], other studies found no such evidence in healthy [41] and infertile men [42]. By the way, several studies published in the last 5 years have confirmed the detrimental effect of cigarettes smoking on sperm vitality both in infertile men and in general population [34, 36, 43–51]. As a further demonstration, sperm vitality significantly increases after smoking cessation [35]. Notably, the studies that support the detrimental effects of smoking on sperm viability mention that duration and frequency of the smoking act [38].

Alcohol

Alcohol consumption negatively affects sperm parameters by an adverse effect on testosterone metabolism and spermatogenesis [52]. Alcohol intake induces spermatogenetic arrest, Sertoli-cell-only syndrome [53], and modifies the ratio between free oestradiol and free testosterone [54]. Surprisingly, the only study evaluating the effects of alcohol consumption on sperm vitality in the last 10 years is the one by Ramírez et al., who retrospectively collected data regarding lifestyle factors of 9464 subjects evaluated for couple infertility. Interestingly, the authors observed better overall semen quality in men with daily alcohol intake of 1–2 glasses/day than non-drinkers, but mean sperm vitality was not different between non-drinkers (83.05%) and men with alcohol intake of 1–2 or >3 glasses/day (83.79% and 82.99%, respectively) [30]. Thus, the effects of alcohol consumption on sperm vitality need to be clarified.

Overweight and Metabolic Syndrome

Dysregulation of fatty acids' metabolism in the testis [55], scrotal hyperthermia [56], OS, decreased testosterone levels, altered spermatogenesis [57], and sperm abnormal maturation during transit through the epididymis [57] may be the consequences of overweight on sperm parameters, including sperm vitality.

Metabolic syndrome (METS) is a condition associate with high cardiovascular risk and defined by the simultaneous presence of obesity, atherogenic dyslipidemia, hypertension, dysglycemia, and/or diabetes mellitus (DM) [58]. In patients with METS, hormonal changes, increased levels of ROS, presence of pro-inflammatory cytokines leads to dysregulation of mitochondrial function and DNA damage [59].

Patients with METS have significant reduced sperm vitality when compared to the control group ($P = 0.002$; $67.0 \pm 16.0\%$ and $47.2 \pm 25\%$, respectively) [59], and a similar decrease has been observed in men with DM [60, 61]. Comparable results were reported when comparing sperm vitality in obese and non-obese men

(P = 0.0172; 45.0 ± 26.1% and 62.6 ± 18.1%, respectively) [62]. Moreover, body mass index (BMI) was negatively associated with sperm vitality [55]. This has been recently confirmed both for patients with extreme obesity (BMI >42 kg/m^2) [30] and overweight men [63, 64]. On the other hand, no association between obesity and decreased sperm vitality was observed by other authors when comparing normal, overweight, and obese patients [65, 66].

Endocrinopathies

Endocrinopathies, such as hypogonadotropic or hypergonadotropic hypogonadism, androgen or oestrogen excess, hyperprolactinemia, insulin disorders, affect male reproduction by increasing or decreasing hormonal levels, or by affecting the spermatogenesis and semen parameters directly [67].

Dysfunction of thyroid may affect spermatogenesis due to increased oestradiol levels and decreased total testosterone [68, 69]. Additionally, dysfunction of thyroid hormones may lead to alterations in basal luteinizing hormone and follicle-stimulating hormone levels and in their response to gonadotropin-releasing hormone stimulation, and changes in sex steroid binding due to elevated levels of sex hormone binding globulin (SHBG) [70].

Although necrozoospermia has been reported in almost half of the patients with hyperthyroidism in Grave's disease [70], to date no other studies have investigate the effects of thyroid dysfunction or other endocrinopathies on sperm vitality. Further studies are therefore needed.

Medications

The effects of medications on male fertility are often inadequately considered, recognized, and investigated. In particular, very few studies evaluated the effects of different medication on sperm vitality, and most of the current evidence come from in vitro studies. Several factors make it difficult to evaluate the influence of a specific medication on male reproductive system. Medications, in general, can affect fertility by affecting the hypothalamic–pituitary–gonadal hormonal axis and the sperm production, by impairing the sperm function or by reducing the sexual function [71], but most evidence remains anecdotal.

Acetylsalicylic acid, for example, negatively affects sperm parameters by impairing testosterone synthesis, nuclear factor kappa-light-chain-enhancer of activated B cells function, and seminal nitric oxide (NO) production. Moreover, is was observed a decrease in testicular prostaglandins and increased OS [72].

The opioid analgesic tramadol affects sperm vitality by increasing the prolactin levels, which leads to hypogonadotropic hypogonadism and consequent inhibition of testosterone synthesis [73].

Calcium channel blockers prescribed for hypertension and heart failure may affect sperm viability as it has been shown that sperm exposed to calcium channel blockers undergo structural changes at the head and tail regions [74].

Anti-epilepsy drugs may affect sperm parameters because they interact with sex hormones and, in consequence, interfere with the hypothalamic–pituitary–gonadal axis [75]. A study published in 2015 compared three valproate doses and sperm parameters. Sperm vitality in patients receiving valproate 1000 mg/day for 4 months and in those receiving valproate 1500 mg/day for 2 years was reduced when comparing with patients receiving valproate 500 mg/day for 6 years (20%, 20%, and 55%, respectively). Moreover, the sperm vitality increased considerably 9 months after patients stopped the treatment (70%) [76]. High doses of the antibiotic amoxicillin impaired sperm viability in vitro [77], and lithium carbonate diminished sperm vitality after 3 weeks of continuous therapy in vivo [78].

Taken together, these data suggest that medication may impair sperm vitality, but systematic investigations should be conducted to fully understand which drugs may be more harmful for male fertility.

Radiofrequencies and Radiations

Studies analysing the influence of radiofrequency on male fertility showed contradictory results. Some studies affirm that radiofrequency is associated with a decrease in sperm viability due to reduced membrane fluidity that is linked to the increase in free radicals or superoxide anion which in turn leads to the oxidation of membrane phospholipids [79–82]. Radioactivity exposure also increases the levels or ROS, which affect sperm viability [83].

A meta-analysis including 321 samples concluded that sperm vitality is affected by mobile phone radiation [84]. Additionally, a systematic review and meta-analysis that included data on viability from five studies (816 samples) also concluded that mobile phone exposure was associated with reduced sperm vitality [85]. There was one study denying the correlation between mobile phone radiation exposure and sperm vitality [86]. In a recent in vitro study, the exposure to near infrared radiation (750–1100 nm) led to a decrease in sperm vitality from $66.2 \pm 5\%$ to $41.3 \pm 8\%$ and, at the same time, an increase of lipid peroxidation coupled with reduction of superoxide dismutase activity, suggesting OS-related damage [87].

Since radiofrequencies and radiations are commonly encountered by men during most of their lives, their effects on reproductive health deserve more investigation.

Environmental and Occupational Pollutants

Heavy metals exposure increases levels of ROS which leads to lipid peroxidation and DNA damage [88]. Consequently, sperm parameters including vitality will be affected by the pollutants. It has been shown that environmental and occupational exposures were associated with reduced of sperm vitality [89]. A recent meta-analysis confirmed lower sperm vitality in subjects exposed to air pollution compared with unexposed men (standardized mean difference elevated to −0.78 (95%CI −0.96 to −0.5; $P < 0.0001$)) [90].

Carbon disulphide is a widespread environmental chemical present in various industrial processes such as extracting oil and vulcanizing rubber. Workers exposed to carbon disulphide had lower sperm vitality when compared with the control unexposed group [91]. Bisphenol A (BPA) is a derivative of polycarbonate plastic and resins production which present estrogenic effects and endocrine-disrupting properties and its urinary concentration negatively correlates with sperm vitality [92].

Genital Infections

Necrozoospermia is observed in about 40% of male genital infections [93]. In such cases, sperm vitality is reduced as a result of damages at intratesticular level and/or lesions throughout excretory tract [9].

The pathogens most frequently identified as being a potential cause of reduced sperm parameters including vitality are *Escherichia coli*, *Ureaplasma urealyticum*, *Mycoplasma hominis*, *Chlamydia trachomatis*, and *Candida albicans* [9].

Different pathogenetic mechanisms have been proposed and many of them are specific to the microorganism involved. For example, the direct contact with *Escherichia coli* or with its metabolites leads to the increase of phosphatidylserine externalization on the sperm plasma membrane. This mechanism, together with the toxins released by the bacteria induce sperm cell death [9].

The incubation of sperm with the haemolytic *Escherichia coli* strain in a ratio of 1:128 resulted in the decrease of sperm vitality from 90.6% ± 4.8% to 86.2% ± 3.3% when comparing to the control group (sperm incubated without *Escherichia coli*). Sperm incubated with the haemolytic *Escherichia coli* strain in a ratio of 1:2 and 1:16 did not affect sperm vitality. Also, the nonhemolytic strains did not have any detrimental effect on sperm vitality regarding the tested ratio (1:2, 1:16, and 1:128) [94]. On the other hand, another study suggested that uropathogenic *Escherichia coli* isolates did not have any effect of sperm vitality in vitro [95].

Ureaplasma urealyticum may interfere with sperm motility through an immune response or through direct adhesion of the bacteria to the sperm tail [96]. A significant deterioration of sperm vitality was observed in men who had semen specimens positive for genital Ureaplasma [97]. Similarly, another study showed that *Ureaplasma urealyticum* was associated with decrease in sperm vitality in infected patients compared to uninfected men ($P = 0.027$; 30.63%, and 36.47%, respectively) [98].

Infection with *Mycoplasma hominis* may lead to the increase in sperm DNA fragmentation [9]. However, no differences with respect to sperm vitality were identified in patients positive for Mycoplasma compared to control ones [97, 98].

The infection with *Chlamydia trachomatis* leads to increase in ROS production through a CD14 protein whose location is at sperm plasma membrane level [9].

Infection with *Chlamydia trachomatis* leads to urethritis, epididymitis, epididymo-orchitis, prostatitis, and reactive arthritis, and negatively affects sperm viability [99]. It has been proposed that lipopolysaccharide derived from Chlamydia induce sperm to generate ROS, thus affecting sperm motility and viability [100]. However, other studies state no differences with respect to sperm vitality were identified between negative and positive patients for *Chlamydia trachomatis* infection [97, 98]. Recently, both *Chlamydia trachomatis* and *Ureaplasma urealyticum* infection have been found in association with decreased sperm vitality by Liu et al. [101].

Candidiasis is caused by *Candida* spp., the most important sexually transmitted fungal. Infection with Candida leads to mitochondrial membrane potential loss, phosphatidylserines externalization, and formation of sperm DNA fragmentation, leading to sperm cell apoptosis [9]. As confirmed by a recent in vitro study, the infection of both *Candida albicans* and *Candida glabrata* has detrimental effects on semen quality, leading to a significant decrease in sperm vitality [102].

Systemic Infections

Infections, in general, may lead to the formation of sperm antibodies with detrimental effects on sperm function and motility. Moreover, a defective spermatogenesis and the decrease in sperm vitality stimulates leukocyte phagocytose and the elimination of defective sperms [103]. Consequently, there is an accumulation of ROS and cytokines, leading to impairment of sperm cells [104–107]. Human immunodeficiency virus (HIV), hepatitis B and C viruses (HBV and HCV), and human papillomavirus (HPV) are pathogens causing systematic infections which may impair semen quality.

In this purpose, some evidence suggest that sperm parameters, including sperm vitality, may be affected due to the increased level of ROS and OS in HIV-infected men [108]. In addition, HIV DNA has been identified in seminal fluid or seminal cells such as spermatozoa, precursors of germ cells, T lymphocytes, macrophages, and epithelial cells. To investigate this hypothesis, sperm viability was compared between men with HIV infection and a control group. Results showed no differences regarding sperm vitality. However, the study included only patients with chronic HIV infection, with undetectable viral load for most of them [109]. Conversely, sperm vitality was significantly lower in HIV patients with CD4+ cell count less or equal to 350/μL, compared to HIV patients with counts of more than 350/μL [110]. Moreover, besides the viral infection, the highly active antiretroviral therapy has also been suggested as a cause of decreased sperm vitality in HIV patients [111, 112].

Regarding HBV and HCV, it should be noted that they are able to integrate their genome into sperm's genetic material, which may lead to sperm genomic instability [109, 113]. In addition, HBV core proteins may interact with histones and decrease the chromosome condensation level, induce local chromosome despiralization, and premature chromosome condensation [113]. During infection, HBV can be found at multiple sites, including male germ cells. Moreover, it has the ability to integrate into the sperm chromosomes and be transmitted vertically via the germ cells. Also, HBV has the ability to induce mutations on sperm chromosomes, leading to genomic instability [114].

In accordance with these data, sperm vitality was observed to be significantly reduced in patients seropositive for HCV and HBV compared to control men ($P < 0.001$), HCV-positive subjects had lower sperm vitality than HIV- and HCV-HIV-infected men ($P < 0.001$), HBV-positive subjects had lower sperm vitality than HIV-seropositive men ($P < 0.001$), and patients infected with both HCV and HIV had lower sperm vitality compared to controls ($P < 0.01$) [109]. This was recently confirmed by Taha et al., who reported that HBV-positive subjects shows decreased sperm vitality compared with HBV-negative subjects (53.7 ± 15.3 vs. 68.6 ± 15.2, $P < 0.05$) [115]. Similarly, sperm vitality was considerably reduced in both HCV patients with primary infertility and HCV patients with secondary infertility when comparing to control subjects ($P < 0.05$) [116].

Finally, HPV has been identified at spermatozoa level in the equatorial region of the sperm head by primary attachment with syndecan-1 in infertile patients [114]. Studies report conflicting data regarding the effect of HPV on sperm parameters [114, 117], but the most recent evidence suggest that the presence of HPV in semen (and not in penile swab) may affect sperm concentration and total sperm count [118]. By the way, since no difference in sperm vitality parameter between HPV-infected and non-infected semen samples has been observed so far [119–121], no firm conclusions can be drawn.

Urological Disease

Chronic bacterial prostatitis may affect sperm parameters. Prostate infection, indeed, lead to ROS and inflammatory cytokines production that can lead to sperm cell impairment, and consequently to sperm vitality reduction. In accordance with this, a meta-analysis of seven case-control studies has concluded that patients with chronic bacterial prostatitis had lower sperm vitality levels when comparing to control group [107]. Conversely, another meta-analysis study identified seven studies (with a broader definition of chronic bacterial prostatitis/chronic pelvic pain) which reported conflicting results on sperm vitality, leading to an overall not significant effect on sperm vitality [122]. Notably, prostatitis may be part of a broader diagnostic category recognized only recently, which is called male accessory gland inflammation (MAGI) and includes several other chronic inflammatory conditions affecting the male genital tract, being involved in 2–18% of male infertility cases [123]. To date, there are no studies that have evaluated the impact of MAGI on sperm viability. The adoption of a unified diagnostic definition of inflammatory diseases of the male urogenital tract may allow this to be clarified in the future.

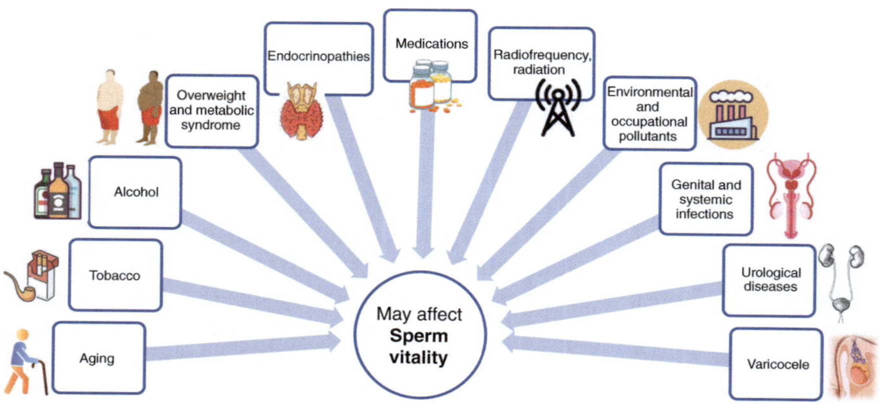

Fig. 6.1 Causes of necrozoospermia

Table 6.1 Causes, degree and reference values of necrozoospermia

Causes	Degree	Reference values
Ageing	Mild to moderate	Linear decrease ($r = -0.219$; $P = 0.01$) [23] after the age of 35, with a 4–5% reduction every 5 years [28, 31, 32]
Tobacco	Mild to moderate	Unclear degree of necrozoospermia and no clear correlation between number of cigarettes/day and severity of necrozoospermia
Alcohol	Unclear	To be defined
Overweight and metabolic syndrome	Mild to severe	A decrease of 20% in sperm vitality is expected for men with METS [59]
Endocrinopathies	Unclear	To be defined
Medications	Unclear	To be defined
Radiofrequency, radiation, pollution	Unclear	To be defined
Environmental and occupational pollutants	Mild to severe	To be defined
Genital infections	Mild	A decrease of 4–6% in sperm vitality is expected for men with genital infections [94, 98]
Systemic infections	Mild	To be defined
Urological disease	Mild	To be defined
Varicocele	Mild	A decrease of 3–20% in sperm vitality is expected for men with varicocele [132, 133]

METS metabolic syndrome

Varicocele

The mechanisms by which varicocele may affect sperm vitality are local hyperthermia, increase of ROS and of DNA damage levels [9, 124, 125]. A significant decrease in sperm vitality has been reported in patients with varicocele by several authors [126–133]. In addition, severity of varicocele may directly affect this parameter, as suggested by the inverse correlation between sperm vitality and diameter of the spermatic vein and degree of reflux [133]. Moreover, varicocele treatment is associated with significant improvement in sperm vitality (see next section) [134].

Causes (Fig. 6.1), degree, and reference values of necrozoospermia are given in Table 6.1.

Sperm Vitality and Planning of Further Investigations

As discussed in previous sections, numerous factors can cause necrozoospermia. Proper investigation, therefore, should start with medical interrogation, which allows identification of lifestyle risk factors (alcohol consumption, smoking, medications, drugs), the presence of systemic diseases affecting fertility, or urologic disorders. Second, physical examination with collection of anthropometric parameters and careful examination of the subject's external genitalia and seminal tract (including digital rectal exploration) can help define the subject's general health status and highlight specific pathological conditions such as varicocele and genital infections.

At this point, specific conditions may require further testing (Fig. 6.2): In suspecting endocrinopathies, gonadal function should be studied from testosterone levels. Although free testosterone is the one that actually reflects the biological activity of this hormone, its assay by routinely used immunometric methods is not reliable [135]. Therefore, if it is not possible to use a reliable method (such as equilibrium dialysis, which is expensive and uncommon), the best option remains to assay total testosterone, which includes both the albumin-bound and SHBG fractions.

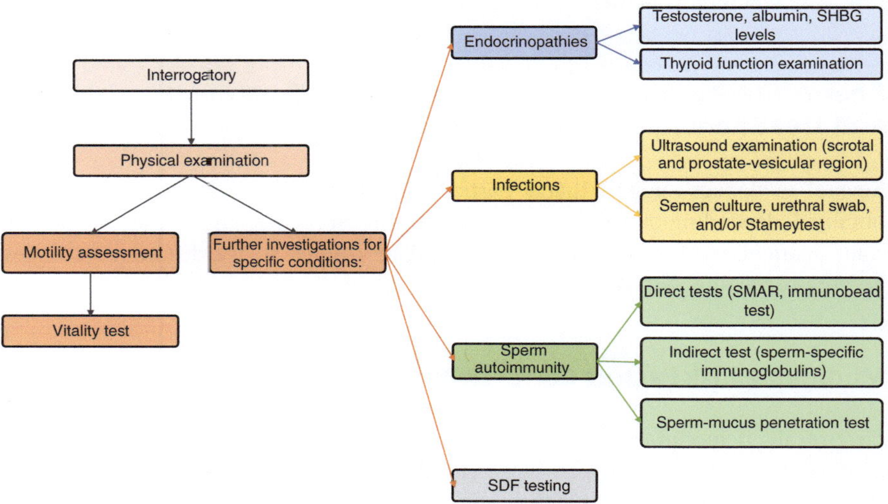

Fig. 6.2 Further testing. *SHBG* sex hormone binding globulin, *SMAR* sperm mixed-agglutination reaction, *SDF* sperm DNA fragmentation

Simultaneous measurement of albumin and SHBG thus allows reliable estimation of free testosterone, which can be done using Vermeulen's formula [136]. Certain conditions, such as obesity and systemic diseases, already seen as a direct cause of necrozoospermia, may associate with reduced testosterone levels leading to depression of the hypothalamic–pituitary–testicle axis known as "functional hypogonadism". Since this is a potential reversible condition, its identification is fundamental in the care pathway of the infertile male [137]. Hyperthyroidism can increase levels of SHBG, which binds testosterone, reducing its bioavailability [69]. Therefore, in the presence of signs of frank hypo- or hyperthyroidism, evaluation of thyroid function is mandated, but it should be kept in mind that some authors suggest that it be done routinely in all infertile subjects [138].

If abnormalities of the male genital tract due to infections, acquired obstruction, or congenital malformations are suspected, the ultrasound examination of the scrotal and prostate-vesicular region is highly recommended not only for diagnostic but also for therapeutic purpose. Indeed, it may help to identify reversible causes of male infertility such as varicocele and prostatic midline cysts, and to guide further testing (semen culture, urethral swab, and/or Stamey test) if signs of genital infection emerge [139].

Finally, antisperm antibodies (ASA) have been pointed out as a possible cause of necrozoospermia [140] and should be assessed, especially if spermatozoa demonstrate agglutination [1]. Direct tests (sperm mixed-agglutination reaction (SMAR) or immunobead test) can be used to detect IgA or IgG on spermatozoa, whereas indirect tests measure sperm-specific immunoglobulins in sperm-free fluids, including semen samples from azoospermic subjects or cervical mucus from the partner [141]. Notably, the presence of sperm antibodies per se is insufficient for diagnosis of sperm autoimmunity, which is classically done by a sperm-mucus penetration test, which demonstrate the severe impairment of sperm function by ASA [1].

Sperm Vitality and Non-ART Management: Treatment and Treatment Response Monitoring

Several evidences suggest that a partial correction of necrozoospermia may be obtained, depending on the causes [9]. For this reason, after an accurate diagnostic route, patients with necrozoospermia could be offered to try different strategies before proceeding with ART.

Modifiable Risk Factors Corrections

First of all, if modifiable risk factors for necrozoospermia are identified through medical interview, etiological treatment should aim to eliminate the source of impaired sperm vitality. This is the case of lifestyle factors such as cigarettes smoking, alcohol consumption, high-calorie diet, and sedentary life. Surprisingly, although theoretically the elimination of these factors should result in improved sperm viability, the scientific evidence for this is scant. To date, indeed, the effects of smoking cessation on sperm vitality have not been elucidated, even if in vitro evidence suggests that antioxidants molecules may contribute to fight the negative effects of tobacco on sperm viability [142]. Similarly, data on alcohol withdrawal and correction of METS-associated risk factors on sperm viability are not currently available. Therefore, although it is always useful to recommend adherence to a healthy lifestyle with adequate diet and regular physical activity, further studies are needed to understand how effective these corrections alone can really be on improving seminal quality.

Repeated Ejaculation

Repeated ejaculation is a simple and cheap method that was proposed over 30 years ago to treat necrozoospermia. According with the first report by Wilton et al. in 1988, frequent ejaculations (two ejaculates per day for 4–5 days) increase the percentage of live motile sperms in the ejaculate. The authors hypothesized that this was due to the lesser time spent in the epididymis and proposed the term "epididymal necrospermia" for this type of male infertility [143]. More recently, Mayorga-Torres et al. reported a significant decrease in intracellular ROS levels after four repeated ejaculations on the same day at 2-h intervals, which might suggest a positive effect on seminal quality, but, unfortunately, the same study showed no significant effects of repeated ejaculations on routine semen parameters including sperm vitality [144]. Taken together, this evidence is too scant to consider repeated ejaculations as a valid treatment in cases of low spermatic vitality.

Antibiotic Therapy

If genital infection emerges during the evaluation of the infertile man, antibiotic therapy should be offered, but data on sperm vitality are controversial, especially if the infection is asymptomatic. Indeed, in a study on 60 infertile men who were diagnosed with leukocytospermia due to asymptomatic genital infection by *Chlamydia trachomatis* or *Ureaplasma urealyticum*, Pjovic et al. administered a single oral dose of 1000 mg azithromycin or a single dose of 2000 mg metronidazole followed by 500 mg erythromycin four times/day for 7 days (for treatment of patients diagnosed with Chlamydia or Ureaplasma infection, respectively). Notably, the authors failed to demonstrate significant effects of antibiotic therapy on sperm vitality [145]. Similarly, a subsequent study from the same authors did not find a significant improvement in sperm vitality from semen samples of men with tobacco-related sterile leukocytospermia treated with a 2-week course of 100 mg doxycycline twice daily [47]. Conversely, the eradication of mixed sexually transmitted infections (*Trichomonas vaginalis, Mycoplasma genitalium,* and *Ureaplasma urealyticum*) led to a significant ($P < 0.05$) increase in sperm vitality (from 38.7 ± 8.4%

at the baseline to 47.9 ± 12.6%, 74.1 ± 11.5%, and 75 ± 10.2% at third, sixth, and ninth month after eradication, respectively) in a study by Yasynetskyi et al. [146].

Varicocele Correction

The European Association of Urology (EAU) 2022 guidelines recommend varicocele repair in men with abnormal semen analysis [147]. In this regard, a recent randomized controlled trial (RCT) by Bryniarski et al. showed a significant improvement in all semen parameters, including sperm vitality ($P < 0.001$) after surgical varicocele correction [128]. Similarly, another study evaluated the effects of varicocele embolization in 47 men, showing a significant improvement in sperm vitality after 3 months (61.88% ± 15.98 to 69.14% ± 14.86; $P = 0.02$) [134]. In addition, evidence of benefits from varicocele correction on sperm vitality exist for adolescents as well [148]. These findings are in line with the results of a recent meta-analysis which provided a high level of evidence in favour of a positive effect of varicocele repair on conventional semen parameters [149]. Taken together, these data make it possible to recommend the correction of clinical varicocele in patients with seminal abnormalities, including necrozoospermia.

Antioxidants

The effects of antioxidants on semen quality have long been debated and their use in the context of male infertility is a cause for discussion among both clinicians and leading scientific societies. Several recent in vitro studies have evaluated the effects of antioxidants on sperm vitality, showing positive impact of various molecules, including α-tocopherol [150], vitamin C [151], vitamin E [152], zinc [153], selenium [154], and L-carnitine [155]. Moreover, different combinations of antioxidants, including L-arginine, coenzyme Q10, vitamin C, vitamin E, Ginseng, inositol, L-carnitine, zinc, selenium, folic acid, and vitamin B12 have shown favourable effects on sperm vitality in vivo [156–158]. However, the heterogeneity among studies and the variable quality of evidence has always dampened enthusiasm about this type of treatment. Very recently, a meta-analysis by Agarwal et al. included 45 RCTs (for a total of 4332 patients) and analysed the effects of antioxidants on conventional semen parameters and spontaneous pregnancy rate, upgrading the level of evidence favouring a recommendation for using antioxidants in male infertility [159]. No doubt, therefore, that in the future the recommendations could be changed and that the use of antioxidants could become one of the cornerstones of the treatment of men with necrozoospermia.

Timing for Reassessment

Since the time required for the sperm to develop is approximately 74 days, the optimal time for repeat semen analysis has been considered at least 1 month [160]. Recently, this timing has been questioned, since 4 weeks may not be ideal and the optimal time depends on the initial results and the specific parameter being evaluated [161]. Since there are no studies focused on viability, at present it seems reasonable to consider 1 month as a baseline, but further studies are needed to determine whether this timing is appropriate and, more importantly, what is the right follow-up time if treatment is given.

Sperm Vitality and ART Management: Guide ART Choice

The vitality testing is necessary to distinguish between absolute asthenozoospermia (100% immotile alive spermatozoa) from almost absolute necrozoospermia. WHO laboratory manual for the examination and processing of human semen recommends use the HOST in infertile men with absolute asthenozoospermia who desire ICSI [2]. If more than 25–30% of spermatozoa are immotile, but alive, it is an indicative of genetic structural defects in the flagellum [2, 5].

Moreover, sperm vitality rates have been correlated with sperm DNA fragmentation rates. There is a relationship of inverse proportionality between the SDF and sperm vitality. Besides this, depending on the test results for sperm vitality and DNA fragmentation, fresh or testicular sperm can be used in ART. Semen samples

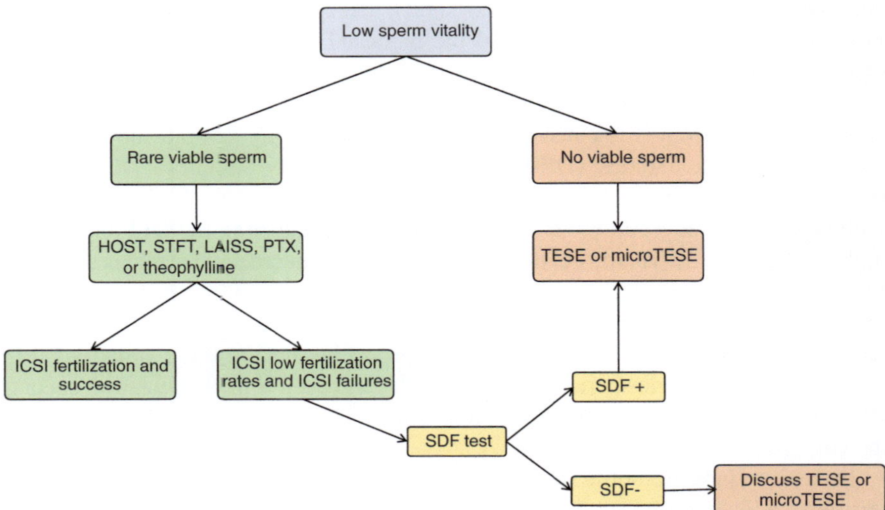

Fig. 6.3 ART management. *HOST* hypo-osmotic swelling test, *STFT* sperm tail flexibility test, *LAISS* laser assisted immotile sperm selection, *PTX* pentoxifylline, *ICSI* intracytoplasmic sperm injection, *SDF* sperm DNA fragmentation, *TESE* testicular sperm extraction

with a very low number of live immotile spermatozoa should be tested for DNA fragmentation in order to decide if ejaculated sperm or testicular sperm extraction (TESE) should be used in ICSI [4]. In case of absolute asthenozoospermia, HOST or sperm motility enhancers should be used to select viable sperm for ICSI. In case of absolute necrozoospermia, SDF of ejaculated live sperm may be tested, or TESE should be chosen (Fig. 6.3) [4].

The source of spermatozoa for ART is decided according to several clinical and diagnostic conditions. With fewer exceptions, such as azoospermia, the first option for ART is the use of fresh ejaculated semen sample. However, studies have highlighted that testicular spermatozoon could bring better ART outcome in patients with poor semen parameters or previous ART failures [162, 163]. This may be because SDF is lower in testicular sperm compared to ejaculated sperm [164]. However, besides the disadvantages of using testicular sperm related to patients' discomfort, there is a higher occurrence of aneuploidy rates in testicular compared to ejaculated spermatozoa in the same patients [165]. In terms of necrozoospermia, if absolute necrozoospermia is confirmed in fresh ejaculated semen sample, there is need to undergo testicular sperm extraction to obtain live spermatozoa for ART [4].

Several mechanisms, such as OS, abortive apoptosis and chromatin condensation defects, could lead to a decrease in the number of viable spermatozoa, which is an important semen parameter associated with fertility. In OS conditions, ROS penetrate the sperm membrane, attack DNA, and trigger the apoptotic cascade. In consequence, the sperm motility and membrane integrity are reduced, and necrozoospermia occurs [166, 167]. The presence of abnormal sperm parameters, such as necrozoospermia, may be due to impaired sperm DNA integrity, which in turn, affects sperm structure and the pregnancy outcome [168]. DNA fragmentation is an indicator of sperm deteriorating function. It has been shown that sperm DNA damage was higher in patients with necrozoospermia and the highest DNA fragmentation value was observed in those with necrozoospermia exceeding 80% [3].

The use of initially immotile and probably dead spermatozoa results in low fertilization rates [169]. It is considered that a normal quality sample should have a DNA fragmentation index (DFI) <15%, a good quality sample a DFI ranging between 16% and 29%, and a low quality sample a DFI >30% [170]. In patients with severe necrozoospermia (>80% non-viable spermatozoa), the DFI tends to be higher than 30% [3]. Therefore, the presence of severe necrozoospermia is a predictive factor for higher SDF, and SDF testing is recommended in patients with high levels of necrozoospermia before ICSI [3]. Sperm DNA testing represents an important step for samples with few living spermatozoa because in these situations it is difficult to select viable sperm from the sample, and even if the fertilization occurs, there is a high incidence of mitotic spindle defects which affects the development of the embryo [171].

In case of viable immotile sperm, apart from E-N staining, there are a few laboratory tests which can be performed to assess sperm viability and chose sperm for ICSI: HOST, STFT, LAISS, PTX, or theophylline. The HOST [171, 172] and STFT [16, 172, 173] have been proven to work when fresh ejaculated semen, and fresh and frozen-thawed TESE samples are used. The techniques are not suitable for cryopreserved and thawed testicular sperm because flagellum could spontaneously curl after freezing-thawing [174]. On the other hand, chemical substances [171, 172, 175, 176] and LAISS [172] can be used to select spermatozoa for ICSI from all sample types: fresh and cryopreserved ejaculated and testicular spermatozoa.

As it was previously discussed, E-N staining cannot be used to identify and select viable sperm during ART because of the potential toxic exposure of spermatozoa to the dyes used for this method.

HOST is a reliable and recommended technique for both diagnostic and therapeutic. This technique can be used for fresh ejaculate, TESE spermatozoa (fresh or frozen), or immotile cilia syndrome [177]. This technique is used when there are no motile spermatozoa present during the microscopic examination. HOST is a time-consuming method, and an experimented laboratory personnel is needed, as the time of spermatozoa exposure to the media must be minimal (no more than 5 min) [2]. Moreover, HOST is not possible to be performed on banking sperm (freeze and thaw) because the preservation method itself may lead to flagella swelling [177]. Another disadvantage of the technique is that sperm selected may have a non-functional membrane, even if it is alive. There are no clear recommendations regarding and several modifications of the basic protocol have been implemented throughout the years [172, 178, 179].

STFT can be used on both fresh ejaculate and TESE sperm (fresh or frozen). The advantages of the technique are that no substances are used, the structural integrity of sperm is not changed, sperm can immediately be injected, to possible toxic effect to the embryo and offspring. However, it is not suitable for cryopreserved ejaculated spermatozoa and false positive results may occur for frozen sperm. There is need of a very experienced laboratory personnel to perform STFT and an optical microscope [177].

The results obtained by LAISS were comparable with those obtained by using HOST. LAISS is an easy, quick, and safe technique (no chemicals are used) with no side effects. However, the instrument is expensive and experienced laboratory personnel is needed [177]. LAISS can be used when HOST does not give enough information. It is time-effective regarding the preparation time for ICSI and the time sperm is exposed. It has been shown that sperm membrane or DNA integrity are not affected by the laser [180, 181].

The use of activating substances such as PTX or theophylline has not yet been proven to be superior over HOST and conflicting results have been published [177]. Even if several studies showed that the use of this method improve the ART outcomes, there are still concerns regarding the safety for the offspring. The disadvantage of using substances for sperm motility activation is the potential toxicity of the substances used upon offspring [182, 183].

The advantage of birefringence evaluation is the possibility of selecting sperm without affecting their vitality of motility. However, there is need of an expensive equipment [18, 19].

Two Clinical Scenarios

Clinical Scenario #1

A 28-year-old patient was referred for reproductive counselling with primary couple infertility after 13 months of regular, unprotected, intercourse. The patient did not report any problems with sexual function and did not suffer from systemic diseases. He was slightly overweight (BMI = 26 kg/m^2) and reported moderate alcohol consumption and smoking habit of about 15 cigarettes/day. The female partner was 26 years old, had regular menstrual cycles, and had already had a gynaecological evaluation that showed no pathological elements. The patient had provided a semen sample that showed a reduction in total motility (15%). The eosin-nigrosin test performed had shown a marked reduction in the percentage of viable sperm (about 10%). The seminologist also reported a high concentration of leukocytes ($>1 \times 10^6$/mmc).

How Should the Patient Be Managed?

Solution: The patient presents with a condition of necrozoospermia. From a diagnostic point of view, conducting a comprehensive medical examination, collecting the medical history, performing hormonal tests (including follicle-stimulating hormone, luteinizing hormone, total testosterone, and SHBG), and performing an ultrasound examination of the genital tract may be helpful in highlighting potentially reversible causes of necrozoospermia.

On medical examination, there was evidence of tension and modest pain on palpation of the epididymis, which was shown to be enlarged in the proximal portion on scrotal ultrasound. Questioned about any irritative complaints during urination or ejaculation, the patient denied it. Bacteriological tests and HPV DNA search on seminal fluid were then performed, but all were negative. Therefore, it was concluded that necrozoospermia could represent the outcome of inflammation of the seminal tract, which is hypothesized to persist even after resolution of an infectious episode as a functional alteration of the male accessory sex glands. Given the young age of the couple, a non-ART approach aimed at improving the chances of spontaneous reproduction was recommended: discontinuing cigarette smoking, limiting alcohol consumption, and weight loss. A commercial combination of antioxidant molecules was also suggested. Further indication was to repeat the seminal fluid examination after 3 months.

Clinical Scenario #2

A 38-year-old patient was referred for reproductive counselling after 3 years of regular, unprotected, intercourse. The female partner was 39 years old, had a 10-year-old son from a previous marriage and had been taking oral contraceptives for about 5 years after. She also referred regular menstrual cycles and no health issues. The patient had no lifestyle risk factors for infertility, in particular he was a non-smoker, consumed minimal alcohol, and exercised regularly. The semen sample provided by the patient showed complete lack of motile sperm in the ejaculate, without significant alterations in either sperm concentration or sperm morphology. The eosin-nigrosin test performed had shown a marked reduction in the percentage of viable sperm (about 5%).

How Should the Patient Be Managed?

Solution: the couple received careful counselling about therapeutic options in their situation. Given the age of the female partner and the almost complete absence of viable spermatozoa, they were immediately started on a course of ART with ICSI technique. An SDF test was then performed on the seminal fluid, which showed a high DFI. In light of this, the use of TESE was proposed with the subsequent use of HOST to identify viable spermatozoa for ICSI.

Take Home Messages

- Sperm vitality testing is included in the sixth edition of the *WHO Laboratory Manual for the Examination and Processing of Human Semen* and could be routinely conducted in all cases of sperm motility less than 40% using E-N staining to distinguish between live and dead immobile spermatozoa. Low sperm viability values (<25–30%) are compatible with necrozoospermia, whereas normal values suggest the presence of a ciliary defect of genetic origin.
- In the presence of necrozoospermia, careful clinical investigation of the patient based on objective examination, medical history, and ultrasound of the male genital tract may allow recognition and removal of known causes of necrozoospermia.
- In the event that removal of the causes of necrozoospermia is not sufficient, the clinician can choose between non-ART or ART management, based on the clinical characteristics of the infertile couple.
- Among the non-ART choices, repeated ejaculations, antibiotic therapy, varicocele correction, and antioxidants are the most studied and can be offered.
- In case the couple undergoes ART, SDF can provide additional guidance for choosing to use sperm from ejaculate or retrieved at the testicular level, while additional methods of viable sperm selection, such as HOST, STFT, and LAISS (but not E-N), can be used to increase the chances of successful ICSI.

References

1. World Health Organization. WHO laboratory manual for the examination and processing of human semen. 6th ed. Geneva: World Health Organization; 2021.
2. World Health Organization. WHO laboratory manual for the examination and processing of human semen. 5th ed. Geneva: World Health Organization; 2010.

3. Brahem S, Jellad S, Ibala S, Saad A, Mehdi M. DNA fragmentation status in patients with necrozoospermia. Syst Biol Reprod Med. 2012;58(6):319–23. https://doi.org/10.310 9/19396368.2012.710869.

4. Agarwal A, Sharma RK, Gupta S, et al. Sperm vitality and necrozoospermia: diagnosis, management, and results of a global survey of clinical practice. World J Mens Health. 2022;40(2):228–42. https://doi.org/10.5534/wjmh.210149.

5. Afzelius BA, Eliasson R, Johnsen O, Lindholmer C. Lack of dynein arms in immotile human spermatozoa. J Cell Biol. 1975;66(2):225–32. https://doi.org/10.1083/jcb.66.2.225.

6. Correa-Pérez JR, Fernández-Pelegrina R, Aslanis P, Zavos PM. Clinical management of men producing ejaculates characterized by high levels of dead sperm and altered seminal plasma factors consistent with epididymal necrospermia. Fertil Steril. 2004;81(4):1148–50. https://doi.org/10.1016/j.fertnstert.2003.09.047.

7. Cortés-Gutiérrez EI, Crespo F, Gosálvez A, Davila-Rodriguez MI, López-Fernández C, Gosalvez J. DNA fragmentation in frozen sperm of Equus asinus: Zamorano-Leones, a breed at risk of extinction. Theriogenology. 2008;69(8):1022–32.

8. Aitken RJ, De Iuliis GN. On the possible origins of DNA damage in human spermatozoa. Mol Hum Reprod. 2010;16(1):3–13.

9. Boursier A, Dumont A, Boitrelle F, et al. Necrozoospermia: the tree that hides the forest. Andrology. 2022;10(4):642–59. https://doi.org/10.1111/andr.13172.

10. Björndahl L, Söderlund I, Kvist U. Evaluation of the one-step eosin-nigrosin staining technique for human sperm vitality assessment. Hum Reprod. 2003;18(4):813–6. https://doi.org/10.1093/humrep/deg199.

11. Agarwal A, Gupta S, Sharma R. Eosin-nigrosin staining procedure BT. In: Agarwal A, Gupta S, Sharma R, editors. Andrological evaluation of male infertility: a laboratory guide. Springer; 2016. p. 73–7. https://doi.org/10.1007/978-3-319-26797-5_8.

12. Ramu S, Jeyendran RS. The hypo-osmotic swelling test for evaluation of sperm membrane integrity. Methods Mol Biol. 2013;927:21–5. https://doi.org/10.1007/978-1-62703-038-0_3.

13. Barbăroşie C, Agarwal A, Henkel R. Diagnostic value of advanced semen analysis in evaluation of male infertility. Andrologia. 2021;53(2):e13625. https://doi.org/10.1111/and.13625.

14. Kızılay F, Altay B. Sperm function tests in clinical practice. Turk J Urol. 2017;43(4):393–400. https://doi.org/10.5152/tud.2017.96646.

15. Hossain AM, Rizk B, Barik S, Huff C, Thorneycroft IH. Time course of hypo-osmotic swellings of human spermatozoa: evidence of ordered transition between swelling subtypes. Hum Reprod. 1998;13(6):1578–83. https://doi.org/10.1093/humrep/13.6.1578.

16. Soares JB, Glina S, Antunes NJ, Wonchockier R, Galuppo AG, Mizrahi FE. Sperm tail flexibility test: a simple test for selecting viable spermatozoa for intracytoplasmic sperm injection from semen samples without motile spermatozoa. Rev Hosp Clin Fac Med Sao Paulo. 2003;58(5):250–3. https://doi.org/10.1590/s0041-87812003000500003.

17. Aktan TM, Montag M, Duman S, Gorkemli H, Rink K, Yurdakul T. Use of a laser to detect viable but immotile spermatozoa. Andrologia. 2004;36(6):366–9. https://doi.org/10.1111/j.1439-0272.2004.00636.x.

18. Petersen CG, Vagnini LD, Mauri AL, et al. Relationship between DNA damage and sperm head birefringence. Reprod Biomed Online. 2011;22(6):583–9. https://doi.org/10.1016/j.rbmo.2011.03.017.

19. Gianaroli L, Magli MC, Collodel G, Moretti E, Ferraretti AP, Baccetti B. Sperm head's birefringence: a new criterion for sperm selection. Fertil Steril. 2008;90(1):104–12. https://doi.org/10.1016/j.fertnstert.2007.05.078.

20. Terriou P, Hans E, Cortvrindt R, et al. Papaverine as a replacement for pentoxifylline to select thawed testicular or epididymal spermatozoa before ICSI. Gynecol Obstet Fertil. 2015;43(12):786–90. https://doi.org/10.1016/j.gyobfe.2015.10.007.

21. Neri QV, Lee B, Rosenwaks Z, Machaca K, Palermo GD. Understanding fertilization through intracytoplasmic sperm injection (ICSI). Cell Calcium. 2014;55(1):24–37. https://doi.org/10.1016/j.ceca.2013.10.006.

22. Simopoulou M, Gkoles L, Bakas P, et al. Improving ICSI: a review from the spermatozoon perspective. Syst Biol Reprod Med. 2016;62(6):359–71. https://doi.org/10.1080/1939636 8.2016.1229365.
23. Brahem S, Mehdi M, Elghezal H, Saad A. The effects of male aging on semen quality, sperm DNA fragmentation and chromosomal abnormalities in an infertile population. J Assist Reprod Genet. 2011;28(5):425–32. https://doi.org/10.1007/s10815-011-9537-5.
24. Verón GL, Tissera AD, Bello R, et al. Impact of age, clinical conditions, and lifestyle on routine semen parameters and sperm kinematics. Fertil Steril. 2018;110(1):68–75.e4. https://doi.org/10.1016/j.fertnstert.2018.03.016.
25. Siddighi S, Chan CA, Patton WC, Jacobson JD, Chan PJ. Male age and sperm necrosis in assisted reproductive technologies. Urol Int. 2007;79(3):231–4. https://doi.org/10.1159/000107955.
26. Collodel G, Ferretti F, Masini M, Gualtieri G, Moretti E. Influence of age on sperm characteristics evaluated by light and electron microscopies. Sci Rep. 2021;11(1):4989. https://doi.org/10.1038/s41598-021-84051-w.
27. Rubes J, Sipek J, Kopecka V, et al. The effects of age on DNA fragmentation, the condensation of chromatin and conventional semen parameters in healthy nonsmoking men exposed to traffic air pollution. Heal Sci Rep. 2021;4(2):e260. https://doi.org/10.1002/hsr2.260.
28. Oliveira JBA, Petersen CG, Mauri AL, Vagnini LD, Baruffi RLR, Franco JGJ. The effects of age on sperm quality: an evaluation of 1,500 semen samples. JBRA Assist Reprod. 2014;18(2):34–41. https://doi.org/10.5935/1518-0557.20140002.
29. Elhanbly S, El-Saied MA, Fawzy M, El-Refaeey A, Mostafa T. Relationship of paternal age with outcome of percutaneous epididymal sperm aspiration-intracytoplasmic sperm injection, in cases of congenital bilateral absence of the vas deferens. Fertil Steril. 2015;104(3):602–6. https://doi.org/10.1016/j.fertnstert.2015.06.020.
30. Ramírez N, Estofán G, Tissera A, et al. Do aging, drinking, and having unhealthy weight have a synergistic impact on semen quality? J Assist Reprod Genet. 2021;38:2985. https://doi.org/10.1007/s10815-021-02274-2.
31. Nazari A, Ketabchi AA, Pakmanesh H, Rahnama A, Fard A, Kharazmi F. What is the optimum age of male fertility in infertile couples? J Kerman Univ Med Sci. 2019;26(2):161–8. https://doi.org/10.22062/JKMU.2019.89208.
32. Demirkol MK, Barut O, Dogan NT, Hamarat MB, Resim S. At what age threshold does the decline in semen parameters begin? J Coll Physicians Surg Pak. 2021;31(1):4–7. https://doi.org/10.29271/jcpsp.2021.01.4.
33. Kaarouch I, Bouamoud N, Madkour A, et al. Paternal age: negative impact on sperm genome decays and IVF outcomes after 40 years. Mol Reprod Dev. 2018;85(3):271–80. https://doi.org/10.1002/mrd.22963.
34. Mostafa RM, Nasrallah YS, Hassan MM, Farrag AF, Majzoub A, Agarwal A. The effect of cigarette smoking on human seminal parameters, sperm chromatin structure and condensation. Andrologia. 2018;50(3):e12910. https://doi.org/10.1111/and.12910.
35. Prentki Santos E, López-Costa S, Chenlo P, et al. Impact of spontaneous smoking cessation on sperm quality: case report. Andrologia. 2011;43(6):431–5. https://doi.org/10.1111/j.1439-0272.2010.01089.x.
36. Hamad MF, Dayyih WAA, Laqqan M, AlKhaled Y, Montenarh M, Hammadeh ME. The status of global DNA methylation in the spermatozoa of smokers and non-smokers. Reprod Biomed Online. 2018;37(5):581–9. https://doi.org/10.1016/j.rbmo.2018.08.016.
37. Harlev A, Agarwal A, Gunes SO, Shetty A, du Plessis SS. Smoking and male infertility: an evidence-based review. World J Mens Health. 2015;33(3):143–60. https://doi.org/10.5534/wjmh.2015.33.3.143.
38. Taha EA, Ez-Aldin AM, Sayed SK, Ghandour NM, Mostafa T. Effect of smoking on sperm vitality, DNA integrity, seminal oxidative stress, zinc in fertile men. Urology. 2012;80(4):822–5. https://doi.org/10.1016/j.urology.2012.07.002.
39. Zhang ZH, Zhu HB, Li LL, Yu Y, Zhang HG, Liu RZ. Decline of semen quality and increase of leukocytes with cigarette smoking in infertile men. Iran J Reprod Med. 2013;11(7):589–96.

40. Taha EA, Ezz-Aldin AM, Sayed SK, Ghandour NM, Mostafa T. Smoking influence on sperm vitality, DNA fragmentation, reactive oxygen species and zinc in oligoasthenoteratozoospermic men with varicocele. Andrologia. 2014;46(6):687–91. https://doi.org/10.1111/and.12136.

41. Jeng HA, Chen Y-L, Kantaria KN. Association of cigarette smoking with reproductive hormone levels and semen quality in healthy adult men in Taiwan. J Environ Sci Health A Tox Hazard Subst Environ Eng. 2014;49(3):262–8. https://doi.org/10.1080/1093452 9.2014.846195.

42. Yu B, Qi Y, Liu D, et al. Cigarette smoking is associated with abnormal histone-to-protamine transition in human sperm. Fertil Steril. 2014;101(1):51–57.e1. https://doi.org/10.1016/j.fertnstert.2013.09.001.

43. Pinto-Pinho P, Matos J, Arantes-Rodrigues R, et al. Association of lifestyle factors with semen quality: a pilot study conducted in men from the Portuguese Trás-os-Montes and Alto Douro region followed in fertility support consultations. Andrologia. 2020;52(4):1–10. https://doi.org/10.1111/and.13549.

44. Asare-Anane H, Bannison SB, Ofori EK, et al. Tobacco smoking is associated with decreased semen quality. Reprod Health. 2016;13(1):90. https://doi.org/10.1186/s12978-016-0207-z.

45. Shelko N, Hamad MF, Montenarh M, Hammadeh ME. The influence of cigarette smoking on sperm quality and sperm membrane integrity. Curr Womens Health Rev. 2016;12(1):58–65. https://doi.org/10.2174/1573404812666160113234853.

46. Zhang M, Zhang Q-S, Zheng H-S, et al. Clinical, demographic and psychological characteristics of infertile male smokers in Northeast China. J Int Med Res. 2016;44(1):75–80. https://doi.org/10.1177/0300060515606285.

47. Pajovic B, Pajovic L, Vukovic M. Effectiveness of antibiotic treatment in infertile patients with sterile leukocytospermia induced by tobacco use. Syst Biol Reprod Med. 2017;63(6):391–6. https://doi.org/10.1080/19396368.2017.1373158.

48. Balasundaram S, Ranganathan P, Rao KA. Tea poly phenol-zinc oxide nano particle effects on infertile smoker's spermatozoa—a short report. Res J Pharm Technol. 2018;11(2):667. https://doi.org/10.5958/0974-360X.2018.00125.7.

49. Saha R. A comparative assessment of semen quality in smokers and non-smokers including sperm BPDE-DNA adduct formation and acrosome status. J Microbiol Biotechnol Food Sci. 2018;8(1):741–4. https://doi.org/10.15414/jmbfs.2018.8.1.741-744.

50. De Brucker S, Drakopoulos P, Dhooghe E, et al. The effect of cigarette smoking on the semen parameters of infertile men. Gynecol Endocrinol. 2020;36(12):1127–30. https://doi.org/10.1080/09513590.2020.1775195.

51. Ou Z, Wen Q, Deng Y, Yu Y, Chen Z, Sun L. Cigarette smoking is associated with high level of ferroptosis in seminal plasma and affects semen quality. Reprod Biol Endocrinol. 2020;18(1):55. https://doi.org/10.1186/s12958-020-00615-x.

52. Ricci E, Al Beitawi S, Cipriani S, et al. Semen quality and alcohol intake: a systematic review and meta-analysis. Reprod Biomed Online. 2017;34(1):38–47. https://doi.org/10.1016/j.rbmo.2016.09.012.

53. Pajarinen J, Karhunen PJ, Savolainen V, Lalu K, Penttilä A, Laippala P. Moderate alcohol consumption and disorders of human spermatogenesis. Alcohol Clin Exp Res. 1996;20(2):332–7. https://doi.org/10.1111/j.1530-0277.1996.tb01648.x.

54. Hansen ML, Thulstrup AM, Bonde JP, Olsen J, Håkonsen LB, Ramlau-Hansen CH. Does last week's alcohol intake affect semen quality or reproductive hormones? A cross-sectional study among healthy young Danish men. Reprod Toxicol. 2012;34(3):457–62. https://doi.org/10.1016/j.reprotox.2012.06.004.

55. Andersen JM, Rønning PO, Herning H, Bekken SD, Haugen TB, Witczak O. Fatty acid composition of spermatozoa is associated with BMI and with semen quality. Andrology. 2016;4(5):857–65. https://doi.org/10.1111/andr.12227.

56. Garolla A, Torino M, Miola P, et al. Twenty-four-hour monitoring of scrotal temperature in obese men and men with a varicocele as a mirror of spermatogenic function. Hum Reprod. 2015;30(5):1006–13. https://doi.org/10.1093/humrep/dev057.

57. Martin LJ. Implications of adiponectin in linking metabolism to testicular function. Endocrine. 2014;46(1):16–28. https://doi.org/10.1007/s12020-013-0102-0.
58. Eckel RH, Grundy SM, Zimmet PZ. The metabolic syndrome. Lancet. 2005;365(9468):1415–28. https://doi.org/10.1016/S0140-6736(05)66378-7.
59. Leisegang K, Udodong A, Bouic PJD, Henkel RR. Effect of the metabolic syndrome on male reproductive function: a case-controlled pilot study. Andrologia. 2014;46(2):167–76. https://doi.org/10.1111/and.12060.
60. Lu X, Huang Y, Zhang H, Zhao J. Effect of diabetes mellitus on the quality and cytokine content of human semen. J Reprod Immunol. 2017;123(August):1–2. https://doi.org/10.1016/j.jri.2017.08.007.
61. Imani M, Talebi AR, Fesahat F, Rahiminia T, Seifati SM, Dehghanpour F. Sperm parameters, DNA integrity, and protamine expression in patients with type II diabetes mellitus. J Obstet Gynaecol. 2021;41(3):439–46. https://doi.org/10.1080/01443615.2020.1744114.
62. Leisegang K, Bouic PJD, Menkveld R, Henkel RR. Obesity is associated with increased seminal insulin and leptin alongside reduced fertility parameters in a controlled male cohort. Reprod Biol Endocrinol. 2014;12:34. https://doi.org/10.1186/1477-7827-12-34.
63. Taha EA, Sayed SK, Gaber HD, et al. Does being overweight affect seminal variables in fertile men? Reprod Biomed Online. 2016;33(6):703–8. https://doi.org/10.1016/j.rbmo.2016.08.023.
64. Oliveira JBA, Petersen CG, Mauri AL, et al. Association between body mass index and sperm quality and sperm DNA integrity. A large population study. Andrologia. 2018;50(3):e12889. https://doi.org/10.1111/and.12889.
65. Martini AC, Tissera A, Estofán D, et al. Overweight and seminal quality: a study of 794 patients. Fertil Steril. 2010;94(5):1739–43. https://doi.org/10.1016/j.fertnstert.2009.11.017.
66. Fariello RM, Pariz JR, Spaine DM, Cedenho AP, Bertolla RP, Fraietta R. Association between obesity and alteration of sperm DNA integrity and mitochondrial activity. BJU Int. 2012;110(6):863–7. https://doi.org/10.1111/j.1464-410X.2011.10813.x.
67. Sengupta P, Dutta S, Karkada IR, Chinni SV. Endocrinopathies and male infertility. Life (Basel). 2021;12(1):10. https://doi.org/10.3390/life12010010.
68. Krassas GE, Poppe K, Glinoer D. Thyroid function and human reproductive health. Endocr Rev. 2010;31(5):702–55. https://doi.org/10.1210/er.2009-0041.
69. La Vignera S, Vita R, Condorelli RA, et al. Impact of thyroid disease on testicular function. Endocrine. 2017;58(3):397–407. https://doi.org/10.1007/s12020-017-1303-8.
70. Abalovich M, Levalle O, Hermes R, et al. Hypothalamic-pituitary-testicular axis and seminal parameters in hyperthyroid males. Thyroid. 1999;9(9):857–63. https://doi.org/10.1089/thy.1999.9.857.
71. Samplaski MK, Nangia AK. Adverse effects of common medications on male fertility. Nat Rev Urol. 2015;12(7):401–13. https://doi.org/10.1038/nrurol.2015.145.
72. Banihani SA. Effect of aspirin on semen quality: a review. Andrologia. 2020;52(1):e13487. https://doi.org/10.1111/and.13487.
73. Farag AGA, Basha MA, Amin SA, et al. Tramadol (opioid) abuse is associated with a dose- and time-dependent poor sperm quality and hyperprolactinaemia in young men. Andrologia. 2018;50(6):e13026. https://doi.org/10.1111/and.13026.
74. Kanwar U, Anand RJ, Sanyal SN. The effect of nifedipine, a calcium channel blocker, on human spermatozoal functions. Contraception. 1993;48(5):453–70. https://doi.org/10.1016/0010-7824(93)90135-t.
75. Herzog AG, Seibel MM, Schomer DL, Vaitukaitis JL, Geschwind N. Reproductive endocrine disorders in men with partial seizures of temporal lobe origin. Arch Neurol. 1986;43(4):347–50. https://doi.org/10.1001/archneur.1986.00520040035015.
76. Kose-Ozlece H, Ilik F, Cecen K, Huseyinoglu N, Serim A. Alterations in semen parameters in men with epilepsy treated with valproate. Iran J Neurol. 2015;14(3):164–7.
77. Hargreaves CA, Rogers S, Hills F, Rahman F, Howell RJ, Homa ST. Effects of co-trimoxazole, erythromycin, amoxycillin, tetracycline and chloroquine on sperm function in vitro. Hum Reprod. 1998;13(7):1878–86. https://doi.org/10.1093/humrep/13.7.1878.

78. Levin RM, Amsterdam JD, Winokur A, Wein AJ. Effects of psychotropic drugs on human sperm motility. Fertil Steril. 1981;36(4):503–6.

79. Veerachari SB, Vasan SS. Mobile phone electromagnetic waves and its effect on human ejaculated semen: an in vitro study. Int J Infertil Fetal Med. 2012;3(1):15–21.

80. Agarwal A, Desai NR, Makker K, et al. Effects of radiofrequency electromagnetic waves (RF-EMW) from cellular phones on human ejaculated semen: an in vitro pilot study. Fertil Steril. 2009;92(4):1318–25. https://doi.org/10.1016/j.fertnstert.2008.08.022.

81. Agarwal A, Deepinder F, Sharma RK, Ranga G, Li J. Effect of cell phone usage on semen analysis in men attending infertility clinic: an observational study. Fertil Steril. 2008;89(1):124–8. https://doi.org/10.1016/j.fertnstert.2007.01.166.

82. Kesari KK, Agarwal A, Henkel R. Radiations and male fertility. Reprod Biol Endocrinol. 2018;16(1):118. https://doi.org/10.1186/s12958-018-0431-1.

83. Kumar D, Salian SR, Kalthur G, et al. Semen abnormalities, sperm DNA damage and global hypermethylation in health workers occupationally exposed to ionizing radiation. PLoS One. 2013;8(7):e69927. https://doi.org/10.1371/journal.pone.0069927.

84. Dama MS, Bhat MN. Mobile phones affect multiple sperm quality traits: a meta-analysis. F1000Res. 2013;2:40. https://doi.org/10.12688/f1000research.2-40.v1.

85. Adams JA, Galloway TS, Mondal D, Esteves SC, Mathews F. Effect of mobile telephones on sperm quality: a systematic review and meta-analysis. Environ Int. 2014;70:106–12. https://doi.org/10.1016/j.envint.2014.04.015.

86. Gorpinchenko I, Nikitin O, Banyra O, Shulyak A. The influence of direct mobile phone radiation on sperm quality. Cent Eur J Urol. 2014;67(1):65–71. https://doi.org/10.5173/ceju.2014.01.art14.

87. Highland H, Rajput N, Sharma R, George LB. Differential sensitivity of the human sperm cell to near infrared radiation. J Photochem Photobiol B Biol. 2018;183:119–26. https://doi.org/10.1016/j.jphotobiol.2018.04.027.

88. Sukhn C, Awwad J, Ghantous A, Zaatari G. Associations of semen quality with non-essential heavy metals in blood and seminal fluid: data from the Environment and Male Infertility (EMI) study in Lebanon. J Assist Reprod Genet. 2018;35(9):1691–701. https://doi.org/10.1007/s10815-018-1236-z.

89. Wijesekara GUS, Fernando DMS, Wijerathna S, Bandara N. Environmental and occupational exposures as a cause of male infertility. Ceylon Med J. 2015;60(2):52–6. https://doi.org/10.4038/cmj.v60i2.7090.

90. Pizzol D, Foresta C, Garolla A, et al. Pollutants and sperm quality: a systematic review and meta-analysis. Environ Sci Pollut Res. 2021;28(4):4095–103. https://doi.org/10.1007/s11356-020-11589-z.

91. Ma J-Y, Ji J-J, Ding Q, et al. The effects of carbon disulfide on male sexual function and semen quality. Toxicol Ind Health. 2010;26(6):375–82. https://doi.org/10.1177/0748233710369127.

92. Kranvogl R, Knez J, Miuc A, Vončina E, Vončina DB, Vlaisavljević V. Simultaneous determination of phthalates, their metabolites, alkylphenols and bisphenol A using GC-MS in urine of men with fertility problems. Acta Chim Slov. 2014;61(1):110–20.

93. Nduwayo L, Barthélémy C, Lansac J, Tharanne MJ, Lecomte P. Management of necrospermia. Contracept Fertil Sex. 1995;23(11):682–5.

94. Boguen R, Treulen F, Uribe P, Villegas JV. Ability of Escherichia coli to produce hemolysis leads to a greater pathogenic effect on human sperm. Fertil Steril. 2015;103(5):1155–61. https://doi.org/10.1016/j.fertnstert.2015.01.044.

95. Boguen R, Uribe P, Treulen F, Villegas JV. Distinct isolates of uropathogenic Escherichia coli differentially affect human sperm parameters in vitro. Andrologia. 2014;46(8):943–7. https://doi.org/10.1111/and.12167.

96. Liu H, Yang K, He L, et al. Risk prediction of Ureaplasma urealyticum affecting sperm quality based on mathematical model and cross-sectional study. Comput Math Methods Med. 2022;2022:2498306. https://doi.org/10.1155/2022/2498306.

97. Rybar R, Prinosilova P, Kopecka V, et al. The effect of bacterial contamination of semen on sperm chromatin integrity and standard semen parameters in men from infertile couples. Andrologia. 2012;44(Suppl 1):410–8. https://doi.org/10.1111/j.1439-0272.2011.01198.x.

98. Liu J, Wang Q, Ji X, et al. Prevalence of Ureaplasma urealyticum, Mycoplasma hominis, Chlamydia trachomatis infections, and semen quality in infertile and fertile men in China. Urology. 2014;83(4):795–9. https://doi.org/10.1016/j.urology.2013.11.009.

99. Mackern-Oberti JP, Motrich RD, Breser ML, Sánchez LR, Cuffini C, Rivero VE. Chlamydia trachomatis infection of the male genital tract: an update. J Reprod Immunol. 2013;100(1):37–53. https://doi.org/10.1016/j.jri.2013.05.002.

100. Hosseinzadeh S, Pacey AA, Eley A. Chlamydia trachomatis-induced death of human spermatozoa is caused primarily by lipopolysaccharide. J Med Microbiol. 2003;52(Pt 3):193–200. https://doi.org/10.1099/jmm.0.04836-0.

101. Liu K-S, Mao X-D, Pan F, Chen Y-J. Application of leukocyte subsets and sperm DNA fragment rate in infertile men with asymptomatic infection of genital tract. Ann Palliat Med. 2021;10(2):1021. https://doi.org/10.21037/apm-19-597.

102. Castrillón-Duque EX, Puerta Suárez J, Cardona Maya WD. Yeast and fertility: effects of in vitro activity of Candida spp. on sperm quality. J Reprod Infertil. 2018;19(1):49–55.

103. Henkel R, Offor U, Fisher D. The role of infections and leukocytes in male infertility. Andrologia. 2021;53(1):e13743. https://doi.org/10.1111/and.13743.

104. Kang X, Xie Q, Zhou X, et al. Effects of hepatitis B virus S protein exposure on sperm membrane integrity and functions. PLoS One. 2012;7(3):e33471. https://doi.org/10.1371/journal.pone.0033471.

105. Boeri L, Capogrosso P, Ventimiglia E, et al. High-risk human papillomavirus in semen is associated with poor sperm progressive motility and a high sperm DNA fragmentation index in infertile men. Hum Reprod. 2019;34(2):209–17. https://doi.org/10.1093/humrep/dey348.

106. Zhou J-F, Xiao W-Q, Zheng Y-C, Dong J, Zhang S-M. Increased oxidative stress and oxidative damage associated with chronic bacterial prostatitis. Asian J Androl. 2006;8(3):317–23. https://doi.org/10.1111/j.1745-7262.2006.00144.x.

107. Shang Y, Liu C, Cui D, Han G, Yi S. The effect of chronic bacterial prostatitis on semen quality in adult men: a meta-analysis of case-control studies. Sci Rep. 2014;4(1):7233. https://doi.org/10.1038/srep07233.

108. Savasi V, Oneta M, Laoreti A, et al. Effects of antiretroviral therapy on sperm DNA integrity of HIV-1-infected men. Am J Mens Health. 2018;12(6):1835–42. https://doi.org/10.1177/1557988318794282.

109. Lorusso F, Palmisano M, Chironna M, et al. Impact of chronic viral diseases on semen parameters. Andrologia. 2010;42(2):121–6. https://doi.org/10.1111/j.1439-0272.2009.00970.x.

110. Wang D, Li L, Xie Q, et al. Factors affecting sperm fertilizing capacity in men infected with HIV. J Med Virol. 2014;86(9):1467–72. https://doi.org/10.1002/jmv.23991.

111. Pavili L, Daudin M, Moinard N, et al. Decrease of mitochondrial DNA level in sperm from patients infected with human immunodeficiency virus-1 linked to nucleoside analogue reverse transcriptase inhibitors. Fertil Steril. 2010;94(6):2151–6. https://doi.org/10.1016/j.fertnstert.2009.12.080.

112. Frapsauce C, Grabar S, Leruez-Ville M, et al. Impaired sperm motility in HIV-infected men: an unexpected adverse effect of efavirenz? Hum Reprod. 2015;30(8):1797–806. https://doi.org/10.1093/humrep/dev141.

113. Huang J-M, Huang T-H, Qiu H-Y, et al. Effects of hepatitis B virus infection on human sperm chromosomes. World J Gastroenterol. 2003;9(4):736–40. https://doi.org/10.3748/wjg.v9.i4.736.

114. Garolla A, Pizzol D, Bertoldo A, Menegazzo M, Barzon L, Foresta C. Sperm viral infection and male infertility: focus on HBV, HCV, HIV, HPV, HSV, HCMV, and AAV. J Reprod Immunol. 2013;100(1):20–9. https://doi.org/10.1016/j.jri.2013.03.004.

115. Taha EA, Mekky MA, Gaber HD, et al. Impact of chronic hepatitis B virus infection on semen parameters of fertile men. Future Virol. 2019;14(8):515–22. https://doi.org/10.2217/fvl-2019-0039.

116. La Vignera S, Condorelli RA, Vicari E, D'Agata R, Calogero AE. Sperm DNA damage in patients with chronic viral C hepatitis. Eur J Intern Med. 2012;23(1):e19–24. https://doi.org/10.1016/j.ejim.2011.08.011.

117. Gizzo S, Ferrari B, Noventa M, et al. Male and couple fertility impairment due to HPV-DNA sperm infection: update on molecular mechanism and clinical impact—systematic review. Biomed Res Int. 2014;2014:230263. https://doi.org/10.1155/2014/230263.

118. Jaworek H, Koudelakova V, Oborna I, et al. Impact of human papillomavirus infection on semen parameters and reproductive outcomes. Reprod Biol Endocrinol. 2021;19(1):156. https://doi.org/10.1186/s12958-021-00840-y.

119. Foresta C, Garolla A, Zuccarello D, et al. Human papillomavirus found in sperm head of young adult males affects the progressive motility. Fertil Steril. 2010;93(3):802–6. https://doi.org/10.1016/j.fertnstert.2008.10.050.

120. Foresta C, Pizzol D, Moretti A, Barzon L, Palù G, Garolla A. Clinical and prognostic significance of human papillomavirus DNA in the sperm or exfoliated cells of infertile patients and subjects with risk factors. Fertil Steril. 2010;94(5):1723–7. https://doi.org/10.1016/j.fertnstert.2009.11.012.

121. Garolla A, Pizzol D, Bertoldo A, De Toni L, Barzon L, Foresta C. Association, prevalence, and clearance of human papillomavirus and antisperm antibodies in infected semen samples from infertile patients. Fertil Steril. 2013;99(1):125–131.e2. https://doi.org/10.1016/j.fertnstert.2012.09.006.

122. Fu W, Zhou Z, Liu S, et al. The effect of chronic prostatitis/chronic pelvic pain syndrome (CP/CPPS) on semen parameters in human males: a systematic review and meta-analysis. PLoS One. 2014;9(4):e94991. https://doi.org/10.1371/journal.pone.0094991.

123. La Vignera S, Crafa A, Condorelli RA, et al. Ultrasound evaluation of patients with male accessory gland inflammation: a pictorial review. Andrology. 2021;9(5):1298–305. https://doi.org/10.1111/andr.13011.

124. Jellad S, Hammami F, Khalbous A, et al. Sperm DNA status in infertile patients with clinical varicocele. Prog Urol. 2021;31(2):105–11. https://doi.org/10.1016/j.purol.2020.07.241.

125. Cho C-L, Esteves SC, Agarwal A. Novel insights into the pathophysiology of varicocele and its association with reactive oxygen species and sperm DNA fragmentation. Asian J Androl. 2016;18(2):186–93. https://doi.org/10.4103/1008-682X.170441.

126. Vivas-Acevedo G, Lozano JR, Camejo MI. Effect of varicocele grade and age on seminal parameters. Urol Int. 2010;85(2):194–9. https://doi.org/10.1159/000314226.

127. Alargkof V, Kersten L, Stanislavov R, Kamenov Z, Nikolinakos P. Relationships between sperm DNA integrity and bulk semen parameters in Bulgarian patients with varicocele. Arch Ital Urol Androl. 2019;91(2). https://doi.org/10.4081/aiua.2019.2.125.

128. Bryniarski P, Taborowski P, Rajwa P, Kaletka Z, Życzkowski M, Paradysz A. The comparison of laparoscopic and microsurgical varicocoelectomy in infertile men with varicocoele on paternity rate 12 months after surgery: a prospective randomized controlled trial. Andrology. 2017;5(3):445–50. https://doi.org/10.1111/andr.12343.

129. Gual-Frau J, Abad C, Amengual MJ, et al. Oral antioxidant treatment partly improves integrity of human sperm DNA in infertile grade I varicocele patients. Hum Fertil (Camb). 2015;18(3):225–9. https://doi.org/10.3109/14647273.2015.1050462.

130. Xue J, Yang J, Yan J, et al. Abnormalities of the testes and semen parameters in clinical varicocele. Nan Fang Yi Ke Da Xue Xue Bao. 2012;32(4):439–42.

131. Collodel G, Moretti E, Longini M, Pascarelli NA, Signorini C. Increased F(2)-isoprostane levels in semen and immunolocalization of the 8-iso prostaglandin F(2α) in spermatozoa from infertile patients with varicocele. Oxidative Med Cell Longev. 2018;2018:7508014. https://doi.org/10.1155/2018/7508014.

132. Gill K, Kups M, Harasny P, et al. The negative impact of varicocele on basic semen parameters, sperm nuclear DNA dispersion and oxidation-reduction potential in semen. Int J Environ Res Public Health. 2021;18(11):5977. https://doi.org/10.3390/ijerph18115977.

133. Li K, Liu X, Huang Y, Liu X, Song Q, Wang R. Evaluation of testicular spermatogenic function by ultrasound elastography in patients with varicocele-associated infertility. Am J Transl Res. 2021;13(8):9136–42.

134. Prasivoravong J, Marcelli F, Lemaître L, et al. Beneficial effects of varicocele embolization on semen parameters. Basic Clin Androl. 2014;24:9. https://doi.org/10.1186/2051-4190-24-9.

135. Keevil BG, Adaway J. Assessment of free testosterone concentration. J Steroid Biochem Mol Biol. 2019;190:207–11. https://doi.org/10.1016/j.jsbmb.2019.04.008.

136. Agretti P, Pelosini C, Bianchi L, et al. Importance of total and measured free testosterone in diagnosis of male hypogonadism: immunoassay versus mass spectrometry in a population of healthy young/middle-aged blood donors. J Endocrinol Investig. 2021;44(2):321–6. https://doi.org/10.1007/s40618-020-01304-7.

137. Grossmann M, Matsumoto AM. A perspective on middle-aged and older men with functional hypogonadism: focus on holistic management. J Clin Endocrinol Metab. 2017;102(3):1067–75. https://doi.org/10.1210/jc.2016-3580.

138. La Vignera S, Vita R. Thyroid dysfunction and semen quality. Int J Immunopathol Pharmacol. 2018;32:2058738418775241. https://doi.org/10.1177/2058738418775241.

139. Lotti F, Maggi M. Ultrasound of the male genital tract in relation to male reproductive health. Hum Reprod Update. 2015;21(1):56–83. https://doi.org/10.1093/humupd/dmu042.

140. Silva AF, Ramalho-Santos J, Amaral S. The impact of antisperm antibodies on human male reproductive function: an update. Reproduction. 2021;162(4):R55–71. https://doi.org/10.1530/REP-21-0123.

141. Gupta S, Sharma R, Agarwal A, et al. Antisperm antibody testing: a comprehensive review of its role in the management of immunological male infertility and results of a global survey of clinical practices. World J Mens Health. 2022;40(3):380–98. https://doi.org/10.5534/wjmh.210164.

142. Goss D, Oyeyipo IP, Skosana BT, Ayad BM, du Plessis SS. Ameliorative potentials of quercetin against cotinine-induced toxic effects on human spermatozoa. Asian Pac J Reprod. 2016;5(3):193–7. https://doi.org/10.1016/j.apjr.2016.03.005.

143. Wilton LJ, Temple-Smith PD, Baker HW, de Kretser DM. Human male infertility caused by degeneration and death of sperm in the epididymis. Fertil Steril. 1988;49(6):1052–8. https://doi.org/10.1016/s0015-0282(16)59960-9.

144. Mayorga-Torres JM, Agarwal A, Roychoudhury S, Cadavid A, Cardona-Maya WD. Can a short term of repeated ejaculations affect seminal parameters? J Reprod Infertil. 2016;17(3):177–83.

145. Pajovic B, Radojevic N, Vukovic M, Stjepcevic A. Semen analysis before and after antibiotic treatment of asymptomatic Chlamydia- and Ureaplasma-related pyospermia. Andrologia. 2013;45(4):266–71. https://doi.org/10.1111/and.12004.

146. Yasynetskyi M, Banyra O, Nikitin O, et al. Mixed sexually transmitted infections in infertile couples: empirical treatment and influence on semen quality. Recent Adv Antiinfect Drug Discov. 2021;16(3):227–36. https://doi.org/10.2174/2772434416666211129105145.

147. Minhas S, Bettocchi C, Boeri L, et al. European Association of Urology guidelines on male sexual and reproductive health: 2021 update on male infertility. Eur Urol. 2021;80(5):603–20. https://doi.org/10.1016/j.eururo.2021.08.014.

148. Pajovic B, Radojevic N. Prospective follow up of fertility after adolescent laparoscopic varicocelectomy. Eur Rev Med Pharmacol Sci. 2013;17(8):1060–3.

149. Agarwal A, Cannarella R, Saleh R, et al. Impact of varicocele repair on semen parameters in infertile men: a systematic review and meta-analysis. World J Mens Health. 2022;41:289. https://doi.org/10.5534/wjmh.220142.

150. Zerbinati C, Caponecchia L, Fiori C, et al. Alpha- and gamma-tocopherol levels in human semen and their potential functional implications. Andrologia. 2020;52(4):1–8. https://doi.org/10.1111/and.13543.

151. Fanaei H, Khayat S, Halvaei I, et al. Effects of ascorbic acid on sperm motility, viability, acrosome reaction and DNA integrity in teratozoospermic samples. Iran J Reprod Med. 2014;12(2):103–10.

152. Ghafarizadeh AA, Malmir M, Naderi Noreini S, Faraji T, Ebrahimi Z. The effect of vitamin E on sperm motility and viability in asthenoteratozoospermic men: in vitro study. Andrologia. 2021;53(1):e13891. https://doi.org/10.1111/and.13891.

153. Wu J, Wu S, Xie Y, et al. Zinc protects sperm from being damaged by reactive oxygen species in assisted reproduction techniques. Reprod Biomed Online. 2015;30(4):334–9. https://doi.org/10.1016/j.rbmo.2014.12.008.

154. Ghafarizadeh AA, Vaezi G, Shariatzadeh MA, Malekirad AA. Effect of in vitro selenium supplementation on sperm quality in asthenoteratozoospermic men. Andrologia. 2018;50(2). https://doi.org/10.1111/and.12869.

155. Naderi Noreini S, Malmir M, Ghafarizadeh A, Faraji T, Bayat R. Protective effect of L-carnitine on apoptosis, DNA fragmentation, membrane integrity and lipid peroxidation of spermatozoa in the asthenoteratospermic men. Andrologia. 2021;53(2):e13932. https://doi.org/10.1111/and.13932.

156. Micic S, Lalic N, Djordjevic D, et al. Double-blind, randomised, placebo-controlled trial on the effect of L-carnitine and L-acetylcarnitine on sperm parameters in men with idiopathic oligoasthenozoospermia. Andrologia. 2019;51(6):1–9. https://doi.org/10.1111/and.13267.

157. Gambera L, Stendardi A, Ghelardi C, Fineschi B, Aini R. Effects of antioxidant treatment on seminal parameters in patients undergoing in vitro fertilization. Arch Ital Urol Androl. 2019;91(3):187–90. https://doi.org/10.4081/aiua.2019.3.187.

158. Delbarba A, Arrighi N, Facondo P, Cappelli C, Ferlin A. Positive effect of nutraceuticals on sperm DNA damage in selected infertile patients with idiopathic high sperm DNA fragmentation. Minerva Endocrinol. 2020;45(2):89–96. https://doi.org/10.23736/S0391-1977.20.03188-0.

159. Agarwal A, Cannarella R, Saleh R, et al. Impact of antioxidant therapy on natural pregnancy outcomes and semen parameters in infertile men: a systematic review and meta-analysis of randomized controlled trials. World J Mens Health. 2022;41:14. https://doi.org/10.5534/wjmh.220067.

160. Male Infertility Best Practice Policy Committee of the American Urological Association, Practice Committee of the American Society for Reproductive Medicine. Report on optimal evaluation of the infertile male. Fertil Steril. 2006;86(5 Suppl 1):S202–9. https://doi.org/10.1016/j.fertnstert.2006.08.029.

161. Punjani N, Wald G, Al-Hussein Alwamlh O, Feliciano M, Dudley V, Goldstein M. Optimal timing for repeat semen analysis during male infertility evaluation. F S Rep. 2021;2(2):172–5. https://doi.org/10.1016/j.xfre.2021.04.010.

162. Ben-Ami I, Raziel A, Strassburger D, Komarovsky D, Ron-El R, Friedler S. Intracytoplasmic sperm injection outcome of ejaculated versus extracted testicular spermatozoa in cryptozoospermic men. Fertil Steril. 2013;99(7):1867–71. https://doi.org/10.1016/j.fertnstert.2013.02.025.

163. Esteves SC, Sánchez-Martín F, Sánchez-Martín P, Schneider DT, Gosálvez J. Comparison of reproductive outcome in oligozoospermic men with high sperm DNA fragmentation undergoing intracytoplasmic sperm injection with ejaculated and testicular sperm. Fertil Steril. 2015;104(6):1398–405. https://doi.org/10.1016/j.fertnstert.2015.08.028.

164. Kendall Rauchfuss LM, Kim T, Bleess JL, Ziegelmann MJ, Shenoy CC. Testicular sperm extraction vs. ejaculated sperm use for nonazoospermic male factor infertility. Fertil Steril. 2021;116(4):963–70. https://doi.org/10.1016/j.fertnstert.2021.05.087.

165. Moskovtsev SI, Alladin N, Lo KC, Jarvi K, Mullen JBM, Librach CL. A comparison of ejaculated and testicular spermatozoa aneuploidy rates in patients with high sperm DNA damage. Syst Biol Reprod Med. 2012;58(3):142–8. https://doi.org/10.3109/19396368.2012.667504.

166. Muratori M, Marchiani S, Tamburrino L, Baldi E. Sperm DNA fragmentation: mechanisms of origin. Adv Exp Med Biol. 2019;1166:75–85. https://doi.org/10.1007/978-3-030-21664-1_5.

167. Homa ST, Vassiliou AM, Stone J, et al. A comparison between two assays for measuring seminal oxidative stress and their relationship with sperm DNA fragmentation and semen parameters. Genes (Basel). 2019;10(3):236. https://doi.org/10.3390/genes10030236.

168. Kadioglu A, Ortac M. The role of sperm DNA testing on male infertility. Transl Androl Urol. 2017;6(Suppl 4):S600–3. https://doi.org/10.21037/tau.2017.03.82.
169. Nagy ZP, Liu J, Joris H, et al. Andrology: the result of intracytoplasmic sperm injection is not related to any of the three basic sperm parameters. Hum Reprod. 1995;10(5):1123–9. https://doi.org/10.1093/oxfordjournals.humrep.a136104.
170. Sergerie M, Laforest G, Bujan L, Bissonnette F, Bleau G. Sperm DNA fragmentation: threshold value in male fertility. Hum Reprod. 2005;20(12):3446–51. https://doi.org/10.1093/humrep/dei231.
171. Mangoli V, Mangoli R, Dandekar S, Suri K, Desai S. Selection of viable spermatozoa from testicular biopsies: a comparative study between pentoxifylline and hypoosmotic swelling test. Fertil Steril. 2011;95(2):631–4. https://doi.org/10.1016/j.fertnstert.2010.10.007.
172. Esteves SC, Varghese AC. Laboratory handling of epididymal and testicular spermatozoa: what can be done to improve sperm injections outcome. J Hum Reprod Sci. 2012;5(3):233–43. https://doi.org/10.4103/0974-1208.106333.
173. de Oliveira NM, Vaca Sánchez R, Rodriguez Fiesta S, et al. Pregnancy with frozen-thawed and fresh testicular biopsy after motile and immotile sperm microinjection, using the mechanical touch technique to assess viability. Hum Reprod. 2004;19(2):262–5. https://doi.org/10.1093/humrep/deh083.
174. Hossain A, Osuamkpe C, Hossain S, Phelps JY. Spontaneously developed tail swellings (SDTS) influence the accuracy of the hypo-osmotic swelling test (HOS-test) in determining membrane integrity and viability of human spermatozoa. J Assist Reprod Genet. 2010;27(2–3):83–6. https://doi.org/10.1007/s10815-009-9375-x.
175. Taşdemir I, Taşdemir M, Tavukçuoğlu S. Effect of pentoxifylline on immotile testicular spermatozoa. J Assist Reprod Genet. 1998;15(2):90–2. https://doi.org/10.1007/BF02766832.
176. Yovich JM, Edirisinghe WR, Cummins JM, Yovich JL. Preliminary results using pentoxifylline in a pronuclear stage tubal transfer (PROST) program for severe male factor infertility. Fertil Steril. 1988;50(1):179–81. https://doi.org/10.1016/s0015-0282(16)60030-4.
177. Nordhoff V. How to select immotile but viable spermatozoa on the day of intracytoplasmic sperm injection? An embryologist's view. Andrology. 2015;3(2):156–62. https://doi.org/10.1111/andr.286.
178. Sallam HN, Farrag A, Agameya A-F, El-Garem Y, Ezzeldin F. The use of the modified hypo-osmotic swelling test for the selection of immotile testicular spermatozoa in patients treated with ICSI: a randomized controlled study. Hum Reprod. 2005;20(12):3435–40. https://doi.org/10.1093/humrep/dei249.
179. Liu J, Tsai YL, Katz E, Compton G, Garcia JE, Baramki TA. High fertilization rate obtained after intracytoplasmic sperm injection with 100% nonmotile spermatozoa selected by using a simple modified hypo-osmotic swelling test. Fertil Steril. 1997;68(2):373–5. https://doi.org/10.1016/s0015-0282(97)81533-6.
180. Montag M, Rink K, Delacrétaz G, van der Ven H. Laser-induced immobilization and plasma membrane permeabilization in human spermatozoa. Hum Reprod. 2000;15(4):846–52. https://doi.org/10.1093/humrep/15.4.846.
181. Ebner T, Moser M, Tews G. Possible applications of a non-contact 1.48 microm wavelength diode laser in assisted reproduction technologies. Hum Reprod Update. 2005;11(4):425–35. https://doi.org/10.1093/humupd/dmi009.
182. Tournaye H, Van der Linden M, Van den Abbeel E, Devroey P, Van Steirteghem A. Effect of pentoxifylline on implantation and post-implantation development of mouse embryos in vitro. Hum Reprod. 1993;8(11):1948–54. https://doi.org/10.1093/oxfordjournals.humrep.a137966.
183. Tournaye H, Van der Linden M, Van den Abbeel E, Devroey P, Van Steirteghem A. Effects of pentoxifylline on in-vitro development of preimplantation mouse embryos. Hum Reprod. 1993;8(9):1475–80. https://doi.org/10.1093/oxfordjournals.humrep.a138282.

Sperm Morphology

7

Cătălina Zenoaga-Barbăroşie ⓘ and Marlon Martinez ⓘ

Introduction

The assessment of morphology is an important step in the evaluation of sperm quality. Sperm morphology is one of the basic parameters assessed during a routine semen analysis and it is recommended by the World Health Organization (WHO) Laboratory Manual for the Examination and Processing of Human Semen [1]. The evaluation of morphology is done on fixed and stained spermatozoa and whole sperm cell is considered for evaluation [2]. Assessment of sperm morphology is complex, challenging, and difficult. Sperm morphology assessment is not a standard validated test due to the existence of several classifications and high inter-observer variability when performing the technique. The classification of morphologically "normal" spermatozoa has been redefined across the years and debates are still ongoing in relation to the role played by sperm morphology as an indicator of male fertility and success with ART.

This chapter describes in brief the methodology and relevance of sperm morphology testing, and the importance of sperm morphology in the diagnosis of infertile patients. Moreover, etiological diagnosis of male reproductive functions and dysfunctions are discussed. Sperm morphology and both ART (assisted reproduction techniques) and non-ART management are discussed. At the end, we provide two clinical scenarios.

C. Zenoaga-Barbăroşie (✉)
Department of Genetics, Faculty of Biology, University of Bucharest, Bucharest, Romania

M. Martinez
Section of Urology. Department of Surgery, University of Santo Tomas Hospital, Manila, Philippines

© The Author(s), under exclusive license to Springer Nature Switzerland AG 2024
A. Agarwal et al. (eds.), *Human Semen Analysis*,
https://doi.org/10.1007/978-3-031-55337-0_7

Physiology: Methodology of Sperm morphology Testing

Human sperm morphology gives valuable information regarding the functional state of the reproductive organs, especially the testicles and epididymis. Additionally, sperm morphology plays an important role in the prognosis of fertility in case of both spontaneous and ART pregnancies [1]. Since the term "normal" is controversial, specialists have suggested the use of the word "typical" instead of "normal" to describe the shape of sperm. A wide variety of morphological abnormalities have been identified affecting, solely or simultaneously, the sperm head, neck, midpiece, and tail. When discussing about sperm morphology, both the proportion of typical sperm and the specific morphology of the sperm are important [3].

Sperm morphology assessment is a basic examination which consists in following up a systematic approach, considering all functional regions of the spermatozoon: the sperm head, midpiece, tail, and cytoplasmic residue. The "typical" sperm head should be smooth, contoured and oval, with the acrosomal region comprising between 40% and 70% of the sperm head. The acrosomal region is visible, well-defined and may contain two small vacuoles, but no large vacuoles. No vacuoles should be observed in the post-acrosomal region. The midpiece is characterized by a slender and regular shape, and should have the same length as the sperm head. The major axis of the sperm head and midpiece should be aligned. The sperm tail should be thin, without sharp angulation, and with a uniform length which exceeds ten times the length of the head. No cytoplasmic residues should be present at the midpiece or tail level. The cytoplasmic droplets should not exceed more than 1/3 of sperm's head [1].

The laboratory protocol consists of the preparation of the smear by placing a drop of the sperm suspension onto a slide and left to air-dry. Next, slides are fixed and stained by Papanicolaou, Shorr, or Diff-Quik. These three different stains differ in terms of osmotic concentration, thus leads to obtaining sperm cells with different sizes [1].

The modified Papanicolaou staining for sperm morphology assessment is the technique recommended by the WHO. This is a validated staining method using the Tygerberg Strict Criteria. Papanicolaou is a basophilic/acidophilic stain, therefore, stains the acrosomal region in pale blue, the post-acrosomal region in dark blue, the midpiece in red, the tail in blue or reddish, and the excess residual cytoplasm appears in green (if reddish means other abnormalities). At least 200 spermatozoa should be analyzed per sample [1].

Shorr stain is an alternative morphology staining technique, but it is not validated and evaluated using strict criteria. Additionally, several rapid staining methods such as Diffquick are available and the advantage of using them is obtaining the result on the same day. However, the smear quality is lower and the size of the sperm head differ in comparison with the validated method [1, 4].

Morphology is one of the sperm parameters that mostly reacts to stress coming from the body and environment. Abnormal sperm morphology results from negative stressors which may not affect the overall health. Assessment of sperm morphology may help with the diagnosis, treatment or in choosing between ART techniques when a genetic cause for sperm abnormality is identified [5].

Among all sperm parameters, morphology assessment is the most subjective and difficult to standardize. Throughout the years, the classification of sperm morphology and the cut-off for typical forms have significantly changed. The first approach for sperm morphological abnormalities was described in 1951 by MacLeod and Gold [6]. They used a liberal approach in which spermatozoa without well-defined abnormalities were considered normal or typical. Therefore, morphologically normal sperm were identified by default [7]. The first and second editions of the WHO manual adopted the liberal approach. However the cut-off for morphological normal sperm in the first WHO edition was stipulated as 80.5% [8], while in the second WHO edition the value was decreased to 50%. Additional information regarding the evaluation criteria for morphology was added in the second WHO manual [9].

In 1987 the Tygerberg strict criteria was described by Menkveld [10] and applied in vitro by Kruger et al. [11]. Any slightly abnormal borderline feature of a sperm was classified as abnormal morphology. Later, the classification was supported and confirmed by other studies [12]. The third edition of WHO manual adopted Tygerberg strict criteria. Moreover, the cut-off for normal forms was lowered down to 30%. A description of the morphological classification of human sperm was provided in the manual [13].

In the fourth edition of WHO manual the Tygerberg strict criteria was completely adopted, the cut-off of normal forms was reduced even more to 14% and a list of sperm morphological abnormalities was provided, however with no accurate description [14]. The lowest cut-off for normal morphological sperm was published in the fifth edition of the WHO manual and it was set to 4%, and indications regarding different abnormalities and a clearer definition were provided [15, 16]. In the sixth edition of the WHO manual, no changes were made regarding sperm morphology [1].

Sperm Morphology and Diagnosis of Fertility and Infertility

The reference cut-off for normal forms used by the WHO has been decreased by 95% from a value of 80.5% [8] to 4% in the last 30 years [1, 16]. Researchers have come up with three possible explanations for the decrease of the value for normal forms. Firstly, it is believed that the normal value was decreased because of the implementation of strict criteria and the introduction of a stricter definition for normal form. Secondly, additional criteria for sperm morphological abnormalities were introduced. Lastly, a decreasing trend in human semen parameters due to the negative environmental factors [5, 15, 17, 18].

The 4% (3.0–4.0) threshold for normal forms was calculated based on the fifth centile of data combined from several studies which included populations of fertile men [19]. Therefore, based on this cut-off, most fertile men will have a percentage of normal morphological spermatozoa higher than 4% [5].

The 4% cut-off value helps specialists to choose the best assisted reproduction technique (ART) procedure for couples with fertility problems. Intrauterine insemination (IUI) or IVF is preferred when normal forms exceed or is equal to 4%. However, if the percentage of normal forms is below the limit, ICSI may be the preferred option [12, 20, 21].

Sperm Morphology and Etiological Diagnosis of Male Reproductive Functions and Dysfunctions

There are a variety of etiologies (Table 7.1) causing sperm morphological abnormalities including environmental factors and clinical conditions. There are defects associated with functional anomalies including defects in chromatin condensation and acrosome reaction, tail motility, and enhanced apoptosis and necrosis. Others may have genetic causes and the following are part of this category: globozoospermia, sperm macrocephaly syndrome, multiple tail abnormalities, and headless spermatozoa [12].

Tobacco and Cannabis

Exposure to specific environmental factors such as tobacco and cannabis may be linked to reduced normal forms [12]. Around 4000 chemicals and 40 metals are released during the act of smoking and a number of mutagenic compounds have been linked to decrease sperm parameters such as nicotine, carbon monoxide, and cadmium. These compounds affect the mitochondrial activity and chromatin structure of the sperm, leading to poor fertilization capacity and one of the sperm parameter affected is the morphology [22]. Smoking increases oxidative stress (OS) levels, which in turn, cause sperm DNA fragmentation (SDF) [23]. A meta-analysis including 5865 participants, concluded that the exposure to cigarette smoking was associated with a decreased morphology with a mean difference of 1.37% [22]. Morphological defects of sperm were significantly higher at head,

Table 7.1 Varied etiologies of teratozoospermia

Etiologies affecting sperm morphology	References
Tobacco and cannabis	[12, 22–31]
Alcohol consumption	[25, 32]
Overweight/obesity	[33–38]
Environmental and occupational pollutants	[39–41]
Varicocele	[42–49]
Infections	[50–58]
Testicular cancer	[59–61]
Diabetes	[62, 63]
Genetic causes	[64–66]

neck, and tail level in smokers compared to control group [24]. A recent study done on 48 heavy smokers and 70 non-smokers concluded that heavy smokers had significantly reduces sperm morphology compared to control subjects ($P < 0.0001$) [25]. However, other study showed no influence of smoking on sperm morphology [26]. The contradictory results may be due to many factors, including study population, the number of smoked cigarettes per day, and the time of tobacco exposure.

Cadmium, which is one of the substances released during smoking, was negatively correlated with sperm morphology in infertile smokers [23, 27].

Cannabis is one of the most used recreational drugs and it has been linked to decreased sperm parameters. Cannabis may affect sperm morphology by binding to the cannabinoid receptors present in sperm [28].

Moderate users of marijuana, a drug derived from the hemp plant *Cannabis sativa*, were 3.4 times more likely to be assessed with abnormal sperm morphology [29]. Moreover, in a systematic review and meta-analysis, Pacey et al., compared sperm morphology of 318 cannabis users and 1652 non-users. The authors concluded that the use of cannabis 3 months prior to sperm sample collection in young men represents a risk factor for poor sperm morphology [30]. However, another systematic review and meta-analysis, which included 1158 cannabis users and 2856 non-users, concluded that cannabis use did not impair sperm morphology or semen quality in general [31].

Alcohol Consumption

Alcohol can have an adverse effect on testosterone metabolism and spermatogenesis, thus affecting sperm morphology [32]. A meta-analysis published in 2017 included 12 studies and has concluded that alcohol consumption had a detrimental effect on sperm normal morphology ($P = 0.003$) [32]. Another recent study done on 52 heavy drinkers and 41 non-drinkers concluded that heavy drinkers had significantly reduced sperm morphology compared to control subjects ($P = 0.001$) [25].

Overweight/Obesity

Increased body mass index may dysregulate the metabolism of fatty acids and lead to scrotal hyperthermia, OS, alteration of testosterone levels and alter spermatogenesis [33–35], and may affect sperm normal morphology. A meta-analysis published in 2021 indicated that overweight and obese patients had significantly decreased normal forms in the ejaculate [36]. However, in the general population obesity was not found to influence the percentage of normal sperm morphology [37]. Additionally, no association between overweight and decreased sperm morphology was identified when comparing obese and normal weight men [38].

Environmental and Occupational Pollutants

Exposure to heavy metals increases the level of reactive oxygen species which, in turn, leads to lipid peroxidation and DNA damage [39]. Therefore, heavy metals affect sperm parameters, including sperm morphology. Wijesekara et al. concluded that sperm normal morphology was significantly reduced in the group exposed to environmental or occupational pollution compared to control subjects ($P = 0.029$). Particle matter is the most important air pollutant and a study revealed that the level of normal forms was decreased in individuals exposed to fine particle matter ($PM_{2.5}$), and every increment of 5 $\mu g/m^3$ in a 2-year average $PM_{2.5}$ was significantly associated with a decrease of 1.29% in sperm normal forms [40]. On the other hand, a study published recently stated that the environment has minor impact on sperm morphology and it may be indirectly influenced by other existing factors [41].

Varicocele

Varicocele is one of the most common causes of primary and secondary male factor infertility and is found in 35% and 80% of cases, respectively [42, 43]. The mechanisms by which varicocele may affect sperm vitality are local hyperthermia, increased reactive oxygen species (ROS) and DNA damage levels [44–46]. Percentage of normal forms are significantly decreased in patients with varicocele, though sperm morphology was less affected in the patients with right varicocele compared to patients with left varicocele [47]. A systematic review and meta-analysis assessing the impact of varicocele on percentage of sperm morphology included 1092 subjects and concluded that varicocele was a risk factor for reduced sperm morphology in 7 of 8 studies [48]. Nork et al. in their meta-analysis reported similar results regarding the negative impact of varicocele, with a reduction in sperm normal forms [49].

Infections

Sperm parameters, including sperm morphology, are reduced following male genital tract infections as a result of damages at intratesticular level and/or lesions throughout excretory tract.

The presence of bacteria and leukocytes in the seminal fluid can compromise sperm quality [50]. The percentage of spermatozoa with normal morphology was statistically lower in men with positive bacterial cultures compared to control group. Teratozoospermia (81.17%) was the most commonly observed abnormality in infertile men subjected to culture using a standard bacteriological technique. The most common organisms isolated in this set of patients were *Enterococcus faecalis* (30%), Staphylococcus (43.33%), and *Escherichia coli* (10%) [51]. In a recent systematic review and meta-analysis, leukocytospermia, a possible marker of seminal tract infection, was significantly associated with reduced normal sperm morphology. The increased levels of ROS, cytokines, and proteases secreted by activated white blood cells were potulated to lead to lipid peroxidation and DNA fragmentation, culminating with sperm damage [52].

Sperm genetic instability may be a consequence of the integration of hepatitis B virus (HBV) and hepatitis C virus (HCV) genome into the genetic material of the spermatozoa [53–55]. HBV infection affects the spermatozoa chromosome condensation [55]. Another virus, the human papillomavirus (HPV) may affect sperm parameters because it binds to the equatorial region of the sperm head [53]. Some studies showed that infection with HPV, HCV, and HBV reduced normal sperm morphology [54, 56] while other studies did not [57, 58].

Testicular Cancer

Testicular cancer decreases semen quality because of its detrimental effect on the hypothalamic–pituitary–gonadal axis. The severity of the effects on sperm parameters depends on the disease stage and type of seminoma [59]. Patients with testicular cancer had higher rates of sperm head abnormalities compared to infertile men [60]. A systematic review and meta-analysis compared sperm parameters, including sperm morphology, in patients with testicular cancer before and after orchiectomy and all included studies showed increased sperm morphology abnormalities prior to orchiectomy [61].

Diabetes

Hyperglycemia and insulin deficiency, characteristic parameters in diabetes mellitus, may have a detrimental effect on gonadal axis, sperm production, and sperm parameters. Diabetic infertile men had significantly lower number of sperm with normal morphology compared to nondiabetic fertile men [62]. In a meta-analysis which comprised diabetic men ($n = 380$) and controls ($n = 434$), the former had significantly lower percentage of normal sperm morphology [63].

Genetic Causes

Male fertility problems are often due to multifactorial causes, with both genetic and extrinsic factors. However, severe cases of male fertility problems are likely to have a predominant genetic etiology. Sperm morphology defects such as globozoospermia, sperm macrocephaly syndrome, multiple tail abnormalities, and headless spermatozoa can be caused by identified gene mutations. Mutations in *AURKC, PICK, ZPBP, SPATA16, DPY19L2* genes have been associated with sperm head defects [64] while mutations in *DNAH1, CFAP43, CFAP44, CFAP69, FSIP2, WDR66 (CFAP251), AK7* genes have been associated with sperm tail defects [65].

Teratozoospermia was associated with an increased rate of aneuploidy of the sperm which could impede ICSI outcome. Compared to controls, a significant higher proportion of 18, XY, XX, and YY disomies in men with severe teratozoo-spermia compared with control group. In addition, significant increase in the mean frequency of total diploidy was observed in the same set of patients [66].

Sperm Morphological Abnormalities

Sperm can present with different morphologic abnormalities (Fig. 7.1). Monomorphic teratozoospermia is the condition when more than 85% of spermatozoa display a unique morphological abnormality and it affects less than 1% of male infertility. There are two forms of monomorphic teratozoospermia: macrozoospermia and globozoospermia. Polymorphic teratozoospermia is the condition in which there is excess of more than one type of sperm morphological abnormality [67].

Globozoospermia

Globozoospermia is a very rare condition (affecting less than 0.1% of infertile males) characterized by sperm with small and rounded heads which lacked an acrosome. It can be categorized as type I or total globozoospermia (all sperm showing the same defect) and type II or partial globozoospermia in which there is a combination of sperm with the defect (up to 90% of total sperm) and normal morphologically sperm [68].

Several gene mutations have been associated with globozoospermia, and these include *SPATA16*, *PICK1*, *DPY19L2*. Mutations may lead to amino acid or missense substitutions, deletions, or the introduction of a premature stop codon and thus, affecting the original function of the protein [67].

Globozoospermia was associated with sperm DNA damage as patients with globozoospermia had statistically significant increase in the sperm DNA fragmentation rate compared to fertile control group (40% ± 3.55% and 8.9% ± 1.3%,

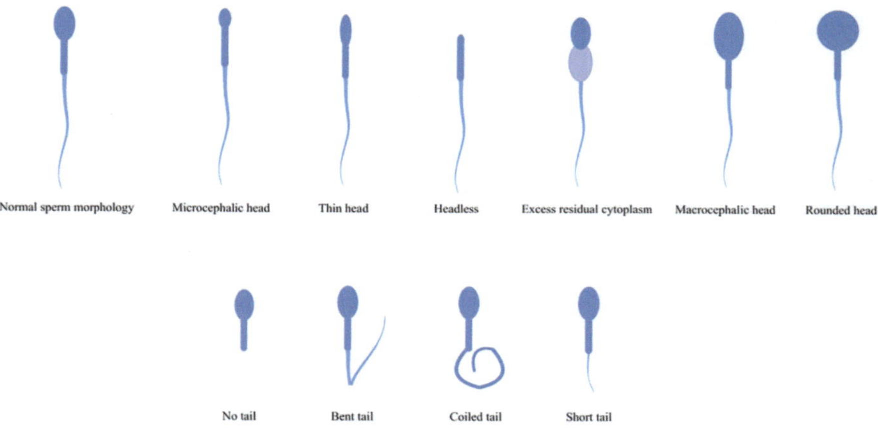

Fig. 7.1 Different sperm morphological abnormalities

respectively) [69]. Moreover, aneuploidy rate was found to be higher in globozoospermia sperm [70]. The forementioned defects lead to decrease of fertilizing ability, leading to a decrease in natural and ART pregnancies. ICSI combined to oocyte activation are recommended n cases of complete globozoospermia [21].

Macrozoospermia

Macrozoospermia or large-headed multiflagellar sperm is a very rare morphological disorder defined as the condition when sperm appear with an oversized irregular head, abnormal midpiece and acrosome, and multiple flagella [16, 71]. In this condition almost all spermatozoa are abnormal. A classification system comprising six types of macrozoospermia, based on sperm deformities, has been suggested to aid in deciding the feasibility of ART [72]. A statistically significant correlation between the rate of macrocephalic forms and the rate of aneuploidy was found. Moreover, this condition has been associated with apoptosis-related DNA strand breaks. Mutations in *AURKC* gene have been associated with macrozoospermia, leading to deletions or the introduction of a premature stop codon, affecting the cell mitosis [67]. Patients with macrozoospermia have a poor prognosis for ICSI and genetic analysis is recommended to determine the ploidy of spermatozoa [21].

Microcephalic and Thin Heads

Sperm with head dimension of less than 3.5 μm in length and 2.5 μm in width are classified as microcephalic head spermatozoa and are commonly associated with acrosome defects [5] and high SDF [73]. Spermatozoa with thin heads are commonly seen in men with varicoceles. In a study including 47 men with high-grade varicocele, the presence of thin sperm heads was present in 14.03 ± 13.09%. Moreover, the proportion of spermatozoa with thin head decreased significantly (6.35 ± 5.29%) 6 months after retrograde embolization [74]. Selection of a typical sperm form followed by ICSI may improve reproductive outcome [5].

Tapered Sperm Head

Sperm with elongated head were identified in varicocele patients with hyperthermia at testicular region. Additionally, tail defects and raised SDF have been identified. Before trying to conceive, the patients are recommended to undergo varicocelectomy or intracytoplasmic morphologically selected sperm injection (IMSI) [21].

Pinhead/Acephalic/Decapitated Spermatozoa

This morphologic phenotype includes headless spermatozoa (flagella) and sperm heads without flagella [64]. Headless or acephalic or decapitated spermatozoa are the result of a defect in the formation of the connecting piece during the process of spermiogenesis. The familial incidence indicates a genetic origin. In a case series of ten infertile men with acephalic sperm, two of these men were brothers [75]. Mutations in *SUN5* gene have been identified in patients with pinhead spermatozoa. When using pinhead sperm for ICSI procedure, fertilization was not followed by progression to the stage of cleavage [21, 64].

Excess Residual Cytoplasm

A small cytoplasmic droplet around the midpiece is retained after spermiogenesis. This is necessary for a normal sperm physiological function such as hyper activation, capacitation, and acrosome reaction [76]. However, the presence of cytoplasmic droplets that exceeds 1/3 of the sperm head size led to detrimental effects on sperm functions. In addition, this contributes to the generation of large amount ROS and subsequent OS which has a negative impact on male reproductive potential [60]. Sperm with excess residual cytoplasm have been identified in patients with varicocele and in smoking ones. Patients are recommended to undergo varicocelectomy and lifestyle modification for sperm parameters improvement [21].

Sperm Tail Abnormalities

For spermatozoa presenting several defects at flagella level, the term of multiple morphological abnormalities of the flagella (MMAF) is used. The condition is characterized by sperm with absent, bent, coiled, short, and irregular flagellar morphologies [77] which may lead to asthenozoospermia [64]. Sperm tail abnormalities may appear as a result of exposure to toxic and chemical substances [21]. Since flagellar defects can lead to impaired sperm motility, MMAF can cause primary infertility with or without primary ciliary dyskinesia (PCD) [78]. PCD is a hereditary disorder characterized with asthenozoospermia caused by abnormalities in cilia and flagella. Infertile men with PCD can likewise present with rhinitis, sinusitis, recurrent respiratory infections, and situs inversus [79].

The proportion of coiled sperm was significantly correlated with age and alpha glucosidase which is an epididymal secretory marker [80]. In addition, it was associated in men infertile men with varicocele and heavy smokers. Sperm with thick and irregular tails can be associated with periaxonemal defects [81].

Genetic mutations in genes *AKAP3*, *AKAP4*, and *DNAH* have been associated with this condition. The proteins encoded by these genes are part of the fibrous sheath and flagellum organization [64].

Hypo-osmotic swelling test and ICSI with testicular or ejaculated sperm should be performed in patients with sperm tail defects [21].

Sperm Morphology and Planning of Further Investigations

There are several tests which evaluate directly or indirectly the sperm morphology (Fig. 7.2). The routine sperm morphology assessment is based on the recommendations provided by the WHO [16]. Agarwal et al. provided standardization of laboratory procedures for the assessment of sperm morphology [21]. This included the establishment policies for quality control and quality assurance. However, the examination of sperm morphology by routine semen analysis is not enough to determine the extent of its detrimental effect to male fertility potential. In the most recent sixth edition of WHO laboratory manual for semen analysis, the evaluation of OS and ROS were described in the section on advanced examination [1]. On the other hand, the determination of SDF and genetic and genomic tests are considered as

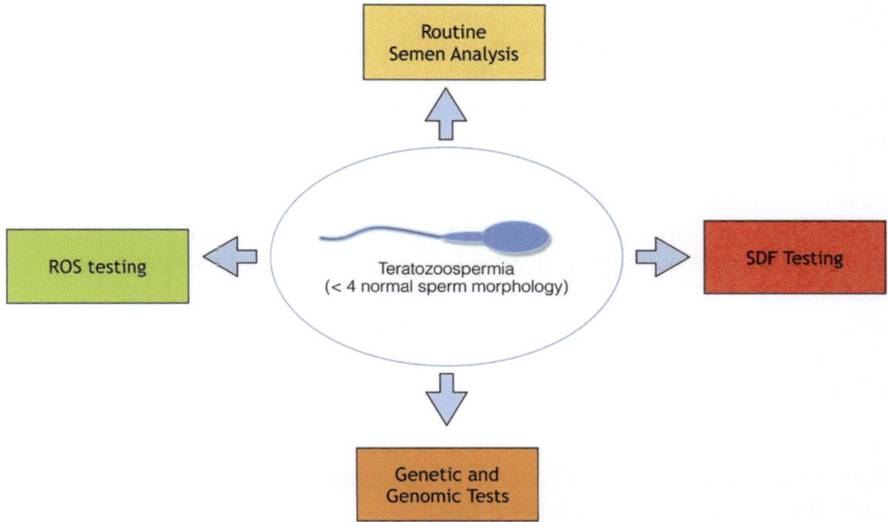

Fig. 7.2 Several tests to evaluate sperm morphological defects directly or indirectly

extended examinations. However, these tests are still not recommended in the initial and routine evaluation of infertile men [82].

In men with isolated teratozoospermia, decreased antioxidant enzymes and high seminal levels of products of lipid peroxidation and ROS are observed [83]. In a study of 69 infertile men with low normal sperm morphology, there was a significant correlation demonstrated between seminal level of glutathione with the percentage of atypical forms and total tail abnormalities. In addition, seminal level of protein sulfhydryl was negatively correlated with multiple anomaly index and total tail abnormalities. There are several tests to measure OS [84–87]. Direct tests, such as chemiluminescence, flow cytometry, electron spin resonance, cytochrome c reduction and nitroblue tetrazolium, measure ROS production and sperm cell oxidation. On the other hand, indirect tests, such as myeloperoxidase, lipid peroxidation, oxidation reduction potential, and total antioxidant capacity evaluate oxidation by measuring the markers of insult from the ROS. Teratozoospermic men had nuclear alterations such as DNA breaks and chromatin decondensation [88, 89]. This sperm DNA damage can be ROS-induced. Compared to control group, teratozoospermic men had significantly higher proportion of sperm with denatured DNA as assessed by acridine orange staining [83]. In another study, men with morphologically abnormal sperm (DFI = 38.86 ± 12.06%) had significantly higher level of SDF measured by TUNEL as compared to control (DFI = 8.14 ± 6.86%) [88]. There was a significant positive correlation between sperm head abnormalities, SDF, DNA denaturation, and hypocondensed chromatin. Indications for SDF testing were proposed based on the available evidences [90]. There are several assays to measure SDF [91]. These can be categorized into tests that measure the susceptibility of DNA integrity after acid denaturation and tests that use probes and dyes to demonstrate

SDF. The most common SDF testing methods used for the assessment of infertile men are sperm chromatin structure assay (SCSA), terminal deoxynucleotidyl transferase dUTP nick end labeling (TUNEL), sperm chromatin dispersion (SCD), and Comet test. These tests are not part of the routine initial evaluation of infertile men, particularly those with low normal sperm morphology [82].

Identification of a major gene responsible for a particular morphologic abnormality is warranted in order to arrive at a complete understanding of genetic anomalies of these infertile men [64]. However, most of the functions and molecular mechanisms of these proteins encoded by a gene are still unknown and undiscovered [65]. Genetic investigation of sperm phenotypes with head, mid piece, and tail defects will offer new insights and new treatment options for these teratozoospermic men [92]. Others may require specific epigenetic profile assessment to identify DNA methylation patterns [93].

Sperm Morphology and Non-ART Management: Treatment and Treatment Response Monitoring

Currently, sperm morphology still lacks a definitive predictive role in reproductive outcomes following ART or natural conception [15]. There is very limited evidence on the impact of sperm morphology on natural pregnancy. Even in men with severe teratozoospermia or total absence of normal forms, alternative treatment options should be offered before proceeding with IVF or ICSI [94]. In a study of 24 men with 0% normal forms, 29.2% of them were able to achieve conception without the aid of IVF after a median follow up of 2.5 years. Of those men, 100% of them had the subsequent child via natural conception [94].

There are several antioxidants which showed improvement of semen parameters, particularly sperm morphology [95]. There was significant correlation between seminal glutathione with the proportion of sperm with atypical forms and those with tail abnormalities. A negative correlation was demonstrated between seminal level of oxidized glutathione with atypical forms. Similar findings were observed when seminal level of total protein sulfhydryl was correlated with multiple anomalies index and total tail abnormalities [83].

Varicocelectomy is recommended in infertile men with palpable varicoceles and abnormal semen parameters [82]. Although the earlier committee opinion in 2014 by the American Society for Reproductive Medicine and the Society for Male Reproduction and Urology recommended against surgical repair of varicocele in infertile men with isolated teratozoospermia [96], it is still a possible option. In 80 men who underwent surgery with a mean postoperative follow-up of 6.8 months, there was significant increase in the mean percentage of sperm with normal morphology (from 0.9% to 3.5%) [97]. In another study of 62 infertile men with isolated teratozoospermia, there was a significant improvement of sperm with normal forms postoperatively (1.15 ± 1.1% versus 2.3 ± 1.8%) [98]. This resulted to natural pregnancy in 31% of men while four men had children through assisted reproduction.

Pacey et al. determined the risk factors for poor sperm morphology [30]. Modifiable risk factor such as the use of cannabis in the past 3 months before semen collection in men aged less than 30 years old was related to having less 4% of sperm with normal forms (odds ratio [OR] = 1.55). There was some of drinking alcohol (OR = 1.51) more than 35 units/week (>456 units over 13 weeks), however, this did not reach statistical significance. Similar finding of a slight increase in risk was observed with smoking (OR 1.20) more than 10 cigarettes/day (>910 over 91 days). Men dealing with poor reproductive potential should be advised to limit exposure to these factors. These lifestyle modifications can help improve the semen quality so that couples can proceed with natural conception or have improved ART outcomes. It is important to address these factors before subjecting patients to a more definitive treatment option.

Sperm Morphology and ART Management: Guiding ART Choices

Have We Become Too Strict?

The adoption of the strict criteria led to the classification of a large number of sperm as abnormal, which would have been regarded as normal by more liberal criteria. Thus, the number of morphologically normal spermatozoa reported has decreased. In this regard, the very low cut-off for percentage of normal forms may have limited its prognostic value [7]. Studies suggest that assessment of sperm morphology may not be a predictor for fertilization, pregnancy, or live birth potential. Almost 30% of patients with 0% normal forms in ejaculate were able to conceive without the help of IVF [94]. A cohort with 0–1% normal forms using the strict criteria reported similar pregnancy rates as the institutional pregnancy rate [99]. However, other studies have supported the predictive value of sperm morphology assessment [100–102].

Additionally, a meta-analysis reported no difference in clinical pregnancy rates following intra-uterine insemination when comparing subjects with normal forms more than 4%, 4% or less, or less than 1% (14.2%,12.1%, and 13.9%, respectively) [103]. Similarly, no differences were reported when comparing pregnancy rates via IVF or ICSI between subjects with normal forms exceeding or under the 4% cut-off [104].

Testicular Versus Ejaculated Sperm

The percentage of normal testicular sperm morphology (4.3%) was lower than of ejaculated sperm (9.6%) [105]. A study analyzing if sperm origin has any effect on embryo morphokinetics suggested that ejaculated sperm is associated with better clinical outcomes compared to testicular sperm [106]. The use of testicular sperm extraction (TESE) has low quality evidence coming from non-randomized studies.

Thus, TESE is not recommended for routine use in patients with oligo-astheno-teratozoospermia and high SDF. In case of two or more ICSI failures in which ejaculated sperm was used, then TESE for ICSI can be considered [107].

The Correlation of Sperm Morphological Profile and Particular Clinical Conditions

The sperm morphological profile is sometimes correlated with particular clinical conditions. However, the sensitivity and specificity are moderate [12]. There are two prognostic categories for patients evaluated with sperm normal forms ≤4%. One prognostic category is composed of patients those sperm morphology defects are unspecified and not genetically determined. Environmental or other stress factor are believed to be the basis of these defects. The sperm morphology can be improved when the source of stress is removed or treated. The second prognostic category encompasses patients with genetically determined sperm defects, including conditions like short tail syndrome, small or large-headed sperm, small or large acrosomes, and globozoospermia. These morphological sperm defects were associated with abnormal sperm function and with poor prognosis [7].

It has been shown that the presence of each abnormal form is slightly higher in infertile men than in fertile [60]. However, WHO does not recommend the assessment of sperm morphology for all samples. One of the reasons may be due to the intraoperator and interoperator variability [12].

On the other hand, some authors still suggest that sperm morphology should be tested using strict criteria and it may have a strong prognostic value [2].

Definition and Types of Multiple Sperm Defects

Three different indices of multiple sperm defects (MSD) have been proposed and defined: the multiple abnormalities index (MAI), the teratozoospermia index (TZI), and the sperm deformity index (DSI). However, data regarding their clinical significance is scarce. The MAI represents the average number of abnormalities per abnormal spermatozoon. The MAI relates to in vivo fertility [12].

When using the TZI, a maximum of four abnormalities per abnormal spermatozoon are counted regardless of the real number of abnormalities per abnormal spermatozoon. The four abnormalities refer to one each for the head, midpiece, principal tail piece, and residual cytoplasm [12]. TZI does not indicate which specific sperm abnormality dominates in a sample. However, patients with a value ≥1.90 for TZI have poor prognosis for IVF and ICSI is recommended [7]. Same as for MAI, the TZI relates to in vivo fertility, but it does not predict spontaneous fertility nor ART outcomes [12].

The SDI represents the number of abnormalities divided by the total number of spermatozoa and it corelates to fertilization rate in conventional IVF [12].

The Clinical Importance of Reporting All of the Morphological Abnormalities

WHO manuals [13, 14] recommended to classify sperm as normal or abnormal and mention if a specific abnormality occured in more than 20% of analyzed spermatozoa.

There are specific situations when it is not enough reporting only the percentages of "normal" and "abnormal" spermatozoa as there are rare sperm morphologic disorders such as primary ciliary dyskinesia, globozoospermia, the presence of headless or macrocephalic spermatozoa, and sperm with oocyte activation deficiency that require specific ART to conceive. However, these sperm morphologic disorders are rare and specific, and can be detected during a routine semen analysis with the possibility to perform a morphology assessment if there is no certainty of the result/diagnosis.

Primary ciliary dyskinesia results in aberrant ultrastructural changes (missing dynein arms, microtubular translocations, lack of radial spokes) in sperm flagella, apart from many other health issues. The diagnostic approach for primary ciliary dyskinesia is limited because the patients phenotypes are not specific [108]. Patients are expected to have low sperm parameters, including morphological abnormalities. Decrease in normal sperm morphology did not reduce IVF or ICSI success [104], but the complete absence of normal form was associated with decreased ICSI success. Genetic testing may be also taken into consideration. Alongside sperm morphology, evaluation of sperm vitality, DNA fragmentation and chromosomal errors are necessary, since poor quality affect reproductive outcomes [109].

If, in addition to primary ciliary dyskinesia, the patients also present situs inversus, then the condition is called Kartagener syndrome. Patients with Kartagener syndrome aiming to conceive can undergo ICSI. There is no morphological criteria for vitality assessment. Therefore, sperm selection methods for assessing vitality can be taken into consideration, namely sperm pentoxifylline activation, hypoosmotic swelling test, the use of laser for sperm viability selection, and sperm tail flexibility test. HOST (hypo osmotic swelling test) does not damage sperm and is compatible with ICSI procedure [110].

Globozoospermia is a sperm defect affecting less than 0.1% of infertile patients. Round-headed spermatozoa lacking acrosome or those in which acrosome is severely malformed are unable to fertilize the oocyte naturally, phenomenon leading to male infertility or sterility. These patients can be given the chance to conceive by using ICSI or IMSI with or without oocyte activation. IMSI is Intracytoplasmic morphologically selected sperm injection, in which sperm undergoes a detailed morphological examination and is selected based on sperm head appearance at a high magnification, thereby, improving reproductive outcomes of these patients [111, 112].

Patients with macrocephalic spermatozoa have a distinct ART management. In patients with macrocephalic sperm syndrome all spermatozoa are macrocephalic with irregular heads and may have abnormal midpiece and acrosome, and multiple tails. *AURKC* gene is predominantly expressed in the testicles and mutations in this gene have been associated with the macrocephalic syndrome. Sperm donation should be taken into consideration by couples when all spermatozoa are affected by an identified *AURKC* mutation. In such cases, ICI is not recommended [12].

Another morphological abnormality that contraindicates intraconjugal ART is the headless spermatozoa. A defect in distal centriole migration results in decapitated sperm syndrome in which sperm do not present heads or have non-inserted tail defects. The use of spermatozoa with defects at head-midpiece level in ICSI leads to fertilization, but pro-nuclear fusion or cleavage does not take place [12].

It is considered that oocyte activation deficiency is directly responsible for 40% of the total fertilization failure cases after ICSI. As the number of ICSI cycles is increasing, it is expected that oocyte activation deficiency will grow proportionally [113]. Several protocols (mechanical, electrical chemical or a combination of these techniques) for assisted oocyte activation have been developed to overcome this issue. However, many physiological, pathological, and ethics aspects of assisted oocyte activation have to be taken in consideration, and further studies are needed to conclude whether the methodology is safe and effective to be used to overcome ICSI fertilization failure [114].

Figure 7.3 summarizes the clinical implications for the morphological sperm defects discussed.

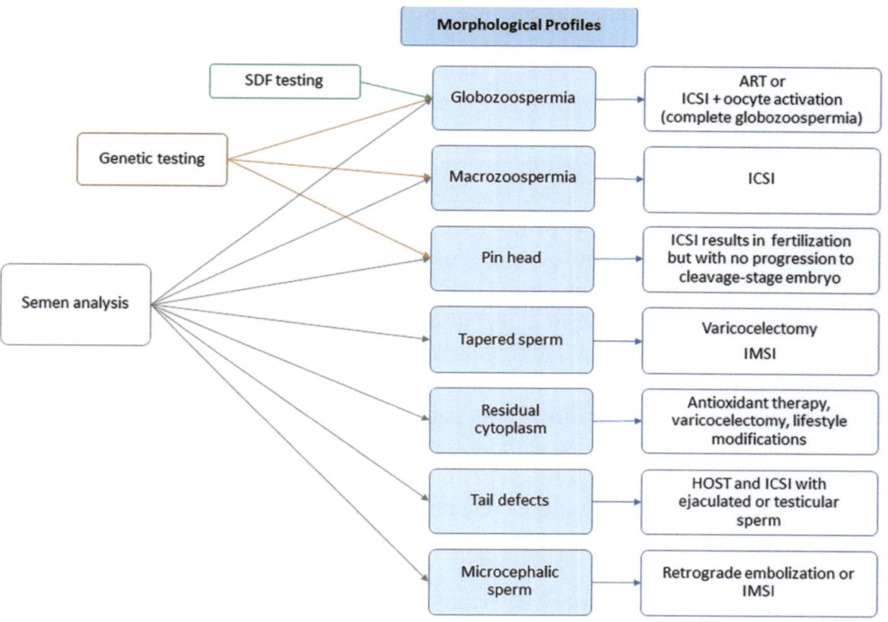

Fig. 7.3 Clinical implications for the morphological sperm defects

Two Clinical Scenarios

Case 1

A 34-year-old man presents with sperm concentration of 34×10^6/mL and progressive motility of 38%. Morphological evaluation revealed all round-headed spermatozoa without acrosome. His 28-year-old partner has normal female evaluation. They underwent ICSI with no fertilisation. Hence, during the second cycle oocyte activation with Ca ionophore was performed and this resulted in a pregnancy and subsequent delivery.

Case 2

A 30-year-old man had bilateral grade 3 varicoceles with sperm concentration of 26×10^6/mL, 38% total motility, and 1% morphology. His wife has normal fertility work up. They had been trying unsuccessfully since 3 years and were considering IVF. However, he first wanted to try for a natural pregnancy so he underwent bilateral microsurgical subinguinal varicocelectomy. Three months after surgery, morphology had improved to 3%, and other parameters had also increased. All semen parameters improved after 3 months. Natural conception was achieved after 1 year.

Take Home Messages

- Sperm morphology evaluation is challenging and difficult because of several reasons, namely the inter-observer variations, manual assessment, and different staining methods used.
- Sperm morphology assessment should be done following a systematic approach that considers all functional regions: the sperm head, midpiece, tail, and cytoplasmic residue.
- The sixth edition of WHO manual recommends the use of strict criteria and 4% as the cut-off for normal forms; however, the specific morphology of head, midpiece and tail, and the presence of cytoplasmic residues are also important in clinical diagnosis.
- Several etiologies cause sperm morphological abnormalities including tobacco and cannabis, alcohol consumption, obesity, varicocele, infections, testicular cancer, diabetes, genetic causes, environmental and occupational pollutants.
- There is need of a more objective and standardized sperm morphology assessment to improve clinical significance.

References

1. WHO. WHO laboratory manual for the examination and processing of human semen. 6th ed. Geneva: WHO Press; 2021.

2. Menkveld R. Sperm morphology assessment using strict (Tygerberg) criteria BT. In: Carrell DT, Aston KI, editors. Spermatogenesis: methods and protocols. Totowa, NJ: Humana Press; 2013. p. 39–50. https://doi.org/10.1007/978-1-62703-038-0_5.

3. Barratt CLR, Mortimer D, Castilla JA, Alvarez JG, Björndahl L, Menkveld R, et al., editors. Basic semen analysis. In: A practical guide to basic laboratory andrology. Cambridge: Cambridge University Press; 2010. p. 33–76. https://www.cambridge.org/core/books/practical-guide-to-basic-laboratory-andrology/basic-semen-analysis/9121211097FBEC464803034E654F3910.

4. Maree L, du Plessis SS, Menkveld R, van der Horst G. Morphometric dimensions of the human sperm head depend on the staining method used. Hum Reprod. 2010;25(6):1369–82.

5. Menkveld R, Holleboom CAG, Rhemrev JPT. Measurement and significance of sperm morphology. Asian J Androl. 2011;13(1):59–68.

6. MacLeod J, Gold RZ. The male factor in fertility and infertility. IV. Sperm morphology in fertile and infertile marriage. Fertil Steril. 1951;2(5):394–414.

7. Menkveld R. Clinical significance of the low normal sperm morphology value as proposed in the fifth edition of the WHO laboratory manual for the examination and processing of human semen. Asian J Androl. 2010;12(1):47–58.

8. WHO. WHO laboratory manual for the examination of human semen and semen-cervical mucus interaction. 1st ed. Singapore: Press Concern; 1980.

9. WHO. WHO laboratory manual for the examination of human semen and semen-cervical mucus interaction. 2nd ed. Cambridge: Cambridge University Press; 1987.

10. Menkveld R. An investigation of environmental influences on spermatogenesis and semen parameters. PhD dissertation, Fac Med Univ Stellenbosch, South Africa; 1987.

11. Kruger TF, Acosta AA, Simmons KF, Swanson RJ, Matta JF, Veeck LL, et al. New method of evaluating sperm morphology with predictive value for human in vitro fertilization. Urology. 1987;30(3):248–51.

12. Gatimel N, Moreau J, Parinaud J, Léandri RD. Sperm morphology: assessment, pathophysiology, clinical relevance, and state of the art in 2017. Andrology. 2017;5(5):845–62.

13. WHO. WHO laboratory manual for the examination of human semen and sperm-cervical mucus interaction. 3rd ed. Cambridge: Cambridge University Press; 1992.

14. WHO. WHO laboratory manual for the examination of human semen and sperm-cervical mucus interaction. 4th ed. Singapore: Cambridge University Press; 1999.

15. Danis RB, Samplaski MK. Sperm morphology: history, challenges, and impact on natural and assisted fertility. Curr Urol Rep. 2019;20(8):43.

16. WHO. WHO laboratory manual for the examination and processing of human semen. Geneva: World Health Organization; 2010.

17. Carlsen E, Giwercman A, Keiding N, Skakkebaek NE. Evidence for decreasing quality of semen during past 50 years. BMJ. 1992;305(6854):609–13. https://www.ncbi.nlm.nih.gov/pubmed/1393072.

18. Menkveld R, Van Zyl JA, Kotze TJ, Joubert G. Possible changes in male fertility over a 15-year period. Arch Androl. 1986;17(2):143–4.

19. Cooper TG, Noonan E, von Eckardstein S, Auger J, Baker HWG, Behre HM, et al. World Health Organization reference values for human semen characteristics. Hum Reprod Update. 2010;16(3):231–45.

20. Zhu D-L, Zhang H-G, Wang R-X, Jiang Y-T, Liu R-Z. Re-evaluation of the value of sperm morphology in classical in vitro fertilization in a Northeastern Chinese population. J Int Med Res. 2019;47(9):4134–42.

21. Agarwal A, Sharma R, Gupta S, Finelli R, Parekh N, Panner Selvam MK, et al. Sperm morphology assessment in the era of intracytoplasmic sperm injection: reliable results require focus on standardization, quality control, and training. World J Mens Health. 2022;40(3):347–60.

22. Sharma R, Harlev A, Agarwal A, Esteves SC. Cigarette smoking and semen quality: a new meta-analysis examining the effect of the 2010 World Health Organization laboratory methods for the examination of human semen. Eur Urol. 2016;70(4):635–45.

23. Ranganathan P, Rao KA, Sudan JJ, Balasundaram S. Cadmium effects on sperm morphology and semenogelin with relates to increased ROS in infertile smokers: an in vitro and in silico approach. Reprod Biol. 2018;18(2):189–97.
24. Bundhun PK, Janoo G, Bhurtu A, Teeluck AR, Soogund MZS, Pursun M, et al. Tobacco smoking and semen quality in infertile males: a systematic review and meta-analysis. BMC Public Health. 2019;19(1):36.
25. Amor H, Hammadeh ME, Mohd I, Jankowski PM. Impact of heavy alcohol consumption and cigarette smoking on sperm DNA integrity. Andrologia. 2022;54(7):e14434.
26. De Brucker S, Drakopoulos P, Dhooghe E, De Geeter J, Uvin V, Santos-Ribeiro S, et al. The effect of cigarette smoking on the semen parameters of infertile men. Gynecol Endocrinol. 2020;36(12):1127–30.
27. De Franciscis P, Ianniello R, Labriola D, Ambrosio D, Vagnetti P, Mainini G, et al. Environmental pollution due to cadmium: measure of semen quality as a marker of exposure and correlation with reproductive potential. Clin Exp Obstet Gynecol. 2015;42(6):767–70.
28. Payne KS, Mazur DJ, Hotaling JM, Pastuszak AW. Cannabis and male fertility: a systematic review. J Urol. 2019;202(4):674–81.
29. Carroll K, Pottinger AM, Wynter S, DaCosta V. Marijuana use and its influence on sperm morphology and motility: identified risk for fertility among Jamaican men. Andrology. 2020;8(1):136–42.
30. Pacey AA, Povey AC, Clyma J-A, McNamee R, Moore HD, Baillie H, et al. Modifiable and non-modifiable risk factors for poor sperm morphology. Hum Reprod. 2014;29(8):1629–36.
31. Belladelli F, Del Giudice F, Kasman A, Kold Jensen T, Jørgensen N, Salonia A, et al. The association between cannabis use and testicular function in men: a systematic review and meta-analysis. Andrology. 2021;9(2):503–10.
32. Ricci E, Al Beitawi S, Cipriani S, Candiani M, Chiaffarino F, Viganò P, et al. Semen quality and alcohol intake: a systematic review and meta-analysis. Reprod Biomed Online. 2017;34(1):38–47.
33. Andersen JM, Rønning PO, Herning H, Bekken SD, Haugen TB, Witczak O. Fatty acid composition of spermatozoa is associated with BMI and with semen quality. Andrology. 2016;4(5):857–65.
34. Garolla A, Torino M, Miola P, Caretta N, Pizzol D, Menegazzo M, et al. Twenty-four-hour monitoring of scrotal temperature in obese men and men with a varicocele as a mirror of spermatogenic function. Hum Reprod. 2015;30(5):1006–13. https://www.ncbi.nlm.nih.gov/pubmed/25779699.
35. Martin LJ. Implications of adiponectin in linking metabolism to testicular function. Endocrine. 2014;46(1):16–28.
36. Salas-Huetos A, Maghsoumi-Norouzabad L, James ER, Carrell DT, Aston KI, Jenkins TG, et al. Male adiposity, sperm parameters and reproductive hormones: an updated systematic review and collaborative meta-analysis. Obes Rev. 2021;22(1):e13082.
37. Wang S, Sun J, Wang J, Ping Z, Liu L. Does obesity based on body mass index affect semen quality?—a meta-analysis and systematic review from the general population rather than the infertile population. Andrologia. 2021;53(7):e14099.
38. Campbell JM, Lane M, Owens JA, Bakos HW. Paternal obesity negatively affects male fertility and assisted reproduction outcomes: a systematic review and meta-analysis. Reprod Biomed Online. 2015;31(5):593–604.
39. Sukhn C, Awwad J, Ghantous A, Zaatari G. Associations of semen quality with non-essential heavy metals in blood and seminal fluid: data from the Environment and Male Infertility (EMI) study in Lebanon. J Assist Reprod Genet. 2018;35(9):1691–701. https://doi.org/10.1007/s10815-018-1236-z.
40. Lao XQ, Zhang Z, Lau AKH, Chan T-C, Chuang YC, Chan J, et al. Exposure to ambient fine particulate matter and semen quality in Taiwan. Occup Environ Med. 2018;75(2):148–54.
41. Olszak-Wasik K, Tukiendorf A, Kasperczyk A, Wdowiak A, Horak S. Environmental exposure to cadmium but not lead is associated with decreased semen quality parameters: quality regionalism of sperm properties. Asian J Androl. 2022;24(1):26–31.

42. Abdel-Maguid A-F, Othman I. Microsurgical and nonmagnified subinguinal varicocelectomy for infertile men: a comparative study. Fertil Steril. 2010;94(7):2600–3.

43. Lai TC-T, Roychoudhury S, Cho C-L. Oxidative stress and varicocele-associated male infertility. Adv Exp Med Biol. 2022;1358:205–35.

44. Jellad S, Hammami F, Khalbous A, Messousi M, Khiari R, Ghozzi S, et al. Sperm DNA status in infertile patients with clinical varicocele. Prog Urol. 2021;31(2):105–11.

45. Cho C-L, Esteves SC, Agarwal A. Novel insights into the pathophysiology of varicocele and its association with reactive oxygen species and sperm DNA fragmentation. Asian J Androl. 2016;18(2):186–93.

46. Boursier A, Dumont A, Boitrelle F, Prasivoravong J, Lefebvre-Khalil V, Robin G, et al. Necrozoospermia: the tree that hides the forest. Andrology. 2022;10(4):642–59.

47. Vivas-Acevedo G, Lozano JR, Camejo MI. Effect of varicocele grade and age on seminal parameters. Urol Int. 2010;85(2):194–9.

48. Agarwal A, Sharma R, Harlev A, Esteves SC. Effect of varicocele on semen characteristics according to the new 2010 World Health Organization criteria: a systematic review and meta-analysis. Asian J Androl. 2016;18(2):163–70.

49. Nork JJ, Berger JH, Crain DS, Christman MS. Youth varicocele and varicocele treatment: a meta-analysis of semen outcomes. Fertil Steril. 2014;102(2):381–7.e6.

50. Fraczek M, Hryhorowicz M, Gill K, Zarzycka M, Gaczarzewicz D, Jedrzejczak P, et al. The effect of bacteriospermia and leukocytospermia on conventional and nonconventional semen parameters in healthy young normozoospermic males. J Reprod Immunol. 2016;118:18–27.

51. Vilvanathan S, Kandasamy B, Jayachandran AL, Sathiyanarayanan S, Tanjore Singaravelu V, Krishnamurthy V, et al. Bacteriospermia and its impact on basic semen parameters among infertile men. Interdiscip Perspect Infect Dis. 2016;2016:2614692.

52. Castellini C, D'Andrea S, Martorella A, Minaldi E, Necozione S, Francavilla F, et al. Relationship between leukocytospermia, reproductive potential after assisted reproductive technology, and sperm parameters: a systematic review and meta-analysis of case-control studies. Andrology. 2020;8(1):125–35.

53. Garolla A, Pizzol D, Bertoldo A, Menegazzo M, Barzon L, Foresta C. Sperm viral infection and male infertility: focus on HBV, HCV, HIV, HPV, HSV, HCMV, and AAV. J Reprod Immunol. 2013;100(1):20–9.

54. Lorusso F, Palmisano M, Chironna M, Vacca M, Masciandaro P, Bassi E, et al. Impact of chronic viral diseases on semen parameters. Andrologia. 2010;42(2):121–6.

55. Huang J-M, Huang T-H, Qiu H-Y, Fang X-W, Zhuang T-G, Liu H-X, et al. Effects of hepatitis B virus infection on human sperm chromosomes. World J Gastroenterol. 2003;9(4):736–40.

56. Wang S, Liu L, Zhang A, Song Y, Kang J, Liu X. Association between human papillomavirus infection and sperm quality: a systematic review and a meta-analysis. Andrologia. 2021;53(5):e14034.

57. Foresta C, Garolla A, Zuccarello D, Pizzol D, Moretti A, Barzon L, et al. Human papillomavirus found in sperm head of young adult males affects the progressive motility. Fertil Steril. 2010;93(3):802–6.

58. Garolla A, Pizzol D, Bertoldo A, De Toni L, Barzon L, Foresta C. Association, prevalence, and clearance of human papillomavirus and antisperm antibodies in infected semen samples from infertile patients. Fertil Steril. 2013;99(1):125–31.e2.

59. Ghasemi B, Mosadegh Mehrjardi A, Jones C, Ghasemi N. Semen analysis of subfertility caused by testicular carcinoma. Int J Reprod Biomed. 2020;18(7):539–50.

60. Auger J, Jouannet P, Eustache F. Another look at human sperm morphology. Hum Reprod. 2016;31(1):10–23.

61. Djaladat H, Burner E, Parikh PM, Beroukhim Kay D, Hays K. The association between testis cancer and semen abnormalities before orchiectomy: a systematic review. J Adolesc Young Adult Oncol. 2014;3:153–9.

62. Bhattacharya SM, Ghosh M, Nandi N. Diabetes mellitus and abnormalities in semen analysis. J Obstet Gynaecol Res. 2014;40(1):167–71.

63. Facondo P, Di Lodovico E, Delbarba A, Anelli V, Pezzaioli LC, Filippini E, et al. The impact of diabetes mellitus type 1 on male fertility: systematic review and meta-analysis. Andrology. 2022;10(3):426–40.

64. Ray PF, Toure A, Metzler-Guillemain C, Mitchell MJ, Arnoult C, Coutton C. Genetic abnormalities leading to qualitative defects of sperm morphology or function. Clin Genet. 2017;91(2):217–32.

65. Nsota Mbango J-F, Coutton C, Arnoult C, Ray PF, Touré A. Genetic causes of male infertility: snapshot on morphological abnormalities of the sperm flagellum. Basic Clin Androl. 2019;29:2.

66. Mehdi M, Gmidène A, Brahem S, Guerin JF, Elghezal H, Saad A. Aneuploidy rate in spermatozoa of selected men with severe teratozoospermia. Andrologia. 2012;44(Suppl 1):139–43.

67. De Braekeleer M, Nguyen MH, Morel F, Perrin A. Genetic aspects of monomorphic teratozoospermia: a review. J Assist Reprod Genet. 2015;32(4):615–23.

68. Anton-Lamprecht I, Kotzur B, Schopf E. Round-headed human spermatozoa. Fertil Steril. 1976;27(6):685–93.

69. Brahem S, Elghezal H, Ghédir H, Landolsi H, Amara A, Ibala S, et al. Cytogenetic and molecular aspects of absolute teratozoospermia: comparison between polymorphic and monomorphic forms. Urology. 2011;78(6):1313–9.

70. Fesahat F, Henkel R, Agarwal A. Globozoospermia syndrome: an update. Andrologia. 2020;52(2):e13459.

71. Nistal M, Paniagua R, Herruzo A. Multi-tailed spermatozoa in a case with asthenospermia and teratospermia. Virchows Arch B Cell Pathol. 1977;26(2):111–8.

72. Guthauser B, Pollet-Villard X, Boitrelle F, Vialard F. Is intracouple assisted reproductive technology an option for men with large-headed spermatozoa? A literature review and a decision guide proposal. Basic Clin Androl. 2016;26:8.

73. Gandini L, Lombardo F, Paoli D, Caponecchia L, Familiari G, Verlengia C, et al. Study of apoptotic DNA fragmentation in human spermatozoa. Hum Reprod. 2000;15(4):830–9. https://doi.org/10.1093/humrep/15.4.830.

74. Prasivoravong J, Marcelli F, Lemaître L, Pigny P, Ramdane N, Peers M-C, et al. Beneficial effects of varicocele embolization on semen parameters. Basic Clin Androl. 2014;24:9.

75. Chemes HE, Puigdomenech ET, Carizza C, Olmedo SB, Zanchetti F, Hermes R. Acephalic spermatozoa and abnormal development of the head–neck attachment: a human syndrome of genetic origin. Hum Reprod. 1999;14(7):1811–8. https://doi.org/10.1093/humrep/14.7.1811.

76. Rengan AK, Agarwal A, van der Linde M, du Plessis SS. An investigation of excess residual cytoplasm in human spermatozoa and its distinction from the cytoplasmic droplet. Reprod Biol Endocrinol. 2012;10(1):92. https://doi.org/10.1186/1477-7827-10-92.

77. Ben Khelifa M, Coutton C, Zouari R, Karaouzène T, Rendu J, Bidart M, et al. Mutations in DNAH1, which encodes an inner arm heavy chain dynein, lead to male infertility from multiple morphological abnormalities of the sperm flagella. Am J Hum Genet. 2014;94(1):95–104.

78. Sha Y, Wei X, Ding L, Ji Z, Mei L, Huang X, et al. Biallelic mutations of CFAP74 may cause human primary ciliary dyskinesia and MMAF phenotype. J Hum Genet. 2020;65(11):961–9. https://doi.org/10.1038/s10038-020-0790-2.

79. Wang W-L, Tu C-F, Tan Y-Q. Insight on multiple morphological abnormalities of sperm flagella in male infertility: what is new? Asian J Androl. 2020;22(3):236–45.

80. Yeung CH, Tüttelmann F, Bergmann M, Nordhoff V, Vorona E, Cooper TG. Coiled sperm from infertile patients: characteristics, associated factors and biological implication. Hum Reprod. 2009;24(6):1288–95.

81. Mitchell V, Sigala J, Ballot C, Jumeau F, Barbotin AL, Duhamel A, et al. Light microscopy morphological characteristics of the sperm flagellum may be related to axonemal abnormalities. Andrologia. 2015;47(2):214–20.

82. Schlegel PN, Sigman M, Collura B, De Jonge CJ, Eisenberg ML, Lamb DJ, et al. Diagnosis and treatment of infertility in men: AUA/ASRM guideline part I. J Urol. 2021;205(1):36–43.

83. Ammar O, Mehdi M, Muratori M. Teratozoospermia: its association with sperm DNA defects, apoptotic alterations, and oxidative stress. Andrology. 2020;8(5):1095–106.

84. Wagner H, Cheng JW, Ko EY. Role of reactive oxygen species in male infertility: an updated review of literature. Arab J Urol. 2018;16(1):35–43.

85. Agarwal A, Roychoudhury S, Sharma R, Gupta S, Majzoub A, Sabanegh E. Diagnostic application of oxidation-reduction potential assay for measurement of oxidative stress: clinical utility in male factor infertility. Reprod Biomed Online. 2017;34(1):48–57.

86. Agarwal A, Parekh N, Panner Selvam MK, Henkel R, Shah R, Homa ST, et al. Male oxidative stress infertility (MOSI): proposed terminology and clinical practice guidelines for management of idiopathic male infertility. World J Mens Health. 2019;37(3):296.

87. Finelli R, Leisegang K, Kandil H, Agarwal A. Oxidative stress: a comprehensive review of biochemical, molecular, and genetic aspects in the pathogenesis and management of varicocele. World J Mens Health. 2022;40(1):87–103.

88. Oumaima A, Tesnim A, Zohra H, Amira S, Ines Z, Sana C, et al. Investigation on the origin of sperm morphological defects: oxidative attacks, chromatin immaturity, and DNA fragmentation. Environ Sci Pollut Res Int. 2018;25(14):13775–86.

89. Ammar O, Haouas Z, Hamouda B, Hamdi H, Hellara I, Jlali A, et al. Relationship between sperm DNA damage with sperm parameters, oxidative markers in teratozoospermic men. Eur J Obstet Gynecol Reprod Biol. 2019;233:70–5.

90. Martinez M, Majzoub A. Best laboratory practices and therapeutic interventions to reduce sperm DNA damage. Andrologia. 2021;53(2):e13736.

91. Agarwal A, Majzoub A, Esteves SC, Ko E, Ramasamy R, Zini A. Clinical utility of sperm DNA fragmentation testing: practice recommendations based on clinical scenarios. Transl Androl Urol. 2016;5(6):935–50.

92. Beurois J, Cazin C, Kherraf Z-E, Martinez G, Celse T, Touré A, et al. Genetics of teratozoospermia: back to the head. Best Pract Res Clin Endocrinol Metab. 2020;34(6):101473.

93. Jenkins TG, Aston KI, Hotaling JM, Shamsi MB, Simon L, Carrell DT. Teratozoospermia and asthenozoospermia are associated with specific epigenetic signatures. Andrology. 2016;4(5):843–9.

94. Kovac JR, Smith RP, Cajipe M, Lamb DJ, Lipshultz LI. Men with a complete absence of normal sperm morphology exhibit high rates of success without assisted reproduction. Asian J Androl. 2017;19(1):39–42.

95. Dutta S, Majzoub A, Agarwal A. Oxidative stress and sperm function: a systematic review on evaluation and management. Arab J Urol. 2019;17:87–97.

96. ASRM & SMRU. Report on varicocele and infertility: a committee opinion. Fertil Steril. 2014;102(6):1556–60.

97. Choe JH, Seo JT. Is varicocelectomy useful for subfertile men with isolated teratozoospermia? Urology. 2015;86(6):1123–8.

98. Ilktac A, Hamidli S, Ersoz C, Dogan B, Akcay M. Efficacy of varicocelectomy in primary infertile patients with isolated teratozoospermia. A retrospective analysis. Andrologia. 2020;52(11):e13875.

99. Lockwood GM, Deveneau NE, Shridharani AN, Strawn EY, Sandlow JI. Isolated abnormal strict morphology is not a contraindication for intrauterine insemination. Andrology. 2015;3(6):1088–93.

100. Kruger TF, Lacquet FA, Sarmiento CA, Menkveld R, Ozgür K, Lombard CJ, et al. A prospective study on the predictive value of normal sperm morphology as evaluated by computer (IVOS). Fertil Steril. 1996;66(2):285–91.

101. Sripada S, Townend J, Campbell D, Murdoch L, Mathers E, Bhattacharya S. Relationship between semen parameters and spontaneous pregnancy. Fertil Steril. 2010;94(2):624–30.

102. Jedrzejczak P, Taszarek-Hauke G, Hauke J, Pawelczyk L, Duleba AJ. Prediction of spontaneous conception based on semen parameters. Int J Androl. 2008;31(5):499–507.

103. Kohn TP, Kohn JR, Ramasamy R. Effect of sperm morphology on pregnancy success via intrauterine insemination: a systematic review and meta-analysis. J Urol. 2018;199(3):812–22. https://www.sciencedirect.com/science/article/pii/S0022534717778822.

104. Hotaling JM, Smith JF, Rosen M, Muller CH, Walsh TJ. The relationship between isolated teratozoospermia and clinical pregnancy after in vitro fertilization with or without intracytoplas-

mic sperm injection: a systematic review and meta-analysis. Fertil Steril. 2011;95(3):1141–5. https://www.sciencedirect.com/science/article/pii/S0015028210025902.

105. Steele EK, McClure N, Lewis S. A comparison of the morphology of testicular, epididymal, and ejaculated sperm from fertile men and men with obstructive azoospermia. Fertil Steril. 2000;73(6):1099–103.

106. Karavani G, Kan-Tor Y, Schachter-Safrai N, Levitas E, Or Y, Ben-Meir A, et al. Does sperm origin—ejaculated or testicular—affect embryo morphokinetic parameters? Andrology. 2021;9(2):632–9.

107. Colpi GM, Francavilla S, Haidl G, Link K, Behre HM, Goulis DG, et al. European Academy of Andrology guideline management of oligo-astheno-teratozoospermia. Andrology. 2018;6(4):513–24.

108. Li Y, Jiang C, Zhang X, Liu M, Sun Y, Yang Y, et al. The effect of a novel LRRC6 mutation on the flagellar ultrastructure in a primary ciliary dyskinesia patient. J Assist Reprod Genet. 2021;38(3):689–96.

109. De Vos A, Van De Velde H, Joris H, Verheyen G, Devroey P, Van Steirteghem A. Influence of individual sperm morphology on fertilization, embryo morphology, and pregnancy outcome of intracytoplasmic sperm injection. Fertil Steril. 2003;79(1):42–8.

110. Montjean D, Courageot J, Altié A, Amar-Hoffet A, Rossin B, Geoffroy-Siraudin C, et al. Normal live birth after vitrified/warmed oocytes intracytoplasmic sperm injection with immotile spermatozoa in a patient with Kartagener's syndrome. Andrologia. 2015;47(7):839–45.

111. Sermondade N, Hafhouf E, Dupont C, Bechoua S, Palacios C, Eustache F, et al. Successful childbirth after intracytoplasmic morphologically selected sperm injection without assisted oocyte activation in a patient with globozoospermia. Hum Reprod. 2011;26(11):2944–9. https://doi.org/10.1093/humrep/der258.

112. Chansel-Debordeaux L, Dandieu S, Bechoua S, Jimenez C. Reproductive outcome in globozoospermic men: update and prospects. Andrology. 2015;3(6):1022–34.

113. Kashir J, Ganesh D, Jones C, Coward K. Oocyte activation deficiency and assisted oocyte activation: mechanisms, obstacles and prospects for clinical application. Hum Reprod Open. 2022;2022(2):hoac003. https://doi.org/10.1093/hropen/hoac003.

114. Anifandis G, Michopoulos A, Daponte A, Chatzimeletiou K, Simopoulou M, Messini CI, et al. Artificial oocyte activation: physiological, pathophysiological and ethical aspects. Syst Biol Reprod Med. 2019;65(1):3–11. https://doi.org/10.1080/19396368.2018.1516000.

Sperm Agglutination

8

Taymour Mostafa ⓘ and Ayad Palani ⓘ

Introduction

Infertility is defined as the inability to conceive within a year of unprotected, healthy coitus [1]. Infertility affects approximately 15% of couples worldwide and the global burden of this condition showed an annual increase in the age-standardized prevalence rate of infertility by 0.370% for females and 0.291% for males [2]. In this context, the male factor is considered as a main or contributing cause in approximately 50% of all infertility issues [3].

Fertilization is a complex process of fusion of the male spermatozoa and female egg and the successful accomplishment of this unity depends on the sperm's ability to pass through the female genital tract [4]. To accomplish this goal, the male partner must have a sufficient number of healthy, progressively motile spermatozoa. Therefore, evaluation of the infertile male is important to identify the cause of impaired sperm function which may be due to internal or external factors [5].

Semen analysis is the basis for evaluating the male's fertilization ability in infertile couples. The World Health Organization (WHO) efforts since the 1970s of producing, updating, editing, and publishing a semen analysis manual has allowed this test to be standardized throughout the world [6]. The latest edition of the WHO manual established reference values of sperm parameters, ≥ 16 million sperms/ml for sperm concentration, $\geq 42\%$ for sperm motility, and $\geq 30\%$ for sperm progressive motility [7]. Sperm parameters below these normal values were considered male factor infertility though the sixth edition of the WHO manual states that such a

T. Mostafa (✉)
Faculty of Medicine, Andrology, Sexology and STIs Department, Cairo University, Cairo, Egypt

A. Palani
College of Medicine, University of Garmian, Kalar, Iraq
e-mail: ayad.palani@garmian.edu.krd

© The Author(s), under exclusive license to Springer Nature Switzerland AG 2024
A. Agarwal et al. (eds.), *Human Semen Analysis*,
https://doi.org/10.1007/978-3-031-55337-0_8

distinction is not valid. The common etiologies are low sperm concentration (oligozoospermia), poor sperm motility (asthenozoospermia), and increased abnormal sperm morphology (teratozoospermia). Other factors that may influence male fertility include; low semen volume, obstruction to spermatozoa in the female genital tract, or defects in the delivery of sperm genetic material into the egg [8].

Sperm agglutination is an important influence that impairs sperm motion and consequently prevents sperm passage through the cervical mucus and the zona pellucida binding. Agglutination is a clumping of motile sperms to each other, head-to-head, tail-to-tail, or in a mixed way. However, sticking of either immotile or motile spermatozoa to cells other than spermatozoa, or to cellular debris, or mucus threads should be differentiated and not be considered agglutination [9]. The presence of sperm agglutination is linked with *the* presence of antisperm antibodies (ASAB), genital tract infection, and/or ascorbic acid deficiency [10].

ASAB are protective proteins that are produced naturally against sperm surface antigens when the body mistakenly triggers the immune system against sperms [11]. These ASABs are present in both female and male bodies and could impair sperm function through several mechanisms, such as reducing sperm motility, preventing cervical mucus penetration, and inhibiting sperm-oocyte fusion. In males, antisperm immunoglobulins can be formed due to the breaking of the blood–testes barrier after some pathological conditions such as; trauma, vasectomy, orchitis, testis biopsy, torsion, or testicular cancer [12].

These immunoglobulins may be present in both blood and seminal plasma in three dissimilar structural classes; IgG, IgA, and IgM. IgA and IgG antibodies are predominantly present in the semen whereas IgM antibodies are rarely present in semen because of their relatively larger size and their main role is in the acute phases of infection [7]. Under normal conditions, the seminal vesicles secrete chemicals that act as reducing agents that prevent sperm agglutination [13]. Both IgA and IgG can be bound to the whole spermatozoon or selectively to the head, middle piece, or tail [14].

The first clinical observation of the presence of ASAB in human semen was by Rümke et al. in 1954 [15]. ASAB has been considered a significant cause in 8.2% of infertility cases with a higher prevalence in infertile men (1–13%) than in fertile men (1–2%) [16]. Vitamin C appears to have a role in sperm agglutination whereas its deficiency has been demonstrated to induce sperm agglutination and its dietary supplementation was linked to improving sperm motility and preventing nonspecific sperm agglutination [17]. Accessory gland infection (MAGI) was found to increase sperm agglutination and using antibiotics could reverse this effect. In this context, different bacterial species, such as *Candida albicans*, *Trichomonas vaginalis*, *Chlamydia trachomatis*, *Helicobacter pylori*, *Escherichia coli*, *Pseudomonas aeruginosa*, *Mycoplasma* spp., *Streptococcus* spp., *Staphylococcus* spp., were demonstrated to reduce sperm motility and increase agglutination via secretion of sperm agglutination factor [18].

Physiology: Methodology of Sperm Agglutinates Testing

During the initial microscopic investigation, it is recommended to report any abnormalities that may be seen beside the basic semen parameters. The presence of motile spermatozoa that stick to each other should be distinguished and recorded for its degree and site of attachment (head to head, midpiece to midpiece, tail to tail, or mixed way). The different types of agglutination degrees were explained and illustrated earlier by Rose et al. [19], and reprinted in the WHO manuals.

There are different causes of sperm agglutination, thus, the occurrence of agglutination is not an adequate indication to assume immunological male infertility. However, sperm agglutination has been always related to ASAB, and since 1970 they are considered to be investigated as the one possible cause contributing to decreasing sperm motility with subsequent male infertility [20].

Therefore, the need to develop a laboratory assay to meet the clinician's need for a diagnostic test for the investigation and treatment of immune-mediated male infertility. Test of sperm antibodies has been recommended by the WHO as a "standard procedure" specifying sperm agglutination as a possible indicator of the presence of ASAB that might be implicated in male infertility [9].

Methods of detection of ASAB have been a subject of concern by the editors of the WHO manual of semen analysis. Hence, during the last decades, several methods have been developed to detect the presence of ASAB. However, the WHO manual recommended both direct and indirect tests to detect and quantitate antisperm immunoglobulin IgG and IgA in human semen [7]. Laboratory tests to quantitate and detect ASAB may be classified into two groups based on the location of the antibodies: direct test (detection of the antibodies on spermatozoa surface) and indirect test (detection of antibodies in the seminal plasma, serum, follicular fluid, or cervical mucus) [21].

Direct Antiglobulin Test

The mixed antiglobulin reaction (MAR) as well as immunobead (IB) are common direct tests used to detect and quantitate ASAB. These tests allow for the detection of ASAB in fresh semen samples by direct mixing with specialized antibody-coated beads. The WHO recommended both tests be applied in andrology laboratories to detect ASAB.

Mixed Antiglobulin Reaction (MAR) Test

MAR test is a simple, sensitive, rapid, and low-cost method but provides less information than the immunobead (IB) test [22]. MAR test was first proposed for the detection of platelet antibodies and then modified in 1978 by Jager et al. [23]. The test is based on the reaction of antibody-coated red blood cells with antisperm antibodies present on the sperm surface. A washed suspension of group O (Rh)-positive RBCs was sensitized and coated with human immunoglobulin (mainly IgG and sometimes IgA). This test is carried out by mixing fresh semen with treated red blood cells. The ASAB on the sperm membrane then bridge with the immunoglobulin-coated erythrocytes after the addition of a suspension of anti-human-IgG and anti-human-IgA [24].

This test was modified later to use artificial latex beads rather than red blood cells and became commercially available as SpermMAR (FertiPro, Beernem, Belgium). This kit is widely used during a routine investigation of male infertility in andrology laboratories, being rapid and applicable to unwashed semen samples. Antibody detection by sperMAR kit is carried out by mixing equal volumes of semen, IgG latex particles, and IgG antiserum on a microscopic slide. The mixture is then covered with a cover slip and the slide is observed using an optical microscope under a 400× or 600× magnification. The presence of ASAB is indicated by agglutinate formation between beads and motile spermatozoa [25]. If the results indicated that 10–39% of the motile sperms are covered by latex beads immunological infertility is suspected, and if ≥40% of the sperms are covered, immunological infertility is highly expected [25].

The Immunobead Test (IB)

IB test is more informative and specific than other ASAB detection methods capable to detect all types of immunoglobulin (IgG, IgA, IgM) and their binding positions on the sperm surface. Additionally, this test requires no specialized equipment [26].

IB test was proposed by Clarke et al. in 1982 allowing rosette-type polyacrylamide beads coated with specific immunoglobulins (IgG, IgM, or IgA) to detect ASAB on sperm surfaces [27]. Currently, the beads are available in the form of Cyanogen bromide-activated Sepharose conjugated with anti-human IgG or IgA. However, with no commercially available immunobead test kit, the beads must be prepared at the laboratory according to manufacturers' protocols [7]. Prepared beads are mixed with washed sperm, and the mixture is observed microscopically for the presence of beads bound to motile spermatozoa indicating the presence of ASAB on the sperm surface.

Indirect Antiglobulin Test

An indirect test is used to detect ASAB in reproductive fluids, i.e., seminal plasma, follicular fluid, and cervical mucus, as well as blood serum. This test is recommended in obstructive azoospermia, oligozoospermia, or asthenozoospermia (alone or in combination with direct test), in case of freezing or saving of semen samples for later testing [21], or when it is not possible to perform the direct tests due to a low percentage of motile spermatozoa in the semen sample [28].

In the indirect test, the fluid is incubated with ASAB-free donor sperm to allow specific antibodies to bind and is then assessed in a direct test (MAR or IB). The test is time-dependent and time is expected to interfere with the results since it may need up to 10 min for mixed agglutination to appear and sperm motility declines with time [29].

Indirect tests for ASAB commonly use the commercially available MAR kits. However, there are also other indirect tests, such as the sperm immobilization test (SIT), tray agglutination test (TAT), and gelatin agglutination test (GAT) that were used in the past but are not so common as antibodies detected with those methods are not necessarily implicated in infertility [30].

A new method of enzyme-linked immunosorbent assays method (ELISA) has been developed to detect IgG, IgA, and IgM antibodies in seminal plasma, cervical mucus, or serum. ELISA method uses sperm surface antigens absorbed on a solid phase. The sample is added to anti-human-immunoglobulin (IgA, IgG, and IgM) conjugated to horseradish peroxidase or alkaline phosphatase enzyme that reacts with its substrate to develop a color that can be measured photometrically [31]. This method is specific, more quantitative, does not require fresh sperm, and is more sensitive and easier than other microscopic methods [32]. Lately, this test is widely accepted in the screening of serum ASAB. The good specificity and the quantitative power of ELISA has allowed this method to be a screening test for ASAB in investigating immune-mediated infertility [28]. However, the disadvantages of this test are that sperm requires fixation that may cause denaturation of sperm antigens or membrane damage leading to false results, high cost, low sensitivity, and inability to determine the ASAB isotype and location on sperm whole body [33].

Limitation of the Test
For routine work, vitality tests need not be carried out unless sperm motility is <40%; MAR tests need not be carried out if there is little agglutination and leukocytes need not be distinguished unless there are many in semen.

ASAB and Male Reproductive Function and Dysfunction

The immune system response is a natural process to counteract the harmful effect of invading foreign bodies that might contact the circulatory system. Sperm proteins are considered foreign antigens being produced in a developmental syncytium protected from recognition by the circulatory system [33]. The body provides two mechanisms to avert immune system reaction against sperms:

1. Testis sequestration of the germ cells in the seminiferous tubules protected from the circulatory and lymphatic systems making it "immune privileged" by the blood–testis and blood–epididymis barriers [34].
2. Induction of active immune suppression by seminal plasma components and suppressor/cytotoxic T-lymphocytes [35].

Despite this, the blood–testis barrier may be breached due to injury or illness, resulting in exposure of sperm antigens to the bloodstream stimulating the male immune system to develop ASAB [36].

Risk Factors of ASAB Formation

Varicocele

Varicocele is a known cause of male infertility estimated to be with an incidence as high as 35–40% [37]. Immune infertility was demonstrated to be linked to varicocele when, its association with ASAB formation was reported in 1959 by Rümke and Hellinka [38]. ASAB have a prevalence of 15% in varicocele patients. Recent studies showed that direct MAR-IgG ($\geq$50%) was thrice more frequent in infertile men as compared to fertile men [39]. However, the data on the possible beneficial effect of varicocele repair on ASAB is conflicting, with clinical studies reporting a positive, negative, or no effect of varicocelectomy on ASAB formation [40–42].

The mechanisms underlying ASAB formation in infertile men with varicocele are unclear. Turner et al. [43] found that the blood–testis barrier was still intact and undamaged in the experimental creation of left unilateral varicocele with a bilateral change in the testicular function. However, others suggested that varicocele was not a direct cause of inducing the immune system response; but it acts as a synergistic factor that increases the risk of ASAB production [44].

Vasectomy

Vasectomy is a surgical intervention for birth control that is used by nearly 42–60 million couples worldwide [45]. Although the method is safe and effective, vasectomy may provoke the immune system to develop ASAB constituting one risk factor for immune infertility in men.

It has been demonstrated that the testes undergo histologic changes after vasectomy due to the hydrostatic back pressure effect resulting from the continuous production of spermatozoa. Such histological changes include; the deposition of collagen in the seminiferous tubule wall basement, Leydig cell hyperplasia, defects in spermatogenesis, distension of the seminiferous tubules, and formation of sperm granulomas [46]. Blockage of the reproductive ducts leads to increased sperm absorption by epididymal endothelial cells and enhanced phagocytosis in the intraluminal place. The reabsorption of the degradation products by the endothelial cells leads to stimulating the immune response against sperm antigens [47].

Infection

Among the risk factors that induce sperm autoimmune is the inflammatory response to the male genital tract infection (MGTI). The main causes of inflammatory disorders of the male genital tract are attributed to sexually transmitted micro-organisms as well as male genital tract pathogens [48]. MGTI has been reported to contribute to 15% of infertility cases [49]. It was suggested that MGTI is linked with a greater risk of developing sperm antibodies [21]. However, while the exact mechanism of ASAB production due to MGTI is still controversial, studies have shown that ASAB formation is significantly linked with genital tract infection [50], while others have declined this association [51].

The mechanism of ASAB formation linked with MGTI proposed that autoimmune reaction could be initiated as a result of local immune dysregulation or local inflammation. The immune system may produce ASAB during cross-immune reactions with foreign antigens of the micro-organisms [52]. In addition, RNA viruses, such as Mumps, Zika, Ebola, Marburg viruses, and Coronavirus can break the blood–testis barrier causing local inflammation [53].

Other Uncommon Risk Factors for ASAB Formation

Other conditions without enough evidence were also reported as risk factors for ASAB formation like testicular torsion, trauma, testicular tumors, testicular sperm extraction, homosexuality, or unsafe sex (anal or oral sex) [52]. However, in many cases, the cause is unknown or defined as idiopathic [21].

Potential Targets of ASAB

The identification and characterization of sperm antibodies involved in fertilization are of great interest, considering that the development of knowledge in this area helps to diagnose and treat immunological infertility [28]. ASAB targets numerous different antigens present mainly upon the sperm surface that could be a part of the internal sperm component [54]. Sperm surface proteins are known by the immune system as foreign antigens that may induce immune reactions following the breaking of the blood–tests barrier, leading to ASAB formation by activated B-lymphocytes [55]. Studies show that carbohydrate moieties of sperm surface and seminal plasma are chief target antigens for ASAB formation [56], but there is no recognized single moiety to interact with all the ASAB [32]. However, several sperm antigens of different sperm components have been identified to be implicated in inducing the immune system, for example, CD52, lactate dehydrogenase (LDHC4), Tektin-2, and triose phosphate isomerase [57, 58]. In female follicular fluid, multiple ASAB can be released by the female immune system against sperm components, and isolated sperm antigens such as; rSMP-B, BE-20, BS-63 (nucleoporin-related), YWK-II, BS-17 (calpastatin), 75-kDa, and HED-2 (zyxin) have been shown to react to follicular fluids ASAB [32]. In addition, ASAB in follicular fluids could interact against proacrosin/acrosin and induce the acrosome reaction leading to blocking sperm–egg fusion [58].

ASAB and Diagnosis of Fertility and Infertility

Landsteiner and Metchnikoff were the first to describe sperm autoimmunity by independent experimental studies in 1899 [59]. However, the role of ASAB in male infertility was not proven until 1954, when Wilson, as well as Rümkeand, independently detected ASAB in the blood and semen of infertile men [60, 61]. Since then, the number of studies have increased progressively and peaked during the period 1980–1990 (Fig. 8.1). In the past years, all studies aimed to develop new methods for the estimation of sperm agglutination or to understand the exact role of sperm auto-immunity in male infertility [62]. In the last two decades the interest in this field has declined gradually due to; (1) the lack of a standard method to calculate the antibody density on the sperm surface, and (2) conflicting reported data regarding the role of ASAB in male infertility. However, the sixth WHO manual that has recommended two tests for the detection of ASAB, and the expected role of COVID-19 in breaking blood–testis barriers, have renewed the interest in this subject again.

Reference Ranges Used by the WHO Manual of Semen Analysis

Although several methods to detect ASAB have developed in the last decades, the latest WHO 6th Edition [7] recommended only two methods:

1. **The MAR test:** To detect sperm IgG and IgA antibodies in fresh semen samples.
2. **The IB test:** To detect sperm IgG and IgA antibodies by direct assessment in washed sperm samples or indirectly in sperm-free fluids.

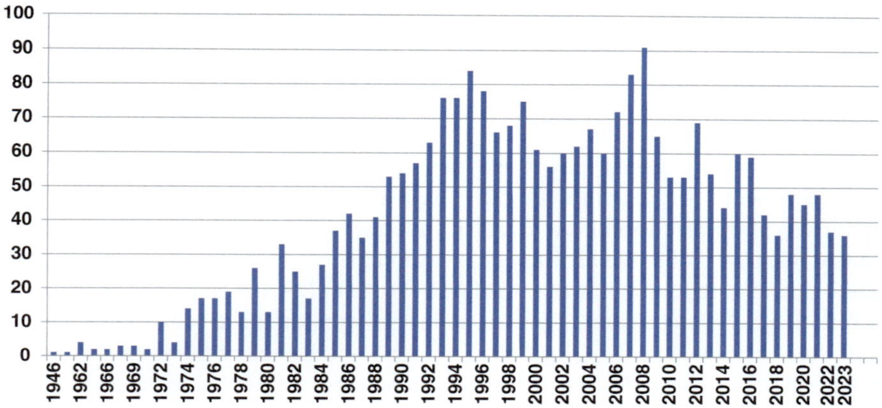

Fig. 8.1 Distribution of studies on ASAB (1946–2023)

The absence of a single validated test for the detection of ASAB brought a conflict in the scoring of the tests and the variation in the results among fertile and infertile men due to the use of different methods. This makes it difficult to establish reference limits for antibody-bound sperms in both MAR and IB tests of semen for fertile men. Hence, each laboratory should delineate its cutoff value by testing an adequate amount of fertile men [7].

In the previous editions of the WHO manual, the diagnosis of immunological infertility was expected if ≥50% of both progressive and non-progressive motile spermatozoa had adherent particles but the suggested cutoff value was based on a small study [63].

Scoring of Agglutination

The presence of sperm agglutination in initial semen analysis is suggestive of the existence of an immunological factor of infertility. Hence, the sticking of motile sperms to each other should be reported in the basic semen analysis report. The WHO manual categorizes agglutination as:

- **Grade 1: isolated:** <10 sperms/agglutinate, large number of free spermatozoa
- **Grade 2: moderate:** 10–50 sperms/agglutinate, moderate number of free spermatozoa
- **Grade 3: large:** >50 sperms/agglutinate, low number of free spermatozoa
- **Grade 4: gross:** All sperms agglutinated and agglutinate interconnected

Report of agglutination in routine semen analysis maybe of uncertain significance [10]. Practically, there is no definite grade that confirms the immunological cause. However, the presence of a large number of agglutinated spermatozoa indicates the need to test for ASAB but it should be noted that:

1. Motile spermatozoa bound to non-sperm cells, debris, or mucus strands, or immotile spermatozoa stuck to each other should be reported as nonspecific aggregation [64].
2. ASAB can be present without sperm agglutination; equally, agglutination can be caused by other factors.

Limitation of the agglutination test

1. Still, there are no standardized methods for the detection of ASAB with determined cutoff levels, and the assessment of their effect on sperm function [58].
2. It is not known exactly what grade of sperm agglutination indicates the need to perform an ASAB assay.
3. The degree of sperm immunobead binding that indicates a significant clinical level of sperm antibodies is not yet established [65].

4. A large size of the agglutinate limits the method's ability to define the region of the sperm to which the antibody type is bound, and limits its utility in estimating the percentage of antibody-bound sperms [26].
5. False positive results may occur due to cross-reaction with antibodies to bacterial antigens not related to infertility [26].

ASAB and Planning of Further Investigations

During the diagnosis of immune infertility, further examinations, in addition to a sperm agglutination test, may be required to identify the etiology behind the breaking of the blood-testis barrier and inducing the immune response (Fig. 8.2). An infection of the genital tract, obstruction or injury to testicles, or varicocele can

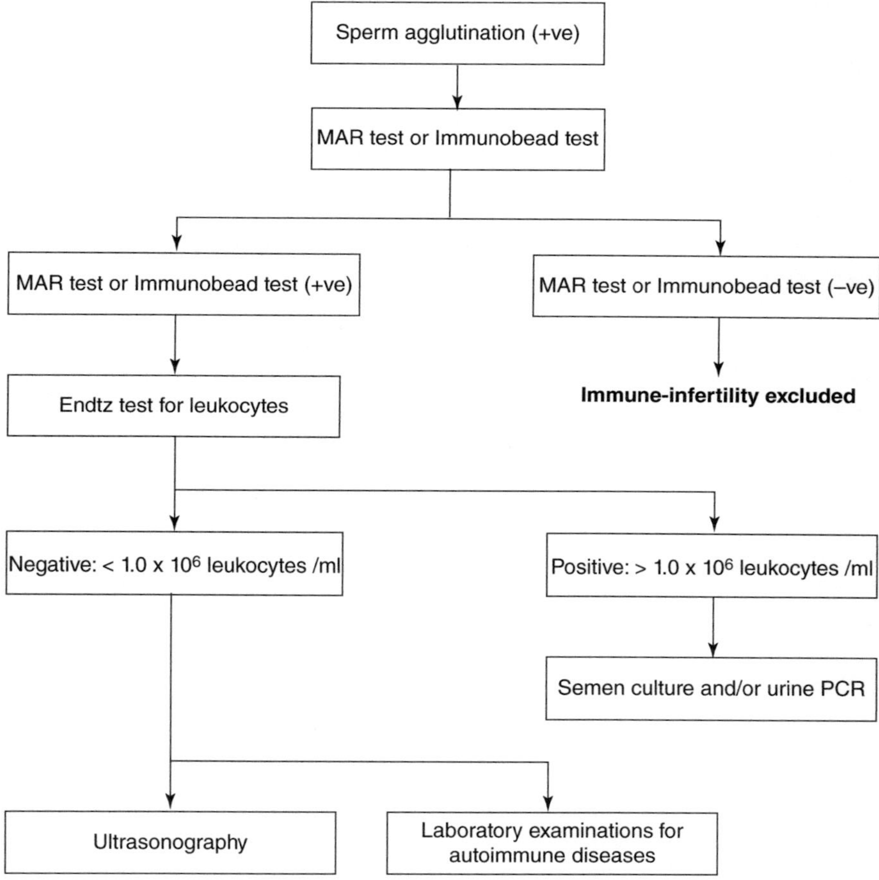

Fig. 8.2 Complementary diagnostic tools to investigate the causes underlying the immune infertility

break the blood–testis barrier and set off an immune response. This can also happen in the course of systemic autoimmune diseases [66].

Infection of the genital tract is an important trigger of an immune response; men who had leukocytospermia linked with bacteriospermia showed a significant increase in sperm agglutination. Leukocytospermia is defined by the WHO as a semen sample containing leukocytes >1.0 × 10^6 cells/ml [7]. Different laboratory methods for WBCs detection are available such as; immunochemistry, elastase, ortho-toluidine, and the Endtz test. The latter is a simple test and provides trustworthy results [67].

A semen culture or urine PCR may be requested to assess for GTI. The EAU and AUA guidelines recommend performing a culture examination when the leukocytes exceed 1 × 10^6 cells/ml of semen., However, the benefit of carrying out semen culture is not clear due to different reasons, i.e., lack of significant differences in the occurrence of positive semen culture between infertile and fertile males, false positive culture results due to contamination in the course of the sample collection, and inability to culture both *Chlamydia trachomatis* and *Ureaplasma urealyticum* which are the two most common GTI bacteria. However, the patient with negative semen culture and leukocytospermia may undergo urine PCR to identify GTI pathogens [67].

Ultrasonography is an important diagnostic tool to evaluate potential testicular abnormalities such as varicocele, cryptorchidism, testicular trauma, the presence of testicular tumors, and evaluation for reproductive tract obstruction [68]. Ultrasound imaging is preferred because it is safe, noninvasive, inexpensive, and allows multiplanes imaging [69].

Management of ASAB

There is no standard medical treatment for immune infertility. The existing approaches include reducing ASAB formation by using immunosuppressives and antibiotics, removing ASAB by sperm washing techniques, and the use of ART, which is the most successful [32, 46].

Immunosuppressive therapy, most commonly, corticosteroids has been used since a long time in an attempt to reduce ASAB formation. Although its use to overcome immunological infertility is still controversial [70], a meta-analysis study of 32 clinical trials of men diagnosed with immunological infertility with significant levels of ASAB revealed that treatment with corticosteroids reduced ASAB formation, and increased sperm motility, sperm concentration, and conception rate [71].

However, there is not enough evidence to support using of immunosuppressive corticosteroids to treat ASAB, as most studies lack appropriate placebo controls, have different doses of different drugs, and have used different laboratory techniques to assay ASAB levels to monitor its effect on sperm quality and the reproductive outcome. These factors make it hard to conclude whether or not corticosteroid therapy is effective in the treatment of immunological infertility [72]. Besides the insufficient evidence of its beneficial effect on reproductive outcomes the potential side effects of steroid therapy have reduced the interest in using corticosteroids for treating immunologic infertility [33].

Infection has also been proposed as a risk factor for ASAB formation. Significant levels of sperm antibodies were observed in patients with orchitis, epididymitis, and chronic prostatitis [73]. These findings have encouraged investigaion of the relationship between infection and ASAB. In this context, inconsistent data have been published during the last few years. A study by Micic et al. found no significant relationship between MGTI and the formation of seminal ASAB [74]. Similar results have been reported by Marconi et al. [47] and Eggert-Kruse et al. [75]. However, others showed that different types of infections such as urethritis, epididymitis, orchitis, and sexually transmitted diseases are significant risk factors for the development of ASAB [73], whereas a high prevalence was reported in patients infected with human papillomavirus [76], Chlamydia trachomatis [77], and Helicobacter pylori in gastroduodenal diseases [78]. Also, it was shown that the number of leukocytes in the seminal plasma of leukocytospermia is proportionally correlated to ASAB level [79].

Antibiotic treatment of leukocytospermia has been shown to ameliorate the harmful effect of invasive pathogens and improve male fecundity [80]; this suggests that a reduction in the level of infectious agents may be necessary for allowing suppression of immunological activity and, thereby, improved sperm quality [71]. Numerous reports have been published on antibiotics and anti-inflammatories therapy, and although reports regarding antibiotic therapy are conflicting, there is a general agreement on the beneficial use of antibiotics in treating of infection-mediated infertility [81].

ASAB and ART Outcome

Still, the impact of ASABs on the IVF/ICSI cycle's reproductive outcomes remains debated. Previously, a few IVF studies have demonstrated that ASABs may adversely impact IVF fertilization and/or pregnancy rates [82–84]. However, several other studies have failed to establish a relationship between ASAB levels and IVF reproductive outcomes [85–87] or show influence of ASAB on fertilization or pregnancy rates following ICSI [88–92]. Meanwhile, some studies showed that ASAB does not have a significant impact on IUI pregnancy rates [93, 94].

Zini et al. identified and analyzed 16 valid studies (10 IVF and 6 ICSI). Though the ASA cutoff values were heterogeneous they reported that the combined OR for failure to achieve a pregnancy using IVF or ICSI in the presence of positive semen ASAB was 1.22 (95% CI: 0.84, 1.77) and 1.00 (95% CI: 0.72, 1.38). The overall (IVF + ICSI) combined OR was 1.08 (95% CI: 0.85, 1.38). These authors concluded that semen ASAs are not related to pregnancy rates after IVF or ICSI, suggesting therefore that IVF or ICSI are viable options for infertile couples with semen ASAB [95].

In another study, Zini et al. pointed out that there was no significant relationship between direct ASAB levels, or sperm parameters and reproductive outcomes after IVF and IVF/ICSI. Clinical pregnancy rates were not significantly different in ASAB-positive (>50% of sperm coated with ASAB) compared with ASA-negative samples (42% vs. 52%, OR: 1.45 (95% CI 0.63, 3.30, $P > 0.05$) [96].

However, in a recent study, Lu et al. indicated lower rates of fertilization (41.7% vs. 54.8%, $P = 0.03$), good embryos (18.9% vs. 35.2%, $P = 0.001$), pregnancy (38.5% vs. 59.4%, $P = 0.00$), and live births (25.8% vs 42.5%, $P = 0.001$) in men of the IVF group with a positive serum ASAB than in men with a negative ASAB. Sperm antibodies were negativity correlated with pregnancy rates ($P = 0.021$, OR: 0.630, 95% CI: 0.425–0.932) and live birth rates ($P = 0.010$, OR: 1.409, 95% CI: 1.084–1.831) after controlling for the female serum FSH level and the couple's ages. Women coupled with ASA-positive men had lower live birth rates with IVF than with ICSI (25.8% and 47.4%, respectively; $P = 0.07$) [97].

Clinical Scenarios

Some clinical scenarios that may be encountered during infertility diagnosis are highlighted:

Case 1

Scenario: A couple presents with primary infertility. Semen analysis was sperm concentration 6.5 $\times 10^6$/ml, total sperm motility 30%, moderate to severe agglutination, with a normal female factor. If this couple selects to undergo ICSI, what specific advice would be given?

Solution: Clinical risk factors for ASAB should be assessed but ASAB testing is not recommended in the case of performing ICSI [95].

Case 2

Scenario: A 34-year-old male has undergone vasectomy reversal. Six months after surgery, semen analysis revealed the results: sperm concentration 4.5 $\times$ 10^6/ml, sperm motility 25%, moderate to severe agglutination (ASAB test showed IgA >50% and IgG >50%, with complete bead attachment to spermatozoa). What is the recommendation(s) for this case?

Solution: Occurrence of ASAB after vasectomy reversal is not uncommon [98]. As the ASAB test report shows >50% agglutination and complete bead attachment, ICSI is advised.

Future Perspectives

There is still no agreement on the implication of sperm autoimmune in male infertility, but it should be considered during the investigation of infertile couples, particularly if other causes of male infertility are absent. MAR and IB tests are the most reliable tests, and the reference value should be determined by the laboratories for each method as the results of both methods are not the same.

There is no proven strategy for the treatment of immune infertility. ASAB-mediated infertility treatment by using corticosteroids has generally declined due to the side effects of their long use and the advent of ART procedures that are unaffected by ASAB levels. However, the inclusion of ASAB testing in the WHO's new edition of the semen manual, and the possible implication of COVID-19 in the breaking of the blood-testis barrier, have increased the interest in ASAB research in the last years. Finally, more research is looked for to establish a standardized method to detect ASAB and to build up a treatment strategies to improve pregnancy outcomes.

Take Home Message

- Sperm autoimmune should be considered during the investigation of male infertility, especially when there is sperm agglutination in routine semen analysis in the absence of other etiological factors.
- Sperm agglutination may occur due to different causes, and it should be distinguished from sperm aggregation due to adherence of sperms to cellular debris or cells other than spermatozoa in the semen. Agglutination is reported when there is adherence of motile spermatozoa to each other.
- Still, the limitation in diagnosing immune infertility is the lack of a standard method of ASAB assay in addition to the absence of a reference value to distinguish infertile patients from fertile men.
- MAR and IB tests are recommended by the WHO in its latest manual [7] as a "standard procedure" for detecting ASAB in human semen. However, the results of both tests are not necessarily similar.
- Different strategies for treating immune infertility are proposed including using immunosuppresses, antibiotics, and ART. As immunosuppressives are not often prescribed due to their unfavorable long-term side effect, IUI, and ICSI are more commonly recommended.

References

1. Agarwal A, Baskaran S, Parekh N, Cho C-L, Henkel R, Vij S, et al. Male infertility. Lancet. 2021;397(10271):319–33.
2. Babakhanzadeh E, Nazari M, Ghasemifar S, Khodadadian A. Some of the factors involved in male infertility: a prospective review. Int J Gen Med. 2020;13:29–41.

3. Agarwal A, Mulgund A, Hamada A, Chyatte MR. A unique view on male infertility around the globe. Reprod Biol Endocrinol. 2015;13(1):1–9.
4. Yoshida M, Kawano N, Yoshida K. Control of sperm motility and fertility: diverse factors and common mechanisms. Cell Mol Life Sci. 2008;65(21):3446–57.
5. Dull RB. Male infertility: an overview of the causes and treatments. US Pharm. 2012;37(6):39–42.
6. Wang C, Swerdloff RS. Limitations of semen analysis as a test of male fertility and anticipated needs from newer tests. Fertil Steril. 2014;102(6):1502–7.
7. WHO, editor. WHO laboratory manual for the examination and processing of human semen. 6th ed. Geneva: WHO; 2021.
8. Kumar N, Singh AK. Trends of male factor infertility, an important cause of infertility: a review of literature. J Hum Reprod Sci. 2015;8(4):191–6.
9. WHO. WHO laboratory manual for the examination and processing of human semen. Geneva: WHO; 2010.
10. Berger GK, Smith-Harrison LI, Sandlow JI. Sperm agglutination: prevalence and contributory factors. Andrologia. 2019;51(5):e13254.
11. Marshburn PB, Kutteh WH. The role of antisperm antibodies in infertility. Fertil Steril. 1994;61(5):799–811.
12. Dhama K, Chakraborty S, Abdul Samad H, Latheef S, Sharun K, et al. Role of antisperm antibodies in infertility, pregnancy, and potential for contraceptive and antifertility vaccine designs: research progress and pioneering vision. Vaccine. 2019;7(3):116.
13. La Vignera S, Vicari E, Condorelli RA, D'Agata R, Calogero AE. Male accessory gland infection and sperm parameters (review). Int J Androl. 2011;34(5):e330–47.
14. Yeh W-R, Acosta AA, Seltman HJ, Doncel G. Impact of immunoglobulin isotype and sperm surface location of antisperm antibodies on fertilization in vitro in the human. Fertil Steril. 1995;63(6):1287–92.
15. Leushuis E, van der Steeg JW, Steures P, Repping S, Schöls W, van der Veen F, et al. Immunoglobulin G antisperm antibodies and prediction of spontaneous pregnancy. Fertil Steril. 2009;92(5):1659–65.
16. Kamphorst K, Faber J, van der Linden PJQ. The presence of antisperm antibodies in semen of subfertile men—positive ASA in subfertile men. Open J Obst Gynecol. 2021;11(02):88–101.
17. Hajjar T, Soleymani F, Vatanchian M. Protective effect of vitamin C and zinc as an antioxidant against chemotherapy-induced male reproductive toxicity. J Med Life. 2020;13(2):138.
18. Oghbaei H, Rastgar Rezaei Y, Nikanfar S, Zarezadeh R, Sadegi M, Latifi Z, et al. Effects of bacteria on male fertility: spermatogenesis and sperm function. Life Sci. 2020;256:117891.
19. Rose NR, Hjort T, Rumke P. Techniques for detection of iso and auto antibodies to human spermatozoa. Clin Exp Immunol. 1976;23(2):175–99.
20. Wakimoto Y, Fukui A, Kojima T, Hasegawa A, Shigeta M, Shibahara H. Application of computer-aided sperm analysis (CASA) for detecting sperm-immobilizing antibody. Am J Reprod Immunol. 2018;79(3):e12814.
21. Gupta S, Sharma R, Agarwal A, Boitrelle F, Finelli R, Farkouh A, et al. Antisperm antibody testing: a comprehensive review of its role in the management of immunological male infertility and results of a global survey of clinical practices. World J Mens Health. 2022;40(3):380–98.
22. Kallen CB, Arici A. Immune testing in fertility practice: truth or deception? Curr Opin Obstet Gynecol. 2003;15(3):225–31.
23. Jager S, Kremer J, van Slochteren-Draaisma T. A simple method of screening for antisperm antibodies in the human male. Detection of spermatozoal surface IgG with the direct mixed antiglobulin reaction carried out on untreated fresh human semen. Int J Fertil. 1978;23(1):12–21.
24. Hendry WF, Stedronska J, Lake RA. Mixed erythrocyte-spermatozoa antiglobulin reaction (MAR test) for IgA antisperm antibodies in subfertile males. Fertil Steril. 1982;37(1):108–12.
25. Agarwal A, Gupta S, Sharma R. Direct SpermMar antibody test. In: Andrological evaluation of male infertility. Cham: Springer; 2016. p. 147–53.
26. Sikka SC, Hellstrom WJ. Tests for antisperm antibodies. Infertil Male. 2019;2019:603–12.

27. Clarke G, Stojanoff A, Cauchi M. Immunoglobulin class of sperm-bound antibodies in semen. In: Bratanov K, editor. Proc Int Symp immunology of reproduction. Bulgaria: Bulgarian Academy of Sciences Press; 1982. p. 492.
28. Silva AF, Ramalho-Santos J, Amaral S. The impact of antisperm antibodies on human male reproductive function: an update. Reproduction. 2021;162(4):R55–71.
29. Agarwal A, Said T. Tests for sperm antibodies. In: Immune infertility. Cham: Springer; 2009. p. 155–64.
30. Windt M-L, Bouic P-J, Lombard C, Menkveld R, Kruger T. Antisperm antibody tests: traditional methods compared to ELISA. Arch Androl. 1989;23(2):139–45.
31. Helmerhorst FM, Finken MJ, Erwich JJ. Antisperm antibodies: detection assays for antisperm antibodies: what do they test? Hum Reprod. 1999;14(7):1669–71.
32. Lu J-C, Huang Y-F, Lu N-Q. Antisperm immunity and infertility. Expert Rev Clin Immunol. 2008;4(1):113–26.
33. Mazumdar S, Levine AS. Antisperm antibodies: etiology, pathogenesis, diagnosis, and treatment. Fertil Steril. 1998;70(5):799–810.
34. Fijak M, Bhushan S, Meinhardt A. The immune privilege of the testis. In: Immune infertility. Cham: Springer; 2017. p. 97–107.
35. Pöllänen P, Cooper T. Immunology of the testicular excurrent ducts. J Reprod Immunol. 1994;26(3):167–216.
36. O'Donnell L, Smith LB, Rebourcet D. Sperm-specific proteins: new implications for diagnostic development and cancer immunotherapy. Curr Opin Cell Biol. 2022;77:102104.
37. Fang Y, Su Y, Xu J, Hu Z, Zhao K, Liu C, et al. Varicocele-mediated male infertility: from the perspective of testicular immunity and inflammation. Front Immunol. 2021;12:729539.
38. Rümke P, Hellinga G. Autoantibodies against spermatozoa in sterile men. Am J Clin Pathol. 1959;32(4):357–63.
39. Bozhedomov VA, Lipatova NA, Alexeev RA, Alexandrova LM, Nikolaeva MA, Sukhikh GT. The role of the antisperm antibodies in male infertility assessment after microsurgical varicocelectomy. Andrology. 2014;2(6):847–55.
40. Djaladat H, Mehrsai A, Rezazade M, Djaladat Y, Pourmand G. Varicocele and antisperm antibody: fact or fiction? South Med J. 2006;99(1):44–8.
41. Bonyadi MR, Madaen SK, Saghafi M. Effects of varicocelectomy on anti-sperm antibody in patients with varicocele. J Reprod Infertil. 2013;14(2):73.
42. Chereshnev V, Pichugova S, Rybina I, Beikin YB. Role of antisperm antibodies in the formation of infertility in varicocele and infertility. Russ J Immunol. 2020;23(3):315–22.
43. Turner T, Jones C, Roddy M. Experimental varicocele does not affect the blood-testis barrier, epididymal electrolyte concentrations, or testicular blood gas concentrations. Biol Reprod. 1987;36(4):926–32.
44. Bozhedomov V, Lipatova N, Rokhlikov I, Alexeev R, Ushakova I, Sukhikh G. Male fertility and varicocoele: role of immune factors. Andrology. 2014;2(1):51–8.
45. Schwarzer JU, Steinfatt H. Current status of vasectomy reversal. Nat Rev Urol. 2013;10(4):195–205.
46. McLachlan RI. Basis, diagnosis and treatment of immunological infertility in men. J Reprod Immunol. 2002;57(1-2):35–45.
47. Marconi M, Weidner W. Site and risk factors of antisperm antibodies production in the male population. In: Immune infertility. Cham: Springer; 2017. p. 133–47.
48. Schuppe H-C, Pilatz A, Hossain H, Diemer T, Wagenlehner F, Weidner W. Urogenital infection as a risk factor for male infertility. Dtsch Arztebl Int. 2017;114(19):339.
49. Burrello N, Salmeri M, Perdichizzi A, Bellanca S, Pettinato G, D'Agata R, et al. Candida albicans experimental infection: effects on human sperm motility, mitochondrial membrane potential and apoptosis. Reprod Biomed Online. 2009;18(4):496–501.
50. Jalal H, Bahadur G, Knowles W, Jin L, Brink N. Mumps epididymo-orchitis with prolonged detection of virus in semen and the development of anti-sperm antibodies. J Med Virol. 2004;73(1):147–50.

51. Marconi M, Pilatz A, Wagenlehner F, Diemer T, Weidner W. Are antisperm antibodies really associated with proven chronic inflammatory and infectious diseases of the male reproductive tract? Eur Urol. 2009;56(4):708–15.
52. Lobo N, Satchi M. The diagnosis and management of men with low sperm motility. Trends Urol Men's Health. 2019;10(5):24–7.
53. Donders GGG, Bosmans E, Reumers J, Donders F, Jonckheere J, Salembier G, et al. Sperm quality and absence of SARS-CoV-2 RNA in semen after COVID-19 infection: a prospective, observational study and validation of the SpermCOVID test. Fertil Steril. 2022;117(2):287–96.
54. Karimi F, Khazaei S, Alaedini F. Serum antisperm antibodies in fertile and infertile individuals. Iran J Med Sci. 2008;33(2):88–93.
55. El-Sherbiny AF, Ali TA, Hassan EA, Mehaney AB, Elshemy HA. The prognostic value of seminal anti-sperm antibodies screening in men prepared for ICSI: a call to change the current antibody-directed viewpoint of sperm autoimmunity testing. Ther Adv Urol. 2021;13:17562872209814 88.
56. Kurpisz M, Alexander NJ. Carbohydrate moieties on sperm surface: physiological relevance. Fertil Steril. 1995;63(1):158–65.
57. Zangbar MS, Keshtgar S, Zolghadri J, Gharesi-Fard B. Antisperm protein targets in azoospermia men. J Hum Reprod Sci. 2016;9(1):47–52.
58. Vazquez-Levin MH, Marin-Briggiler CI, Veaute C. Antisperm antibodies: invaluable tools toward the identification of sperm proteins involved in fertilization. Am J Reprod Immunol. 2014;72(2):206–18.
59. Friberg J. Clinical and immunological studies on sperm-agglutinating antibodies in serum and seminal fluid. Acta Obstet Gynecol Scand. 1974;53(36):1–19.
60. Rumke P. The presence of sperm antibodies in the serum of two patients with oligospermia. Vox Sang. 1954;4:135–40.
61. Wilson L. Sperm agglutinins in human semen and blood. Proc Soc Exp Biol Med. 1954;85(4):652–5.
62. Francavilla F, Santucci R, Barbonetti A, Francavilla S. Naturally-occurring antisperm antibodies in men: interference with fertility and clinical implications. An update. Front Biosci. 2007;12(8):2890–911.
63. Barratt C, Dunphy B, McLeod I, Cooke I. The poor prognostic value of low to moderate levels of sperm surface-bound antibodies. Hum Reprod. 1992;7(1):95–8.
64. Chimote N, Semen analysis. Donald school textbook of human reproductive & gynecological endocrinology. New Delhi: Jaypee Brothers Medical Publishers; 2018. p. 292.
65. Heidenreich A, Bonfig R, Wilbert DM, Strohmaier WL, Engelmann UH. Risk factors for antisperm antibodies in infertile men. Am J Reprod Immunol. 1994;31(2-3):69–76.
66. Chereshnev VA, Pichugova SV, Beikin YB, Chereshneva MV, Iukhta AI, Stroev YI, et al. Pathogenesis of autoimmune male infertility: Juxtacrine, paracrine, and endocrine dysregulation. Pathophysiology. 2021;28(4):471–88.
67. Sharma R, Gupta S, Agarwal A, Henkel R, Finelli R, Parekh N, et al. Relevance of leukocytospermia and semen culture and its true place in diagnosing and treating male infertility. World J Mens Health. 2022;40(2):191–207.
68. Armstrong JM, Keihani S, Hotaling JM. Use of ultrasound in male infertility: appropriate selection of men for scrotal ultrasound. Curr Urol Rep. 2018;19(8):1–9.
69. Mittal PK, Little B, Harri PA, Miller FH, Alexander LF, Kalb B, et al. Role of imaging in the evaluation of male infertility. Radiographics. 2017;37(3):837–54.
70. Mahmoud A, Comhaire F. Immunological causes. Andrology for the clinician. Cham: Springer; 2006. p. 47–52.
71. Skau PA, Folstad I. Does immunity regulate ejaculate quality and fertility in humans? Behav Ecol. 2005;16(2):410–6.
72. Naz RK. Modalities for treatment of antisperm antibody mediated infertility: novel perspectives. Am J Reprod Immunol. 2004;51(5):390–7.
73. Gubin DA, Dmochowski R, Kutteh WH. Multivariant analysis of men from infertile couples with and without antisperm antibodies. Am J Reprod Immunol. 1998;39(2):157–60.

74. Mićić S, Petrovic S, Dotlić R. Seminal antisperm antibodies and genitourinary infection. Urology. 1990;35(1):54–6.
75. Eggert-Kruse W, Rohr G, Probst S, Rusu R, Hund M, Demirakca T, et al. Antisperm antibodies and microorganisms in genital secretions—a clinically significant relationship? Andrologia. 1998;30(S1):61–71.
76. Garolla A, Pizzol D, Bertoldo A, De Toni L, Barzon L, Foresta C. Association, prevalence, and clearance of human papillomavirus and antisperm antibodies in infected semen samples from infertile patients. Fertil Steril. 2013;99(1):125–31.
77. Joki-Korpela P, Sahrakorpi N, Halttunen M, Surcel H-M, Paavonen J, Tiitinen A. The role of Chlamydia trachomatis infection in male infertility. Fertil Steril. 2009;91(4):1448–50.
78. Dimitrova-Dikanarova DK, Lazarov VV, Tafradjiiska-Hadjiolova R, Dimova II, Petkova NU, Krastev ZA. Association between Helicobacter pylori infection and the presence of anti-sperm antibodies. Biotechnol Biotechnol Equip. 2016;31(1):1–8.
79. Wallach EE, Wolff H. The biologic significance of white blood cells in semen. Fertil Steril. 1995;63(6):1143–57.
80. Meares EM Jr. Serum antibody titers in treatment with trimethoprim-sulfamethoxazole for chronic prostatitis. Urology. 1978;11(2):142–6.
81. Keck C, Gerber-Schäfer C, Clad A, Wilhelm C, Breckwoldt M. Seminal tract infections: impact on male fertility and treatment options. Hum Reprod Update. 1998;4(6):891–903.
82. Rajah S, Parslow J, Howell R, Hendry W. The effects on in-vitro fertilization of autoantibodies to spermatozoa in subfertile men. Hum Reprod. 1993;8(7):1079–82.
83. Acosta AA, van der Merwe JP, Doncel G, Kruger TF, Sayilgan A, Franken DR, et al. Fertilization efficiency of morphologically abnormal spermatozoa in assisted reproduction is further impaired by antisperm antibodies on the male partner's sperm. Fertil Steril. 1994;62(4):826–33.
84. van Weert J-M, Repping S, Van Der Steeg JW, Steures P, Van Der Veen F, Mol BW. A prediction model for ongoing pregnancy after in vitro fertilization in couples with male subfertility. J Reprod Med. 2008;53(4):250–6.
85. Sukcharoen N, Keith J. The effect of the antisperm auto-antibody-bound sperm on in vitro fertilization outcome. Andrologia. 1995;27(5):281–9.
86. Culligan PJ, Crane MM, Boone WR, Allen TC, Price TM, Blauer KL. Validity and cost-effectiveness of antisperm antibody testing before in vitro fertilization. Fertil Steril. 1998;69(5):894–8.
87. Vujisić S, Lepej SŽ, Jerković L, Emedi I, Sokolić B. Antisperm antibodies in semen, sera and follicular fluids of infertile patients: relation to reproductive outcome after in vitro fertilization. Am J Reprod Immunol. 2005;54(1):13–20.
88. Nagy Z, Verheyen G, Liu J, Joris H, Janssenswillen C, Wisanto A, et al. Andrology: results of 55 intracytoplasmic sperm injection cycles in the treatment of male-immunological infertility. Hum Reprod. 1995;10(7):1775–80.
89. Clarke GN, Bourne H, Baker HG. Intracytoplasmic sperm injection for treating infertility associated with sperm autoimmunity. Fertil Steril. 1997;68(1):112–7.
90. Mercan R, Oehninger S, Muasher SJ, Toner JP, Mayer J, Lanzendorf SE. Impact of fertilization history and semen parameters on ICSI outcome. J Assist Reprod Genet. 1998;15(1):39–45.
91. Check M, Check J, Katsoff D, Summers-Chase D. ICSI as an effective therapy for male factor with antisperm antibodies. Arch Androl. 2000;45(3):125–30.
92. Esteves SC, Schneider DT, Verza S Jr. Influence of antisperm antibodies in the semen on intracytoplasmic sperm injection outcome. Int Braz J Urol. 2007;33:795–802.
93. Lahteenmaki A, Veilahti J, Hovatta O. Intra-uterine insemination versus cyclic, low-dose prednisolone in couples with male antisperm antibodies. Hum Reprod. 1995;10(1):142–7.
94. Ombelet W, Vandeput H, Janssen M, Cox A, Vossen C, Pollet H, et al. Treatment of male infertility due to sperm surface antibodies: IUI or IVF? Hum Reprod. 1997;12(6):1165–70.
95. Zini A, Fahmy N, Belzile E, Ciampi A, Al-Hathal N, Kotb A. Antisperm antibodies are not associated with pregnancy rates after IVF and ICSI: systematic review and meta-analysis. Hum Reprod. 2011;26(6):1288–95.

96. Zini A, Lefebvre J, Kornitzer G, Bissonnette F, Kadoch IJ, Dean N, et al. Anti-sperm antibody levels are not related to fertilization or pregnancy rates after IVF or IVF/ICSI. J Reprod Immunol. 2011;88(1):80–4.
97. Lu S-M, Li X, Wang S-L, Yang X-L, Xu Y-Z, Huang L-L, et al. Success rates of in vitro fertilization versus intracytoplasmic sperm injection in men with serum anti-sperm antibodies: a consecutive cohort study. Asian J Androl. 2019;21(5):473.
98. Schlegel PN, Sigman M, Collura B, De Jonge CJ, Eisenberg ML, Lamb DJ, et al. Diagnosis and treatment of infertility in men: AUA/ASRM guideline part I. J Urol. 2021;205(1):36–43.

Leukocytospermia and Bacteriospermia 9

Tuncay Toprak

Introduction

Male infertility may be idiopathic or caused by a variety of conditions, such as immunogenic deficiencies, genetic and anatomical conditions, inflammatory and infection issues. Male genital tract infections (MGTIs), that causes an aberrant rise in leukocyte counts in the human ejaculate, account for roughly 15% of cases of male infertility [1–3]. Bacteriospermia is identified when the ejaculate contains more bacteria than 1000 cfu/ml [4, 5]. It is frequently caused by acute or persistent bacterial infections, and it is recognized as a serious medical issue that reduces male fertility [4, 6]. Numerous parts of the male genitourinary system, including the prostate, epididymis, testis, and urethra, are susceptible to bacterial infections [4, 6]. *Escherichia coli*, *Chlamydia trachomatis*, *Ureaplasma urealyticum*, *Mycoplasma*, *Staphylococci*, *Streptococci*, and *Enterococcus faecalis* are the most frequently isolated pathogenic bacteria [4, 7]. Through sexual transmission, these microorganisms can enter the typically sterile GU tract with intracanalicular dissemination of infected urine, or hematogenous spread. These infections can cause local and systemic symptoms. There is evidence that infections of the testis [8], epididymis [9, 10], and prostate [11, 12] can have an adverse effect on spermatogenesis and reproductive potential.

The latest 6th edition of the WHO manual of human semen analysis included the assessment of leukocytes in semen among the "Extended tests of semen" that can be ordered under certain clinical situations [13]. The editors of the latest manual state that "there are currently no evidence-based reference ranges for peroxidase-positive cells in semen from fertile men." However, the manual retains the value of 1.0×10^6 peroxidase-positive cells per ml as a threshold value for clinical significance.

T. Toprak (✉)
Hamidiye Faculty of Medicine, Department of Urology, FSM Health Practice and Research Center, University of Health Sciences, Istanbul, Turkey

This chapter aims to investigate the relationship between bacteriospermia and leukocytospermia, their impact on male reproductive function and assisted reproductive techniques outcomes, the significance of leukocytospermia testing, the methodology of leukocytospermia testing, and the management of bacteriospermia/leukocytospermia.

Relationship of Bacteriospermia and Leukocytospermia

There is inconsistent information regarding the association of leukocytospermia with bacteriospermia, with some research showing a link between bacteriospermia and leukocytospermia [14, 15], while others have found no such link [16–18]. Leukocytospermia has been shown to have limited diagnostic significance in the identification of bacteriospermia, as shown by numerous earlier investigations [19, 20]. According to WHO guidelines, the sensitivity of detecting pathogenic microorganisms in semen with leukocytospermia is just 16–25% [19, 21]. Because, regardless of the presence of leukocytes, bacteriospermia, which is thought to be the result of contamination, can be observed at rates of up to 50% of semen samples [22]. When there are over a million leukocytes per milliliter of ejaculate, current guidelines suggest testing for bacteria in a semen sample. This strategy is based on the hypothesis that bacterial infections would result in an inflammatory reaction that would be easily recognized by an increase in the amount of leukocytes in semen [5] and it is widely acknowledged that leukocytospermia could be a sign of an infection or inflammation of the urogenital tract and male sex glands [2, 23].

Impact of Bacteriospermia on Male Reproductive Function

The study of the effects of bacteriospermia on male reproductive ability has captured scientific attention in recent decades due to the steadily growing number of infertile couples [24]. The relationship between bacteriospermia and seminal parameters has been confirmed through the investigation of several pathophysiologic mechanisms [25]. It is hypothesized that spermatogenesis and semen function are all affected by direct bacterial interaction and involvement of immune capable cells [25, 26]. However, the precise pathophysiologic effects of the various bacteria on semen parameters are still unknown, and the impact of bacteriospermia on semen quality is not entirely understood [25]. When analyzing the bacteriospermia literature, it is difficult to determine which organisms have a significant impact on male fertility potential because there are inconsistent definitions and sample collection techniques for culturing semen, probable contamination from urethral, meatal, and skin organisms, difficulty culturing all potential pathogens, and more [25]. Changes in semen detection methods significantly enhanced the yield of bacteriospermia, particularly when bacterial DNA is detected using polymerase chain reaction assay

[27]. These discrepancies account for the high variability in prevalence of bacteriospermia in the literature, which is reported in 10% to 85% of patients with male factor infertility [25, 28]. Even in the absence of a clinically obvious male accessory gland infection, bacteriospermia is frequently identified in semen samples from infertile men [28–30]. To limit the chance of contaminating the samples with commensal organisms from the skin, the WHO recommendations advise cleaning the hands and penis with soap [31].

The motility of sperm and the ability of sperm to interact with oocytes can be affected by bacterial cellular contacts, adhesion, and/or agglutination [25]. Bacteriospermia can affect sperm function, including the inducibility of the acrosome reaction [32]. Two mechanisms—direct or inflammatory-mediated intratesticular damages and/or post-testicular modifications in the form of excretory tract lesions, such as epididymitis—can both be used to explain the altered sperm viability. A study linked bacteriospermia to elevated DNA fragmentation index (DFI) and reported improvements in DFI following antibiotic administration [17, 33, 34]. There is disagreement about how bacteriospermia affects sperm metrics, DNA integrity, and ROS production in the sperm of subfertile and infertile men, and some research suggested that bacterial infection could not alter sperm parameters [7, 35]. Additionally, Domes et al. demonstrated that bacteria of any kind, such as *E. faecalis*, *E. coli*, group B *Streptococcus*, and *S. aureus*, could not alter the characteristics of semen [7]. It was shown that microorganisms in semen samples had no effect on sperm motility, morphology, or DNA integrity [7, 35]. In a review, it was reported that *Lactobacillus* appears to protect sperm quality, while *Enterococcus faecalis*, *Mycoplasma hominis*, *Ureaplasmaurealyticum*, and *Prevotella* negatively affect semen parameters [36].

Because of host defense, the presence of bacteria causes the migration of white blood cells to the inflammatory region. Later, the activated macrophages and neutrophils create reactive oxygen intermediates (ROI) that have an impact on the spermatozoa [20, 37]. It has been claimed that bacteria and their compounds encourage leukocytes to produce ROI [38]. Studies done to determine the importance of ROI in human semen showed that bacterially contaminated semen samples generated more ROI than uninfected semen samples [39, 40]. According to studies, the attack of free radicals on the sperm membrane reduces the fertility-processing ability of spermatozoa [41–43].

Impact of Leukocytospermia on Male Fertility Potential

Leukocytospermia, which results from bacteriospermia or any other reason, can impair male fertility through a variety of processes, including interference with spermatogenesis, deterioration of sperm function, and genital tract dysfunction [44]. It has been suggested that it serves as a sign of inflammation and genital tract infection. It is described in the WHO manual as having more than 1×10^6

peroxidase-positive leukocytes per milliliter of semen [31]. Leukocytospermia, which affects 10–20% of infertile males, is a poorly understood condition [20]. It can be caused by a variety of factors, including exposure to environmental pollutants, the use of certain drugs, alcohol usage, tobacco use, and vaginal products during sexual activity [45]. Finally, poor sperm viability and abnormal spermatogenesis can cause leukocytospermia because the seminal leukocytes scavenge the defective sperm [3]. The relevance of leukocytes in the semen and their relationship to semen quality is still hotly debated topics in scientific literature. Most experts agree that a rise in seminal leukocytes in ejaculated semen could be a sign of MGTI [2, 30]. However, some research have linked seminal leukocyte increase with degraded semen characteristics, including sperm morphology, motility, and viability, while some have found no negative impacts of leukocytospermia [46, 47]. Kaleli et al. [48] claimed that seminal leukocytes at concentrations between 1 and 3×10^6/ml would be advantageous for sperm function due to effects of scavenging of defective spermatozoa. According to Kiessling et al. [49] it was also reported that semen samples with leukocyte concentrations greater than 2×10^6 ml showed improved sperm motility. According to Lackner et al. [46], the effects of leukocytes on sperm motility and sperm morphology would depend on their concentration. However, a recent meta-analysis that examined 28 case-controlled retrospective studies found no link between leukocytospermia and low male fertilization potential in assisted reproductive programs or poor semen quality in asymptomatic men [50].

According to other researches, genital tract inflammation can reduce sperm function, worsen spermatogenesis, and obstruct the seminal duct in addition to affecting the quality of the semen [51]. In addition to releasing ROS, leukocytes also produce pro-inflammatory cytokines such as tumor necrosis factor-(TNF-), interleukin-1, interleukin-6, or interleukin-8, which triggers an inflammatory response [52], and that may cause the blood–testis barrier to weaken as well as the considerable development of sperm antibodies that can be seen in serum and seminal plasma [53]. Sperm antibodies in the semen may negatively impact sperm function, sperm motility, and the capacity to fertilize [53]. Through a variety of mechanisms, including direct cellular interactions, agglutinations, the release of reactive oxygen species (ROS) and cytokines, the presence of bacteria, and the recruitment of leukocytes in the male genital tract can affect male fertility. These mechanisms not only result in deteriorated spermatogenesis and genital tract dysfunction but also in deteriorated sperm function and integrity [7]. Since the sperm plasma membrane contains an exceptionally high number of poly unsaturated fatty acids [54] and is consequently particularly vulnerable to oxidative damage, ROS can result in lipid peroxidation of the membrane. A rise in sperm DNA fragmentation (SDF) has also been associated to ROS [55]. DNA-damaged spermatozoa can be discovered in any of these locations because oxidative damage can happen in the testis, epididymis, and ejaculate [56]. In addition, leukocytospermic men are more likely to have teratoasthenozoospermia and necrozoospermia than normospermic males [57].

Clinical Significance of Leukocytospermia

Despite the fact that the standard semen analysis described by the WHO [13, 58] includes a leukocyte assessment, there is no agreement on the best practices for its identification, clinical consequences, or therapeutic suggestions. Regarding the clinical importance of leukocytospermia, the EAU believes that it should be regarded as a marker of inflammation rather than a direct indication of bacterial or viral infection of the male genital tract. Clinically, spinal cord damage, smoking, MGTIs, and varicocele may all be linked to leukocytospermia [59]. Leukocytospermia by itself also is not a reliable indicator of a positive semen culture [5]and has limited diagnostic usefulness in identifying bacteriospermia and impaired semen quality [19]. Semen cultures and peroxidase testing together are a more effective clinical technique than the peroxidase test alone [60]. Therefore, using leukocytospermia alone is not sufficient to detect men at risk of semen infection.

In summary, the clinical importance of leukocytospermia and bacteriospermia remains the subject of ongoing debate and warrants future research.

Types of Round Cells

In addition to spermatozoa, other cells can be found in the ejaculate, some of which may be clinically significant. These include epithelial cells, as well as immature germ cells and leukocytes, the latter two collectively referred to as "round cells" [61]. However, by looking at a stained smear at a magnification of ×1000, it is not possible to identify leukocytes and immature germ cells with a high degree of accuracy [62]. A test for leukocytes is recommended if there are more than five round cells per high power field or if there are more than 1×10^6 round cells per mL of sample [59]. Round spermatids and spermatocytes are examples of germ cells; spermatogonia are comparatively uncommon. They can be seen in stained semen smears, albeit it might be challenging to tell them apart from inflammatory cells if the cells are degenerating. In some cases, spermatids and spermatocytes stained with the Papanicolaou method can be distinguished from leukocytes [61]. The color of the stain, the size and shape of the nuclei, the lack of intracellular peroxidase, and absence of leukocyte-specific antigens can all help with identification. Although morphologically similar to polymorphonuclear leukocytes, multinucleated spermatids stain a pinkish color as opposed to the more bluish polymorphonuclear leukocytes [61]. Round spermatids can be recognized using lectins, particular antibodies [63, 64], or stains tailored for the developing acrosome [65].

Methods for Identifying Seminal Leukocytes

Due to the presence of immature germ cells, which cannot be separated from leukocytes, direct counting of round cells in semen is quite incorrect. Leukocytes are difficult to distinguish from immature germ cells visually in semen specimens which have been prepared as wet mounts and examined by manual microscopy. So, confirmatory testing is needed. The peroxidase test, flow cytometry, immunohistochemical staining, and the detection of round cells are currently used to diagnose leukocytospermia [66, 67]. Wet mount microscopy supported by immunohistochemistry is advised by the American Society for Reproductive Medicine (ASRM) and the American Urological Association (AUA) for the diagnosis of leukocytes in a semen sample [68]. They suggest that this might point to an underlying genital tract infection, necessitating additional clinical assessment of this process. In the end, they do not believe that the measurement of leukocytes is necessary for the assessment of male infertility. Immunohistochemical staining with monoclonal antibodies directed against particular WBC subpopulations is the gold standard for evaluating WBCs in semen, but it is costly, time-consuming, and unstandardized [69]. On the other hand, wet mount microscopy verified by peroxidase positive staining is advised by the European Association of Urology (EAU) [70]. The peroxidase test is also advised by the WHO, despite the fact that it only identifies granulocytes and no other WBC sub-types [58].

The leukocyte population in semen can be quantified using a number of different methods. Routine assays of peroxidase activity are helpful as an initial screening tool because peroxidase-positive granulocytes are the most common kind of leukocyte in semen [20, 61]. However, in some cases it is insufficient. Methods for identifying leukocytes are listed below.

Peroxidase Tests

Due to the fact that it is simple to use and inexpensive, peroxidase tests for polymorphonuclear (PMN) leukocytes is frequently employed in clinical laboratories. However, it can only identify PMN granulocytes and not lymphocytes or monocytes. It allows for the separation of PMNs from other round cells and is based on the peroxidase activity in granulocytes. Peroxidase testing is advised by the EAU and WHO to confirm results from wet mount microscopy [70, 71].

Ortho-Toluidine Test

Peroxidase in granulocytes catalyzes the reaction of hydrogen peroxide and ortho-toluidine [71]. Peroxidase-positive cells, such as granulocytes, exhibit a brown staining while peroxidase-negative cells do not.

Endtz Test

The peroxidase approach was adapted by Endtz to distinguish PMN leukocytes from other round cells [72]. The Endtz test can also identify granulocytes that are peroxidase-positive neutrophils and macrophages [73]. In diagnostic andrology laboratories, the Endtz test is the most widely utilized test since it is easy, rapid, and reliable. The granulocytes' peroxidase oxidizes the benzidine derivative, which precipitates and takes on a brown color. This examination identifies granulocytes found in the semen. However, it is unable to distinguish non-peroxidase-rich WBCs.

Immunochemistry

Granulocytes, lymphocytes, and macrophages can all be detected simultaneously using monoclonal antibodies against the common leukocyte antigens CD45 or CD53 [74–76]. The most accurate method for diagnosing leukocytospermia is immunocytology, which is also known as the gold standard. However, it is inconvenient for daily use and relatively expensive when combined with a flow cytometer. Lack of standardization of the precise immunohistological staining method and the precise monoclonal antibodies to be utilized are significant limitations, and manual execution is time-consuming [2, 69, 77]. Immunohistochemistry is advised by both ASRM and AUA as a confirmatory diagnostic test for leukocytospermia [70].

Seminal Granulocyte Elastase Test

Elastase is a protease released by PMN leukocytes during the inflammation [78, 79]. In seminal plasma, it is assessed by immunoassay. An enzyme-linked immunosorbent test (ELISA) assessment of seminal granulocyte elastase enables differentiation between inflammatory and non-inflammatory processes. There is a significant link between leukocytes and elastase because PMN elastase is released during phagocytosis or granulocyte breakdown [80, 81]. It has been demonstrated that elastase concentrations are inversely correlated with sperm morphology, and motility [81]. Granulocyte elastase is also a trustworthy screening test for silent inflammation of the genital tract [82]. However, when employed as a sole measure to screen for subclinical infection or inflammation in males undergoing infertility investigation, the value of routinely determining PMN elastase in semen and/or serum samples is limited [83].

Is the Threshold of 1×10^6 WBC/ml Semen Reliable for Defining Leukocytospermia?

There is debate about whether the WHO's definition of leukocytospermia—more than 1×10^6 leukocytes per milliliter of semen—is a reliable cut-off point. Accordingly, peroxidase-positive cell counts that are higher than or similar to 1 ×

10^6 per ml are regarded as abnormal. Depending on the end-point being evaluated (semen quality, presence of bacteria, IVF results, sperm response to reactive oxygen species), some have found this figure to be too low [20] while others have found it to be too high [21, 84]. Recent research reveals that sperm function can be strongly impacted by the presence of WBCs and the effect of subsequent ROS formation at concentrations as low as 0.1×10^6 WBCs/mL [84, 85]. Other research studies have demonstrated that this crucial point exists at 0.2×10^6 [19, 21, 86] or even 0.5×10^6 WBCs/mL [87]. This shows that many study subjects may have been mischaracterized as leukocytospermia-negative by the criterion of one million, when in reality they may have had decreased fertility due to the presence of numerous WBCs. This would underestimate both the prevalence and the impact of leukocytospermia in comparison to people who are not affected. Additionally, based on these cut-off values, more patients would stand to gain from leukocytospermia evaluation and potential therapy. When predicting aberrant sperm morphology as a result of leukocytospermia, Menkveld and Kruger found that a revised definition of leukocytospermia of $>0.25 \times 10^6$ leukocytes/mL displayed the best sensitivity/specificity [86]. Punab and colleagues also found that a threshold of 0.2×10^6 leukocytes/mL had the best sensitivity and specificity for predicting bacteriospermia [21].

According to Barraud-Lange et al. [88], leukocytospermia appears to be physiologic at moderate levels ($<10^6$/mL). It did not affect the sperm's capacity to fertilize or the clinical pregnancy rates with assisted reproductive technology (ART). According to Wolff et al. [89], a cut-off value for leukocytes in semen in fertile men ranges from 1×10^6 to 2×10^6/ml, which suggests that the clinically significant level for leukocytospermia may be higher than 1×10^6/ml. According to Lackner et al., the role is quite differentiated, with lower concentrations than 0.5×10^6/ml having beneficial effects and greater concentrations having detrimental effects on sperm motility and morphology [46].

As a result, a new assessment of the leukocyte concentration threshold is required, as well as a precise classification of leukocytospermia as a marker of infectious or inflammation.

Management of Leukocytospermia in the Context of Male Infertility

Despite significant effort being invested into determining the optimal course of action for leukocytospermia, a clear approach to management has not been identified. Antibiotics, anti-inflammatory drugs, frequent ejaculation, and antioxidants have all been studied as potential treatments; however, the outcomes have been mixed, and there is still some debate. There is no universal consensus on how to treat leukocytospermia [66]. The current management strategy is on eradicating infection and safeguarding against ROS that are formed as a result of inflammation inside cellular mitochondria [2, 23]. According to the best available research, antibiotics and antioxidants are now the mainstay of treatment for leukocytospermia

[23]. In 2003, a meta-analysis of 12 trials revealed that treating patients with leukocytospermia with wide range antibiotics may enhance sperm motility, concentration, and morphology [90]. EAU recommendations state that although there is no evidence for pregnancy rates following antibiotic therapy of the male partner, antibiotics may improve the general quality of spermatozoa [70].

A systematic review by Jung et al. [66] showed that the present body of research on the efficacy of antibiotics was shown to be conflicting and frequently biased. The promise of antibiotic therapy, however, may be hinted in terms of better semen quality and leukocytospermia resolution. In another review of 11 studies, seven studies examined the use of antibiotics [91–97], one examined the use of antihistamines [98], one examined the use of steroids [99], and two examined the use of nonsteroidal anti-inflammatory drugs (NSAIDs) [57, 100]. Three of the antibiotic therapy comparison groups demonstrated a discernible increase in the rate at which leukocytospermia resolved compared to controls, three showed no discernible differences, and one did not explicitly assess leukocytospermia resolution. In terms of assessment methodology and preferred antibiotic therapy, these researches diverge. Treatment with antibiotics and frequent ejaculation, which was observed in two investigations, was the intervention that was significantly linked to resolution across studies [92, 93]. The length of treatment was another factor that was correlated with effective therapy. In three of the four studies where therapy lasted at least a full month, the resolution rate significantly increased. Four studies also assessed the qualitative and quantitative characteristics of semen parameters. Following antibiotic therapy, two of them displayed a considerable improvement in these measures [96, 97]. The pregnancy rate was compared between antibiotic therapy and control groups in three studies, with one demonstrating a substantial improvement within the treatment group. All three, however, discovered a greater pregnancy rate in the therapy groups, but they lacked the statistical power necessary due to their small sample sizes.

Semen culture may be beneficial for males with leukocytospermia and subclinical asymptomatic infections [30]. When the WBC is more than 1×10^6/mL in the ejaculate, the AUA and EAU recommendations advise doing a semen culture as this could be a sign of an active infection [101]. These suggestions are supported by the idea that bacterial infections might result in an inflammatory reaction, which is demonstrated by a rise in seminal leukocyte concentration [102]. A homogeneous large cohort of white European men presenting with primary infertility was shown to have a prevalence of leukocytospermia (25%) and positive semen culture (10%) [5]. Despite having negative effects on semen quality, leukocytospermia is not a reliable indicator of positive semen cultures [19]. The incidence of positive semen cultures has not been observed to differ between fertile and infertile men [102], and the clinical importance of positive semen cultures is unknown [102, 103]. Prostatic massage may be used to assess the expressed prostate secretion (EPS) in patients with suspected MGTI or those who had a positive semen culture. EPS' cytology is frequently diagnostic and is followed by EPS culture [104, 105].

A course of antibiotics should be given to infertile men who have leukocytospermia and a positive semen culture [106]. Infected semen or pyospermia ejaculates showed an increase in sperm concentration following antibiotic treatment [96]. Similar to this, Ahmadi et al. [107] demonstrated that antibiotic therapy increases sperm concentration in infected semen with *M. genitalium* infection. Leukocytospermia was statistically significantly resolved by antibiotics [91–93, 97, 108], while some investigations did not find a connection [94, 95, 109]. There is inconsistent evidence regarding whether these bacteria induce abnormal semen parameters in vivo and whether treatment improves semen parameters and reproductive potential. As a result, the evidence for employing empiric antibiotics in the clinical setting is debatable. Antibiotics have been also used with caution since animal studies have shown that they can stop spermatogenesis and affect other semen characteristics [110]. To avoid these consequences, care should be made to deliver the proper amount and length of antibiotic therapy.

Leukocytospermia has also been also treated with other medications. Antioxidants, for instance, have been utilized to enhance sperm quality and lower seminal leukocyte ROS generation [2, 23, 111]. Numerous in vitro studies have discovered that a number of antioxidants, including vitamin E, coenzyme Q10, and N-acetyl-L-cysteine, considerably lower ROS in human semen and may be able to improve sperm function [112–114]. Men with leukocytospermia and unexplained infertility were found to benefit from ketotifen, an antihistamine-like medication, in terms of improved sperm motility and morphology [98]. In asthenoteratozoospermic men with leukocytospermia, NSAIDs were also found to improve sperm concentration, motility, and morphology [57, 100]. When taken as a whole, these studies highlight the ongoing disagreement about how to assess and treat leukocytospermia.

In conclusion, it is unclear if leukocytospermia has to be treated or not and the effects of each treatment. In infertile men with leukocytospermia, consistent guidelines for the use of antibiotics and antioxidants should be developed.

Follow-Up of Leukocytospermia Cases

Although a leukocyte assessment is a regular component of semen analysis, there is no agreement on the standards for its diagnosis, clinical implications, or suggested treatments [70]. Combining antibiotic therapy with frequent ejaculation for a minimum of 1 month seems to be the only regimen that has consistently demonstrated a significant improvement in result. To extend the course of antibiotic medication, combine it with frequent ejaculation, and perhaps decrease the leukocytospermia threshold, research-focused studies are required.

A significant concentration of leukocytes in the semen can be caused by varicocele [70]. In comparison to fertile men, subfertile men and men with varicocele have a higher proportion of semen lymphocytes [70]. Despite the fact that the Endtz test only counts granulocytes, flow cytometry measurements have revealed that the varicocele group has considerably more CD4+ helper T-lymphocytes than the control group [115]. This could explain why, despite having normal sperm concentrations, people with varicocele have elevated cytokine levels in the seminal fluid.

In the presence of a pathogen verified following semen culture or PCR testing and antibiotic treatment, what is the optimal timing to re-test and verify whether the antibiotic treatment has cleared the infection? Should we repeat the culture to confirm absence of pathogen? Should we treat by NSAIDs, antibiotics, both?

There is no clear recommendation in the literature on this issue. In a study comparing 102 men with leukocytospermia, Branigan et al. [92] divided the patients into four groups (1) no treatment group, (2) antibiotic treatment alone group, (3) frequent ejaculation alone group, and (4) antibiotic treatment with frequent ejaculation group and examined the resolution of leukocytospermia. They found that significant resolution of leukocytospermia occurred in all treatment groups at 1 month compared with no treatment group, and persisted at months 2 and 3 only in those who received antibiotics and frequently ejaculated. In this context, it can be said that antibiotic treatment, frequent ejaculation and frequent ejaculation and antibiotic treatment treat leukocytospermia immediately after the treatment phase, and only frequent ejaculation with antibiotic treatment is effective until 3 months after the treatment.

In this context, if the patient has only received antibiotic treatment, it may be appropriate to come to the control visit 1 month later and if we made additional recommendations such as frequent ejaculation with antibiotic treatment, it may be appropriate to come to the control visit at the third month unless the patient has any additional complaints. At the control visit, a repeat culture test can be done to understand the eradication of the bacteria, but there is not enough evidence on this subject.

Additional treatments such as antioxidants and NSAIDs may increase the response to the treatment, but there is no evidence yet to offer sufficient advice in this regard.

According to Branigan and Muller [92], frequent ejaculation with antibiotics (at least every 3 days) was more effective than antibiotics alone.

Role of Assisted Reproductive Techniques in the Treatment of Infertile Men with Leukocytospermia

In the context of ART, there are no guidelines for the treatment of leukocytospermia [70]. Some studies demonstrated that high leukocytes counts in semen may affect the outcomes of IVF and ICSI [116, 117]. However, Barraud-Lange [88] hypothesized that seminal leukocytes act as "good Samaritans" for spermatozoa and that high leukocyte concentrations (more than 1×10^6 leukocytes/ml) are related with a higher clinical pregnancy rate. Other studies also reported that the role of leukocytospermia in ART outcomes is uncertain [50, 118, 119]. Leukocytospermic and non-leukocytospermic groups were shown to have similar success rates with ICSI and IVF, according to some studies [34]. Therefore, this might suggest that an antibiotic therapy trial is not required in the context of ART. This can be the result of semen processing carried out before the sample was used. However, many fertility clinics continue to administer brief antibiotic regimens to male sperm donors who have leukocytospermia. According to some studies, therapy is only advised for people who have leukocytospermia and a positive semen culture [66, 102].

Based on studies showing the negative effect of leukocytospermia on ART outcomes [70], WBCs from semen may be removed before sperm is frozen or used in ART operations. There are numerous techniques for eliminating WBCs from semen.

Swim-Up

Swim-up from a washed pellet is the most traditional technique [120]. This method has the advantage of producing a specimen with a very high proportion of motile sperm, a higher proportion of sperm with good morphology and a markedly lower proportion of nonsperm cells, like WBCs.

Glass Wool Filtration

Glass wool filtration can also be used to separate WBCs from semen. Using tightly packed glass wool fibers, this technique separates motile sperm cells from nonsperm cells, such as WBCs [121]. This technique has the advantages of separating sperm from ejaculates with extremely low sperm concentrations and significantly lowering leukocyte and ROS levels. The drawbacks include higher cost compared to swim-up procedure, unclean filtrate, and the presence of debris remains [120].

Mechanical Filtration

Leukocytospermic samples can also be mechanically filtered to separate sperm cells using physical filters like micropore filters. But, the filters easily clog as a result of the large number of WBCs and potential tissues in the sample [122].

Density Gradient Centrifugation

Another technique for isolating WBCs from semen is density gradient centrifugation. It involves centrifugally filtering sperm cells through one or more layers of progressively more concentrated silane-coated silica particles. Highly mobile sperm cells actively travel in the direction of the sedimentation gradient using this technique, and as a result, they are more abundant in the soft pellet at the bottom [120].

This method has the benefit of isolating sperm from ejaculates with extremely low sperm concentrations, significantly lowering WBCs, and significantly lowering ROS. The drawbacks of this method include the fact that it requires more time and expensive than the swim-up method [120].

Microfluidics

Sperm cells may be separated from other cells and cellular waste using microfluidics. With this technique, sperm cells and WBCs are separated using inertial microfluidic technology by being routed into various channels within a spiral chamber. This method allows for the recovery of viable less-motile and non-motile sperm cells in addition to motile sperm while simultaneously lowering the level of WBCs [123].

The final approach for separating WBCs from semen will rely on the tools available in the lab and the general properties of the semen samples. It is recommended to choose spermatozoa with a high degree of motility because this can improve recovery [124].

Impact of Leukocytospermia on ART Outcome

One of the causes of male infertility is leukocytospermia, and there is debate regarding how it may affect the clinical results of ART [50, 116, 119]. Leukocytospermia has been shown to inhibit spermatozoa's ability to fertilize by interfering with the acrosome response and the fusion of sperm and egg [84, 125]. Because of this, having WBCs in seminal plasma is regarded as a significant prognostic factor for unsuccessful IVF and embryo transfer [20]. High amounts of ROS and interferon are produced by leukocytes in seminal fluid, which can impair sperm function and reduce the success rate of IVF [126]. Leukocytes have reportedly been shown to have a deleterious impact on fertilization in IVF cycles [117, 125].

However, a meta-analysis that examined the effects of leukocytospermia in males visiting a reproductive clinic found no links between the disorder and altered semen quality or decreased fertility after ART [50]. Leukocytospermia has been proven in another study to have no effect on the success of IVF or ICSI when leukocyte detection was done using flow cytometry [119]. Leukocytes are removed during sperm preparation, according to some articles, hence leukocytospermia has no effect on the clinical outcomes of IVF or ICSI, nor do various insemination techniques have an impact on the rates of fertilization, clinical pregnancy, or live births [127]. It is unclear if this undifferentiated change is a result of semen optimization, changing semen requirements for ART, or the embryologist's selection of insemination techniques that have improved clinical outcomes. Nevertheless, it is well acknowledged that oxidative stress likely plays a significant role in regulating human sperm function and pregnancy outcomes [128] and many fertility facilities still administer brief antibiotic regimens to male sperm donors who have known leukocytospermia.

Decisional Tree/Clinical Guide for Non-ART and ART Management of Leukocytospermia is presented in Figs. 9.1 and 9.2, Respectively

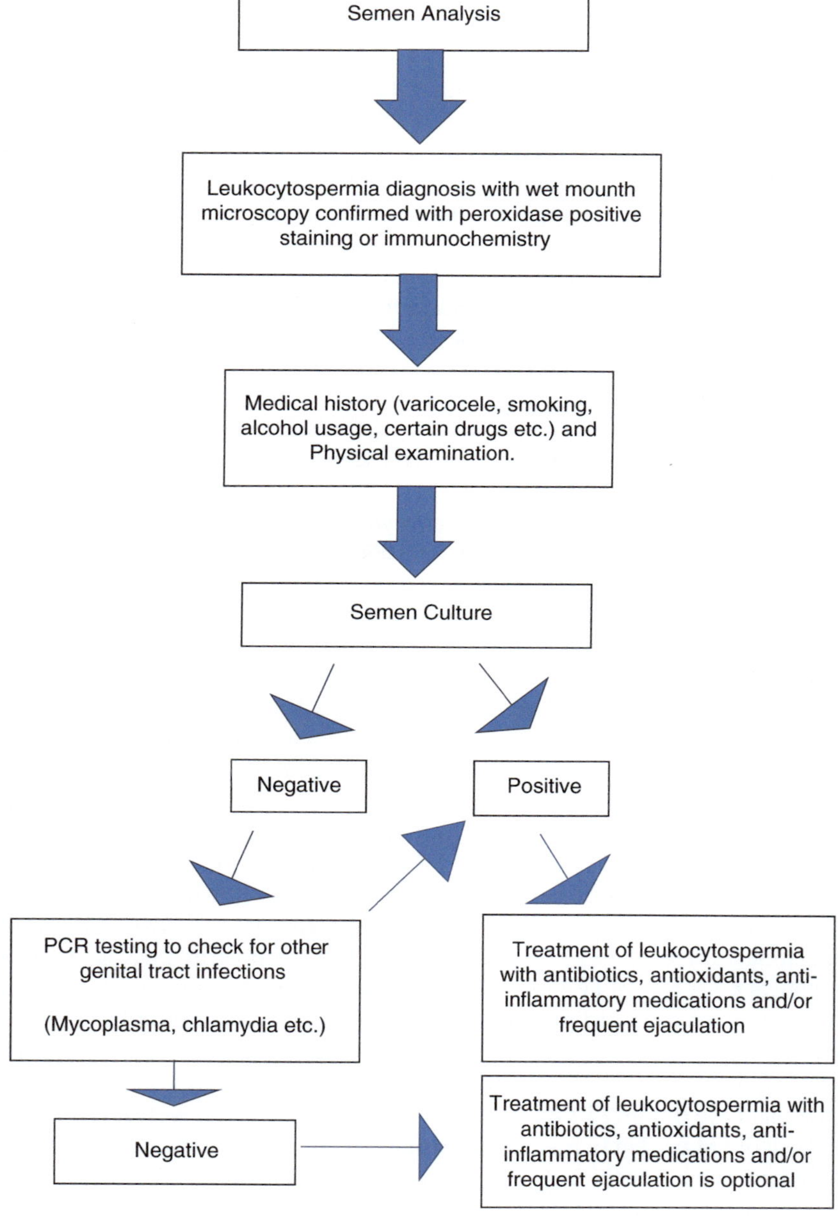

Fig. 9.1 Algorithm for non-ART management of leukocytospermia in infertile men

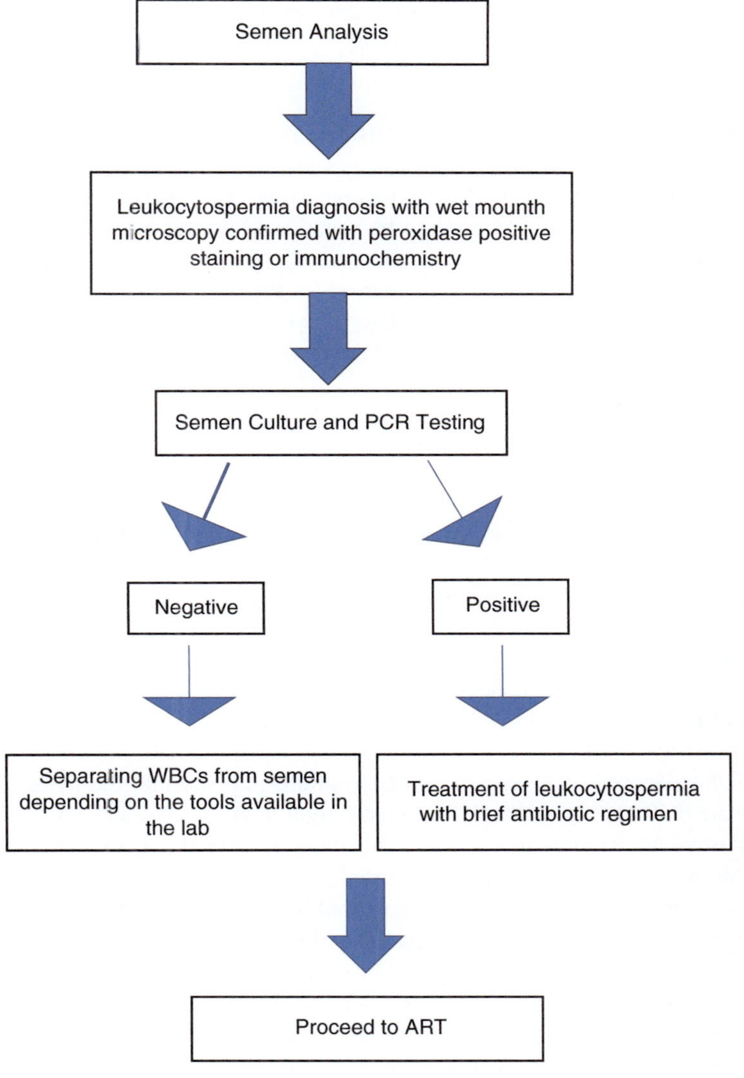

Fig. 9.2 Algorithm for ART management of leukocytospermia in infertile men

Clinical Scenarios

Clinical Scenario 1

A semen analysis and a semen culture are performed on a patient who is being assessed for infertility. Despite the report indicating a positive semen culture, the semen analysis is negative for leukocytospermia. The patient has no clinical complaints. How do you manage this situation?

Solution
To avoid bacterial contamination, the WHO guidelines suggest using good cleanliness measures and urinating before giving a semen sample. It has been observed that when semen was collected with the correct aseptic procedures, false positive semen cultures results will turn out to be negative. However, skin flora contamination can be seen again. In this case, although the effect of bacteriospermia on clinical and pregnancy is controversial, there is a report stating that asymptomatic bacteriospermia has no effect on pregnancy rate [102]. However, if bacteriospermia is accompanied by leukocytospermia, treatment seems to be a more reasonable option.

Clinical Scenario 2

An examination of a patient's semen reveals the following: Sperm concentration of 9×10^6/mL, total motility of 28%, Endtz test value of 6×10^6 WBCs/mL, and negative semen culture. How do you manage this situation?

Solution
This is a case of oligoasthenozoospermia and leukocytospermia. Obtain general medical history (varicocele, smoking, alcohol usage, certain drugs, etc.) and perform physical examination.

Leukocytospermia and negative semen culture indicate that the patient should have urine PCR testing to check for other genital tract infections (i.e., ureaplasma, mycoplasma, and chlamydia). The patient should receive the recommended course of antibiotics if the culture of a semen sample taken avoided any external bacterial contamination [102]. Leukocytospermia could be a sign of a male sex gland infection or inflammation [2, 23]. Leukocytospermia has been treated with broad-spectrum antibiotics that have good prostate penetration [90]. Patients with leukocytospermia have also utilized antioxidants that can lessen ROS produced by semen leukocytes [70, 92]. Nevertheless, there is no agreement on the outcome of each treatment or whether leukocytospermia requires treatment or not. A recent review found that antibiotics may enhance semen parameters, the bacteriologic cure rate, resolution of leukocytospermia, and the pregnancy rate despite some conflicting results [66]. Antibiotics and antioxidants for the treatment of infertile males with leukocytospermia may be effective, but the data are insufficient to draw that conclusion [66].

Take Home Message

- Bacteriospermia and leucocytospermia can negatively affect male fertility.
- The clinical significance of leukocytospermia and bacteriospermia remains a matter of ongoing debate.

- WHO defines leukocytospermia as more than 1×10^6 leukocytes per milliliter of semen. However, some evidence argues that it should be above and below this value.
- Leukocytes and immature germ cells are similar to each other and if there are more than 1×10^6 round cells/mL of sample a test for identification of leukocytes is recommended.
- The peroxidase test, flow cytometry, immunohistochemical staining, and the detection of round cells are currently used to diagnose leukocytospermia.
- Although it is unclear if leukocytospermia needs to be treated, and what is the effects of each treatment, antibiotics and antioxidants are the mainstay of treatment for leukocytospermia.
- The effect of leukocytospermia on ART outcome is not fully known.

References

1. Pellati D, et al. Genital tract infections and infertility. Eur J Obstet Gynecol Reprod Biol. 2008;140(1):3–11.
2. Sandoval JS, Raburn D, Muasher S. Leukocytospermia: overview of diagnosis, implications, and management of a controversial finding. Middle East Fertil Soc J. 2013;18(3):129–34.
3. Barratt C, Bolton A, Cooke I. Functional significance of white blood cells in the male and female reproductive tract. Hum Reprod. 1990;5(6):639–48.
4. Rusz A, et al. Influence of urogenital infections and inflammation on semen quality and male fertility. World J Urol. 2012;30(1):23–30.
5. Ventimiglia E, et al. Leukocytospermia is not an informative predictor of positive semen culture in infertile men: results from a validation study of available guidelines. Hum Reprod Open. 2020;2020:39.
6. Diemer T, et al. Urogenital infection and sperm motility. Andrologia. 2003;35(5):283–7.
7. Domes T, et al. The incidence and effect of bacteriospermia and elevated seminal leukocytes on semen parameters. Fertil Steril. 2012;97(5):1050–5.
8. Andrada J, Von der Walde F, Andrada EC. Immunologic studies of male infertility. Immunol Ser. 1990;52:345–78.
9. Weidner W, et al. Initial therapy of acute unilateral epididymitis using ofloxacin. I. Clinical and microbiological findings. Der Urologe Ausg A. 1990;29(5):272–6.
10. Ludwig G, Haselberger J. Epididymitis and fertility. Treatment results in acute unspecific epididymitis. Fortsch Med. 1977;95(7):397–9.
11. Giamarellou H, et al. Infertility and chronic prostatitis. Andrologia. 1984;16(5):417–22.
12. Henkel R, et al. Chronic pelvic pain syndrome/chronic prostatitis affect the acrosome reaction in human spermatozoa. World J Urol. 2006;24(1):39–44.
13. World Health Organization. WHO laboratory manual for the examination and processing of human semen. 6th ed. Geneva: WHO Press; 2021.
14. Zeyad A, et al. Relationships between bacteriospermia, DNA integrity, nuclear protamine alteration, sperm quality and ICSI outcome. Reprod Biol. 2018;18(1):115–21.
15. Monteiro C, et al. Characterization of microbiota in male infertility cases uncovers differences in seminal hyperviscosity and oligoasthenoteratozoospermia possibly correlated with increased prevalence of infectious bacteria. Am J Reprod Immunol. 2018;79(6):e12838.
16. Fraczek M, et al. In vitro reconstruction of inflammatory reaction in human semen: effect on sperm DNA fragmentation. J Reprod Immunol. 2013;100(1):76–85.
17. Rybar R, et al. The effect of bacterial contamination of semen on sperm chromatin integrity and standard semen parameters in men from infertile couples. Andrologia. 2012;44:410–8.

18. Nasrallah YS, et al. Microbiological profiles of semen culture in male infertility. Hum Androl. 2018;8(2):34–42.

19. Lackner J, et al. Value of counting white blood cells (WBC) in semen samples to predict the presence of bacteria. Eur Urol. 2006;49(1):148–53.

20. Wallach EE, Wolff H. The biologic significance of white blood cells in semen. Fertil Steril. 1995;63(6):1143–57.

21. Punab M, et al. The limit of leucocytospermia from the microbiological viewpoint. Andrologia. 2003;35(5):271–8.

22. Cottell E, et al. Are seminal fluid microorganisms of significance or merely contaminants? Fertil Steril. 2000;74(3):465–70.

23. Pentyala S, et al. Current perspectives on pyospermia: a review. Asian J Androl. 2007;9(5):593–600.

24. Lee HS, et al. Serum and seminal plasma insulin-like growth factor-1 in male infertility. Clin Exp Reprod Med. 2016;43(2):97.

25. Keck C, et al. Seminal tract infections: impact on male fertility and treatment options. Hum Reprod Update. 1998;4(6):891–903.

26. Dieterle S. Urogenital infections in reproductive medicine. Andrologia. 2008;40(2):117–9.

27. Jarvi K, et al. Polymerase chain reaction-based detection of bacteria in semen. Fertil Steril. 1996;66(3):463–7.

28. Fowler JE Jr. Infections of the male reproductive tract and infertility: a selected review. J Androl. 1981;2(3):121–31.

29. Busolo F, et al. Microbial flora in semen of asymptomatic infertile men. Andrologia. 1984;16(3):269–75.

30. Esfandiari N, et al. Positive bacterial culture of semen from infertile men with asymptomatic leukocytospermia. Int J Fertil Womens Med. 2002;47(6):265–70.

31. WHO. WHO laboratory manual for the examination and processing of human semen. Geneva: WHO; 2010.

32. Köhn FM, et al. Influence of urogenital infections on sperm functions. Andrologia. 1998;30(S1):73–80.

33. Moskovtsev SI, et al. Cause-specific treatment in patients with high sperm DNA damage resulted in significant DNA improvement. Syst Biol Reprod Med. 2009;55(2-3):109–15.

34. Zeyad A, Hamad M, Hammadeh M. The effects of bacterial infection on human sperm nuclear protamine P1/P2 ratio and DNA integrity. Andrologia. 2018;50(2):e12841.

35. Hou D, et al. Microbiota of the seminal fluid from healthy and infertile men. Fertil Steril. 2013;100(5):1261–9. e3

36. Farahani L, et al. The semen microbiome and its impact on sperm function and male fertility: a systematic review and meta-analysis. Andrology. 2021;9(1):115–44.

37. Aitken J, Fisher H. Reactive oxygen species generation and human spermatozoa: the balance of benefit and risk. Bioessays. 1994;16(4):259–67.

38. Wang A, et al. Generation of reactive oxygen species by leukocytes and sperm following exposure to urogenital tract infection. Arch Androl. 1997;39(1):11–7.

39. Mazzilli F, et al. Superoxide anion in human semen related to seminal parameters and clinical aspects. Fertil Steril. 1994;62(4):862–8.

40. Vicari E. Seminal leukocyte concentration and related specific reactive oxygen species production in patients with male accessory gland infections. Hum Reprod. 1999;14(8):2025–30.

41. Alvarez JG, et al. Spontaneous lipid peroxidation and production of hydrogen peroxide and superoxide in human spermatozoa Superoxide dismutase as major enzyme protectant against oxygen toxicity. J Androl. 1987;8(5):338–48.

42. Aitken R, Harkiss D, Buckingham D. Relationship between iron-catalysed lipid peroxidation potential and human sperm function. Reproduction. 1993;98(1):257–65.

43. Fraczek M, et al. Peroxidation components of sperm lipid membranes in male infertility. Ginekol Pol. 2001;72(2):73–9.

44. Esmailkhani A, et al. Assessing the prevalence of Staphylococcus aureus in infertile male patients in Tabriz, northwest Iran. Int J Reprod BioMed. 2018;16(7):469.

45. Vickers NJ. Animal communication: when i'm calling you, will you answer too? Curr Biol. 2017;27(14):R713–5.
46. Lackner JE, et al. The association between leukocytes and sperm quality is concentration dependent. Reprod Biol Endocrinol. 2010;8(1):1–6.
47. Aziz N, et al. Novel associations between specific sperm morphological defects and leukocytospermia. Fertil Steril. 2004;82(3):621–7.
48. Kaleli S, et al. Does leukocytospermia associate with poor semen parameters and sperm functions in male infertility? The role of different seminal leukocyte concentrations. Eur J Obstet Gynecol Reprod Biol. 2000;89(2):185–91.
49. Kiessling AA, et al. Semen leukocytes: friends or foes? Fertil Steril. 1995;64(1):196–8.
50. Castellini C, et al. Relationship between leukocytospermia, reproductive potential after assisted reproductive technology, and sperm parameters: a systematic review and meta-analysis of case–control studies. Andrology. 2020;8(1):125–35.
51. Azenabor A, Ekun AO, Akinloye O. Impact of inflammation on male reproductive tract. J Reprod Infertil. 2015;16(3):123.
52. Haidl F, et al. Seminal parameters of chronic male genital inflammation are associated with disturbed sperm DNA integrity. Andrologia. 2015;47(4):464–9.
53. Fijak M, et al. Infectious, inflammatory and 'autoimmune' male factor infertility: how do rodent models inform clinical practice? Hum Reprod Update. 2018;24(4):416–41.
54. Parks JE, Lynch DV. Lipid composition and thermotropic phase behavior of boar, bull, stallion, and rooster sperm membranes. Cryobiology. 1992;29(2):255–66.
55. Alahmar AT. Role of oxidative stress in male infertility: an updated review. J Hum Reprod Sci. 2019;12(1):4.
56. González-Marín C, Gosálvez J, Roy R. Types, causes, detection and repair of DNA fragmentation in animal and human sperm cells. Int J Mol Sci. 2012;13(11):14026–52.
57. Gambera L, et al. Sperm quality and pregnancy rate after COX-2 inhibitor therapy of infertile males with abacterial leukocytospermia. Hum Reprod. 2007;22(4):1047–51.
58. WHO. WHO laboratory manual for the examination and processing of human semen. Geneva: World Health Organization; 2010.
59. Sharma R, et al. Relevance of leukocytospermia and semen culture and its true place in diagnosing and treating male infertility. World J Mens Health. 2022;40(2):191.
60. Cumming JA, Carrell DT. Utility of reflexive semen cultures for detecting bacterial infections in patients with infertility and leukocytospermia. Fertil Steril. 2009;91(4):1486–8.
61. Johanisson E, et al. Evaluation of round cells' in semen analysis: a comparative study. Hum Reprod Update. 2000;6(4):404–12.
62. Freund M. Standards for the rating of human sperm morphology. A cooperative study. Int J Fertil. 1966;11(1):97–180.
63. Ezeh U, et al. Correlation of testicular pathology and sperm extraction in azoospermic men with ejaculated spermatids detected by immunofluorescent localization. Hum Reprod. 1998;13(11):3061–5.
64. Homyk M, et al. Differential diagnosis of immature germ cells in semen utilizing monoclonal antibody MHS-10 to the intra-acrosomal antigen SP-10. Fertil Steril. 1990;53(2):323–30.
65. Couture M, et al. Improved staining method for differentiating immature germ cells from white blood cells in human seminal fluid. Andrologia. 1976;8(1):61–6.
66. Jung JH, et al. Treatment of leukocytospermia in male infertility: a systematic review. World J Men's Health. 2016;34(3):165–72.
67. Lemkecher T, et al. Leucocytospermia, oxidative stress and male fertility: facts and hypotheses. Gynecol Obstet Fertil. 2005;33(1-2):2–10.
68. Jarow J, et al. The optimal evaluation of the infertile male: AUA best practice statement. AUA Best Pract Statement. 2011;39:11.
69. Ricci G, et al. Leukocyte detection in human semen using flow cytometry. Hum Reprod. 2000;15(6):1329–37.
70. Brunner RJ, Demeter JH, Sindhwani P. Review of guidelines for the evaluation and treatment of leukocytospermia in male infertility. World J Men's Health. 2019;37(2):128–37.

71. Esteves SC. Clinical relevance of routine semen analysis and controversies surrounding the 2010 World Health Organization criteria for semen examination. Int Braz J Urol. 2014;40:433–53.

72. Endtz A. A rapid staining method for differentiating granulocytes from "germinal cells" in Papanicolaou-stained semen. Acta Cytol. 1974;18(1):2–7.

73. Endtz A. A direct staining method for moist urinary sediment and moist human sperm. Ned Tijdschr Geneeskd. 1972;116(17):681–5.

74. Wolff H, Anderson DJ. Immunohistologic characterization and quantitation of leukocyte subpopulations in human semen. Fertil Steril. 1988;49(3):497–504.

75. Eggert-Kruse W, et al. Differentiation of round cells in semen by means of monoclonal antibodies and relationship with male fertility. Fertil Steril. 1992;58(5):1046–55.

76. Schöbel W, Schieferstein G, Uchanska-Ziegler B. Immunocytochemical characterization of round cells in human semen using monoclonal antibodies and the APAAP-technique. Andrologia. 1989;21(4):370–6.

77. Khodamoradi K, et al. Laboratory and clinical management of leukocytospermia and hematospermia: a review. Therap Adv Reprod Health. 2020;14:2633494120922511.

78. Fritz H, et al. Granulocyte proteinases as mediators of unspecific proteolysis in inflammation: a review. Folia Histochem Cytobiol. 1986;24(2):99–115.

79. Jochum M, Pabst W, Schill WB. Granulocyte elastase as a sensitive diagnostic parameter of silent male genital tract inflammation. Andrologia. 1986;18(4):413–9.

80. Zorn B, et al. Semen polymorphonuclear neutrophil leukocyte elastase as a diagnostic and prognostic marker of genital tract inflammation–a review. Clin Chem Lab Med. 2003;41(1):2–12.

81. Kopa Z, et al. Role of granulocyte elastase and interleukin-6 in the diagnosis of male genital tract inflammation. Andrologia. 2005;37(5):188–94.

82. Zorn B, Virant-Klun I, Meden-Vrtovec H. Semen granulocyte elastase: its relevance for the diagnosis and prognosis of silent genital tract inflammation. Hum Reprod. 2000;15(9):1978–84.

83. Eggert-Kruse W, et al. Clinical relevance of polymorphonuclear (PMN-) elastase determination in semen and serum during infertility investigation. Int J Androl. 2009;32(4):317–29.

84. Sharma RK, et al. Relationship between seminal white blood cell counts and oxidative stress in men treated at an infertility clinic. J Androl. 2001;22(4):575–83.

85. Henkel R, et al. Effect of reactive oxygen species produced by spermatozoa and leukocytes on sperm functions in non-leukocytospermic patients. Fertil Steril. 2005;83(3):635–42.

86. Menkveld R, Kruger T. Sperm morphology and male urogenital infections. Andrologia. 1998;30(S1):49–53.

87. Thomas J, et al. Increased polymorphonuclear granulocytes in seminal plasma in relation to sperm morphology. Hum Reprod. 1997;12(11):2418–21.

88. Barraud-Lange V, et al. Seminal leukocytes are Good Samaritans for spermatozoa. Fertil Steril. 2011;96(6):1315–9.

89. Wolff H, et al. Impact of clinically silent inflammation on male genital tract organs as reflected by biochemical markers in semen. J Androl. 1991;12(5):331–4.

90. Skau PA, Folstad I. Do bacterial infections cause reduced ejaculate quality? A meta-analysis of antibiotic treatment of male infertility. Behav Ecol. 2003;14(1):40–7.

91. Comhaire F, Rowe P, Farley T. The effect of doxycycline in infertile couples with male accessory gland infection: a double blind prospective study. Int J Androl. 1986;9(2):91–8.

92. Branigan EF, Muller CH. Efficacy of treatment and recurrence rate of leukocytospermia in infertile men with prostatitis. Fertil Steril. 1994;62(3):580–4.

93. Yamamoto M, et al. Antibiotic and ejaculation treatments improve resolution rate of leukocytospermia in infertile men with prostatitis. Nagoya J Med Sci. 1995;58(1-2):41–5.

94. Yanushpolsky EH, et al. Antibiotic therapy and leukocytospermia: a prospective, randomized, controlled study. Fertil Steril. 1995;63(1):142–7.

95. Erel C, et al. Antibiotic therapy in men with leukocytospermia. Int J Fertil Womens Med. 1997;42(3):206–10.

96. Pajovic B, et al. Semen analysis before and after antibiotic treatment of asymptomatic chlamydia-and ureaplasma-related pyospermia. Andrologia. 2013;45(4):266–71.
97. Vicari E. Effectiveness and limits of antimicrobial treatment on seminal leukocyte concentration and related reactive oxygen species production in patients with male accessory gland infection. Hum Reprod. 2000;15(12):2536–44.
98. Oliva A, Multigner L. Ketotifen improves sperm motility and sperm morphology in male patients with leukocytospermia and unexplained infertility. Fertil Steril. 2006;85(1):240–3.
99. Milardi D, et al. Prednisone treatment in infertile patients with oligozoospermia and accessory gland inflammatory alterations. Andrology. 2017;5(2):268–73.
100. Lackner JE, et al. Correlation of leukocytospermia with clinical infection and the positive effect of antiinflammatory treatment on semen quality. Fertil Steril. 2006;86(3):601–5.
101. Jungwirth A, et al. Guidelines on male infertility. Arnhem: European Association of Urology; 2019.
102. Jue JS, Ramasamy R. Significance of positive semen culture in relation to male infertility and the assisted reproductive technology process. Transl Androl Urol. 2017;6(5):916.
103. Moretti E, et al. The presence of bacteria species in semen and sperm quality. J Assist Reprod Genet. 2009;26(1):47–56.
104. Meares EM. Bacterial prostatitis vs prostatosis: a clinical and bacteriological study. JAMA. 1973;224(10):1372–5.
105. Colpi G, et al. Anaerobic and aerobic bacteria in secretions of prostate and seminal vesicles of infertile men. Arch Androl. 1982;9(2):175–81.
106. Schlegel PN, et al. Diagnosis and treatment of infertility in men: AUA/ASRM guideline part I. J Urol. 2021;205(1):36–43.
107. Ahmadi MH, et al. Improvement of semen parameters after antibiotic therapy in asymptomatic infertile men infected with Mycoplasma genitalium. Infection. 2018;46(1):31–8.
108. Lewis-Jones D, et al. Antibiotic treatment of leucospermia in subfertile males. Arch STD/HIV Res. 1996;10:65–72.
109. Krisp A, et al. Treatment with levofloxacin does not resolve asymptomatic leucocytospermia–a randomized controlled study. Andrologia. 2003;35(4):244–7.
110. Schlegel PN, Chang T, Marshall FF. Antibiotics: potential hazards to male fertility. Fertil Steril. 1991;55(2):235–42.
111. Agarwal A, Sekhon LH. The role of antioxidant therapy in the treatment of male infertility. Hum Fertil. 2010;13(4):217–25.
112. Aitken RJ, Clarkson JS. Significance of reactive oxygen species and antioxidants in defining the efficacy of sperm preparation techniques. J Androl. 1988;9(6):367–76.
113. Lewin A, Lavon H. The effect of coenzyme Q10 on sperm motility and function. Mol Asp Med. 1997;18:213–9.
114. Oeda T, et al. Scavenging effect of N-acetyl-L-cysteine against reactive oxygen species in human semen: a possible therapeutic modality for male factor infertility? Andrologia. 1997;29(3):125–31.
115. Mongioì LM, et al. Evaluation of seminal fluid leukocyte subpopulations in patients with varicocele. Int J Immunopathol Pharmacol. 2020;34:2058738420925719.
116. Yilmaz S, et al. Effects of leucocytospermia on semen parameters and outcomes of intracytoplasmic sperm injection. Int J Androl. 2005;28(6):337–42.
117. Lackner JE, et al. Effect of leukocytospermia on fertilization and pregnancy rates of artificial reproductive technologies. Fertil Steril. 2008;90(3):869–71.
118. Cavagna M, et al. The influence of leukocytospermia on the outcomes of assisted reproductive technology. Reprod Biol Endocrinol. 2012;10(1):1–10.
119. Ricci G, et al. Effect of seminal leukocytes on in vitro fertilization and intracytoplasmic sperm injection outcomes. Fertil Steril. 2015;104(1):87–93.
120. Henkel RR, Schill W-B. Sperm preparation for ART. Reprod Biol Endocrinol. 2003;1(1):1–22.
121. Sánchez R, et al. Glass wool filtration reduces reactive oxygen species by elimination of leukocytes in oligozoospermic patients with leukocytospermia. J Assist Reprod Genet. 1996;13(6):489–94.

122. Nash G, et al. Effects of preparative procedures and of cell activation on flow of white cells through micropore filters. Br J Haematol. 1988;70(2):171–6.
123. Son J, et al. Separation of sperm cells from samples containing high concentrations of white blood cells using a spiral channel. Biomicrofluidics. 2017;11(5):054106.
124. Sharma R, et al. Effect of sperm storage and selection techniques on sperm parameters. Syst Biol Reprod Med. 2015;61(1):1–12.
125. Aitken R, West K, Buckingham D. Leukocytic infiltration into the human ejaculate and its association with semen quality, oxidative stress, and sperm function. J Androl. 1994;15(4):343–52.
126. Fedder J. Nonsperm cells in human semen: with special reference to seminal leukocytes and their possible influence on fertility. Arch Androl. 1996;36(1):41–65.
127. Qiao X, et al. Effects of leukocytospermia on the outcomes of assisted reproductive technology. Andrologia. 2022;54:e14403.
128. Aitken RJ. Impact of oxidative stress on male and female germ cells: implications for fertility. Reproduction. 2020;159(4):R189–201.

Part III

Extended Examinations in Clinical Practice

Sperm DNA Fragmentation

10

Armand Zini and Ala'a Farkouh

Introduction

One of the ongoing challenges in infertility is to identify factors that can influence and/or predict natural and assisted reproduction outcomes. The semen analysis and standard sperm parameters (sperm concentration, motility, and morphology) provide us with information on the function of the testicles and reproductive tract. However, a significant disadvantage of this analysis is that conventional sperm parameters are crude indicators of male fertility potential. Moreover, the reference ranges for these parameters are based on a population of fertile couples who have achieved a natural conception, not on a population of infertile men [1]. In addition, sperm parameters cannot be used to reliably predict reproductive outcomes with assisted reproductive technologies (ARTs). As such, we need to identify markers that may allow us to assess male fertility potential and predict reproductive outcomes with ARTs. To date, one of the most promising markers in the evaluation and management of male infertility is sperm DNA integrity or DNA fragmentation.

The advent of ARTs, particularly ICSI (intracytoplasmic sperm injection), has revolutionized the management of the infertile couple. However, despite the success of this technology, we continue to have concerns regarding the safety of ICSI. These concerns are highly pertinent because advanced ARTs bypass the barriers to natural selection, and we know that infertile men have measurable defects in sperm DNA

A. Zini (✉)
McGill University, Montreal, QC, Canada

St. Mary's Hospital, Montreal, QC, Canada
e-mail: armand.zini@mcgill.ca

A. Farkouh
Global Andrology Forum, American Center for Reproductive Medicine,
Moreland Hills, OH, USA

A. Agarwal et al. (eds.), *Human Semen Analysis*,
https://doi.org/10.1007/978-3-031-55337-0_10

integrity [2]. As such, the study of sperm DNA damage becomes highly relevant in the era of ARTs.

The full ramifications of successful fertilization and pregnancy with DNA-damaged spermatozoa are unknown but there is some cause for concern given that sperm DNA damage is common in infertile men and, in experimental studies, sperm DNA damage may be detrimental to the health of the offspring [2, 3]. Reassuringly, in a clinical study, sperm DNA fragmentation has not been associated with measurable adverse effects on the health of the child [4]. However, studies have found that children of fathers that smoked cigarettes pre-conceptually (a habit associated with sperm DNA damage) have a higher risk of developing childhood cancers [5]. Moreover, children of fathers with a history of cancer (a condition associated with sperm DNA damage) have a higher risk of developing a birth defect than a population of children whose fathers do not have cancer [6]. Taken together, these studies suggest a possible link between sperm DNA damage and the subsequent development of childhood diseases, but additional studies are required to corroborate these findings.

Pathophysiology of SDF and Methodology of SDF Testing

The etiology human sperm DNA damage is multifactorial. Human sperm DNA damage and defective sperm function may be due to a primary defect in spermatogenesis (e.g., developmental abnormalities, advanced age) or to extrinsic factors resulting in sperm injury within the testicle or the post-testicular environment (e.g., hyperthermia, varicocele, gonadotoxins) [7].

At the molecular and cellular level, a number of pathways leading to sperm DNA damage have been proposed. These pathways include protamine deficiency (leading to aberrant spermatid chromatin remodeling), oxidative stress, and abortive apoptosis [7]. De Iuliis et al. [8] have suggested a two-step model to explain the development of sperm DNA damage. Based on the model, spermatozoa with poor chromatin compaction resulting from incomplete replacement of histones by protamines (1st step) are susceptible to injury from oxidative stress (second step). This model suggests that primary testicular and post-testicular events may result in sperm DNA damage.

Tests of sperm DNA damage have been designed to detect defects in sperm chromatin compaction and nuclear protein composition as well as defects in DNA integrity. These tests have helped advance our understanding of sperm chromatin architecture and function. The most common tests in clinical practice are the SCSA, TUNEL assay, SCD test, and the COMET assay. Tests of sperm chromatin and DNA damage have also been developed with the hope that these assays may be useful in predicting natural conception and reproductive outcomes with assisted reproduction but their use as specialized biomarkers in the evaluation of the infertile man has not been widely adopted. To date, we have not identified a perfect or best test to detect sperm DNA damage. Generally, SDF measurements provide a more accurate representation of a male's fertility status than conventional semen parameters because these measures have a lower biologic variability than conventional semen parameters [9, 10]. However, considerable inter-laboratory variability exists, influencing the reliability of test results. Moreover, thresholds (or cutoffs) for many of these assays have not been clearly defined.

The **SCSA—sperm chromatin structure assay** is based on the differential staining of chromatin single- and double-strand breaks by acridine orange [11]. SCSA allows the measurement of the extent of sperm DNA fragmentation and sperm chromatin nuclear protein defects, such as poor protamination. Generally, frozen semen samples are thawed and exposed to a 30-s acid denaturation, immediately treated with acridine orange and run through a flow cytometer.

The **COMET assay (single-cell gel electrophoresis)** is a simple method to assess sperm DNA integrity [12]. Briefly, a mix of spermatozoa and agarose is spread on a slide and treated to induce DNA denaturation. The cells are subjected to electrophoresis and, using a fluorescent dye, the DNA forms a structure resembling a comet; the head is intact DNA and the tail is composed of broken DNA, with the intensity of the comet representing the proportion of DNA that has been broken off. The alkaline COMET assay is preferred because it gives a comprehensive measure of DNA damage (i.e., single and double DNA strand breaks). However, minor modifications in test conditions can result in large variations in the results obtained [13] rendering the assay unreliable in clinical practice (WHO 6th edition).

The **TUNEL assay (terminal deoxynucleotidyl transferase-mediated dUTP nick end-labeling)** is a common method to detect DNA breaks. The assay relies on the incorporation and detection of fluorescent UTPs at both blunt and single 3'-OH ends. Although either immunohistochemistry or flow cytometry can be used for this assay [14], greater accuracy is obtained with the FACS assay as far more cells can be analyzed. Briefly, frozen samples are thawed, fixed, permeabilized, stained, and read by flow cytometry. The TUNEL assay is considered a direct approach because it lacks a DNA denaturation steps. However, this feature may reduce effectiveness because of limited access to 3'-OH nicks [15]. Most labs will rely on the Roche Applied Science commercial kit.

The **SCD—sperm chromatin dispersion** assay, also known as the Halo test, is based on the concept that sperm with fragmented DNA do not produce the characteristic halo of dispersed DNA loops that are observed in sperm with non-fragmented DNA following acid denaturation and removal of nuclear proteins. Briefly, agarose-embedded sperm are subjected to a denaturing solution to remove nuclear proteins and expose the damaged DNA (ssDNA, fragmented DNA). Spermatozoa with intact DNA exhibit characteristic loops around the sperm nucleus (creating a halo effect) [16], whereas spermatozoa with DNA damage do not. Halos can be observed via bright field microscope if the staining is done with an eosin and azure B solution. The technique is simple and does not require complex instrumentation. There may be some inter-observer subjectivity when categorizing the halos.

Relationship Between Sperm DNA Test Results and Reproductive Outcomes

Over the past 20 years, investigators have examined the relationship between sperm DNA damage and reproductive outcomes. These studies have shown that sperm DNA damage is associated with lower rates of natural and IUI pregnancies. Couples with sperm DNA damage have low potential for natural fertility and a prolonged time to pregnancy [17]. A recent meta-analysis has shown that sperm DNA damage is associated with lower IUI pregnancy rate (relative risk = 3.2, 95% CI: 1.46–6.79; I2 = 13.1%) but the sperm DNA test has a limited capacity in predicting IUI outcome, and therefore, a limited value in the management of these couples [18]. Systematic reviews and meta-analyses of studies relating DNA damage and assisted reproduction outcomes indicate that sperm DNA damage is associated (albeit weakly) with IVF and IVF/ICSI pregnancy rates [19]. Nonetheless, tests of sperm DNA fragmentation have limited capacity to discriminate between couples who have a low chance to conceive and those who have a high chance to conceive after assisted reproduction [20].

One of the most interesting observations regarding sperm DNA damage and assisted reproduction is the association with increased risk of pregnancy loss after both standard IVF and IVF/ICSI [21]. In line with these findings, numerous reports have shown an association between sperm DNA fragmentation and recurrent miscarriages. A meta-analysis of 13 prospective studies suggests that male partners of women with a history of recurrent pregnancy loss have a significantly higher mean sperm DNA fragmentation level compared to partners of fertile control women (mean difference 11.91, 95% CI 4.97–18.86) [22].

Although the use of sperm DNA fragmentation tests in clinical practice appears promising, testing has not gained wide approval and remains controversial. One of the major concerns regarding these tests is the fact that there are multiple assays, with each assay detecting different sites of sperm DNA damage [23]. Moreover, there are no standardized protocols for many of these assays and little is known about the precision of the assays due to a lack of reproducibility studies (intra- and inter-laboratory). Another important shortcoming is the fact that the clinical thresholds for many of these tests have not been adequately validated. Finally, most of the clinical studies are retrospective, relatively small (many studies reported on 100–200 ART cycles) with heterogeneous study characteristics and most fail to demonstrate the predictive value of these tests.

Based on the observed relationship between DNA damage and reproductive outcomes, some investigators have proposed that tests of sperm DNA fragmentation be used as predictors of natural and ART pregnancies and to guide treatment of infertile couples. There is some evidence that sperm DNA tests are used frequently in the clinical management of infertile couples [24], although the routine application of these tests in clinical practice has not been advocated largely due to the shortcomings of these assays [25]. However, there are specific clinical settings where sperm DNA testing may be useful. Sperm DNA testing may be valuable in couples with recurrent pregnancy loss and in those with unexplained recurrent IVF/ICSI failures to determine if a male factor may be responsible and to provide appropriate therapy in these couples [25, 26]. Sperm DNA testing may also be useful in couples with clinical varicocele and borderline normal semen parameters (to determine whether surgery may help) and those with unexplained infertility [26]. Nonetheless, to date, the level of evidence supporting the use of sperm DNA testing in the management of couple infertility and as a predictor of reproductive outcomes remains modest.

SDF and Etiological Diagnosis of Male Reproductive Functions and Dysfunctions

As research into sperm DNA fragmentation (SDF) and its impact on male reproductive potential has increased over the past several years, many investigators have studied and have attempted to identify the different causes and risks that may be associated with an increase in SDF. These can be classified into: (1) patient conditions, (2) lifestyle factors, and (3) exposures. These are summarized in Fig. 10.1 and are expanded upon in the subsequent text.

Advanced Paternal Age Although there is no general agreement upon the specification of advanced paternal age, it is typically considered at age 40 and above [27]. Studies have shown that an advanced paternal age is associated with adverse reproductive outcomes including reduced fertility after both natural and assisted reproduction, increased miscarriage rates, and increased risk of certain disorders in children [28]. SDF has been found to increase with age. Rybar et al. have shown that age above 40 is significantly correlated with a higher DNA fragmentation index (DFI) ($r = 0.26$, $P < 0.01$) [29]. This was further reinforced by Alshahrani et al. who have evaluated SDF in 472 infertile patients and reported a significantly higher level of DNA damage in men aged 40 and above compared to younger groups (24.4% vs. 16.7%, $P < 0.05$) [30]. Moreover, a retrospective study by Pino et al. grouped men into four groups based on age and found that as age increases, so does the risk of abnormal SDF levels, such that men over 50 are 4.58 times more likely to have high SDF than those aged 21–30 years [31]. Several factors play a role in the rise of SDF as men age. Accumulation of reactive oxygen species (ROS) and an increase in oxidative stress (OS) occurs with aging and contributes to DNA strand breakage

Fig. 10.1 Causes and risk factors leading to elevated sperm DNA fragmentation

Patient Conditions	Lifestyle Factors	Exposures
• Advanced paternal age • Varicocele • Genital tract inflammation and infection • Obesity & Diabetes	• Smoking • Alcohol • Sedentary lifestyle • Dietary factors	• Radiation • Toxic chemicals • Radiomagnetic waves • Heat exposure • Environmental pollutants

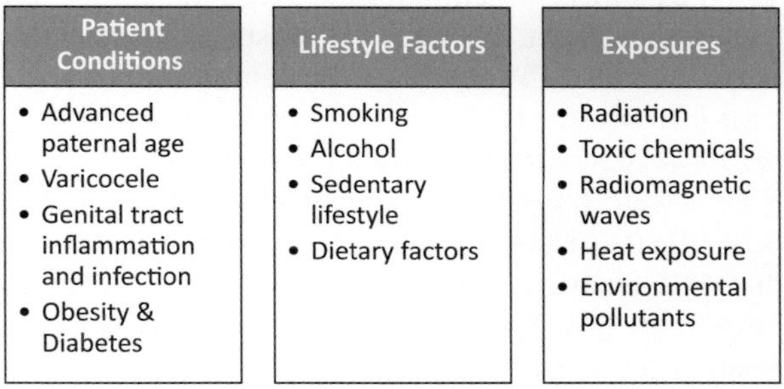

[32]. Poor chromatin packaging has also been reported with aging [33], making DNA more susceptible to breaks. Furthermore, a decline in apoptosis of abnormal spermatozoa that carry damaged DNA compared to younger men, allows sperm with defective DNA to survive and be released [34].

Varicocele Varicocele is a common cause of infertility that can be found in up to 40% of men presenting with primary infertility and up to 80% of men with secondary infertility, and can lead to abnormalities in conventional semen parameters, which typically serve as indications for varicocele repair [35]. Varicocele is also associated with elevated SDF which can further contribute to infertility. A recent meta-analysis included 12 studies which compared DFI between men with clinical varicocele and healthy controls with no varicocele [36]. Pooled analysis compared 845 men with clinical varicocele to 2733 healthy controls and found that clinical varicocele is associated with a significantly higher DFI, with a standard mean difference of 1.40 ($P < 0.0001$). Another study investigated SDF levels among three different groups of men: clinical varicocele with abnormal conventional semen parameters, clinical varicocele with normal conventional semen parameters, and subclinical varicocele [37]. They found that SDF was significantly elevated in men with clinical varicocele when compared to controls, irrespective of changes in conventional semen parameters, however, for men with subclinical varicocele, no significant difference in SDF was found compared to controls. This reinforces the notion that clinical varicocele can lead to infertility by increasing SDF, and this may not be reflected on conventional parameters. The pathophysiology behind varicocele's adverse impact on male fertility involves multiple factors which include increased scrotal temperatures, localized testicular hypoxia, hormonal disruptions, and the reflux of catecholamines and other renal and adrenal metabolites; all of which contribute to impaired spermatogenesis and increase in ROS production, which in turn can lead to increased SDF, increased sperm apoptosis, and impaired sperm function [38].

Genital Tract Inflammation and Infection Infections of the male accessory glands and genital tract lead to activation of the inflammatory response in male reproductive organs as means to eradicate the infection. This leads to recruitment and activation of white blood cells (WBCs), causing leukocytospermia (i.e., $>1 \times 10^6$ WBCs/mL), which in turn increase the production of ROS, causing OS which can damage sperm DNA and impair sperm function, leading to male infertility [39]. Approximately 15% of cases of male infertility are associated with male genital tract infections, with *Chlamydia trachomatis*, *Escherichia coli*, and *Neisseria gonorrhoeae*, being the most common causative microorganisms [39]. In fact, seminal WBCs were found to be significantly positively correlated to seminal ROS ($r = 0.70$, $P < 0.001$) and to SDF levels in spermatozoa ($r = 0.43$, $P = 0.032$), indicating that WBCs may contribute to infertility by increasing OS and SDF [40]. Furthermore, infertile men with confirmed chlamydia and mycoplasma genital infections were found to have 3.2 times higher SDF than fertile controls with no infections ($P <$

0.001) [41]. A recent study investigated the prevalence of genital tract infections among infertile men who either had leukocytospermia, abnormal semen parameters, symptoms or a history of genital tract infections [42]. 34.9% of the participants had a positive semen culture with a single microorganism, while 3.5% had a polymicrobial infection. On further analysis, leukocytospermia was significantly associated with a positive culture (OR = 3.93, $P < 0.001$), and %SDF was significantly higher among infertile men with positive cultures (42.2%), when compared to infertile men with negative cultures (23.5%) and healthy fertile controls (14.3%).

Obesity and Diabetes Obesity is defined as a body mass index of ≥ 30 kg/m^2, which can serve as a risk factor for many serious life-threatening diseases and can also contribute to reduced male fertility potential [43]. Several sequelae of obesity can contribute to male infertility and these include hypogonadism and hormonal imbalance, impaired spermatogenesis and dysregulated spermatogonial apoptosis, epigenetic modifications, and increased sperm DNA damage. The increased SDF with obesity may be attributed to increased ROS production that occurs when adipose tissue accumulates causing more fatty acid oxidation [43]. When SDF was compared between obese men (BMI ≥ 30 kg/m^2) and men with normal BMI (18.5–24.9 kg/m^2), SDF was found to be significantly higher among the obese with a mean difference of 3.9%. On further analysis, obesity was found to be significantly associated with increased SDF, with an OR of 2.5 [44]. The same study did not find a significant elevation of SDF among overweight men (BMI 25–29.9 kg/m^2) compared to normal BMI. Obesity is also a component of the metabolic syndrome, which also includes elevated blood glucose and insulin resistance as part of its definition. A meta-analysis that included four studies comparing SDF levels between men with metabolic syndrome and healthy controls reported significantly higher SDF among those with metabolic syndrome [45]. Diabetes mellitus (DM) can also disrupt male fertility potential and cause elevated SDF and is associated with higher levels of seminal WBCs and OS [46]. Men with type 1 DM were found to have higher SDF and higher 8-hydroxydeoxyguanosine (8-OHdG) levels in sperm DNA, a marker of oxidative damage, which was found to be positively correlated to SDF levels [47]. Infertile men with type 2 DM were also found to have significantly higher SDF (34.2%) compared to nondiabetic controls (18.2%, $P < 0.001$) as well as significantly lower clinical pregnancy rates (28.6% vs. 43.6%, $P < 0.001$) and higher miscarriage rates (50% vs. 24.6%, $P < 0.001$) [48].

Smoking DFI is reported to be significantly higher among infertile smokers compared to infertile non-smokers, and a strong positive correlation between SDF levels with smoking duration and number of cigarettes per day is also documented [49, 50]. The detrimental impact of nicotine on sperm DNA has also been studied in vitro, as spermatozoa were incubated with different concentrations of nicotine and SDF was subsequently measured, revealing a significantly elevated SDF with nicotine and this was also related to concentration [51]. The adverse impact of smoking and the oxidative stress that ensues on sperm DNA has long been studied. Significantly higher sperm DFI as well as ROS and 8-OHdG were found among tobacco users [52]. The higher 8-OHdG in sperm of smokers is also significantly correlated to semen concentration of cotinine, a nicotine metabolite [53]. Moreover, the levels of antioxidants, such as vitamin E, were found to be significantly less in semen of infertile smokers, further contributing to oxidative stress [54]. Chemicals in cigarettes, such as benzopyrene, can directly induce oxidative stress and can also induce DNA damage via the formation of adducts [55]. Elevated white blood cells as well as pro-inflammatory proteins have also been documented in semen of smokers, further adding to oxidative stress [56, 57]. Moreover, heavy metals in cigarettes, such as cadmium, also lead to oxidative DNA damage [58]. Other mechanisms that contribute to DNA damage among smokers include defects in DNA methylation, abnormalities in protamination, DNA mutations, as well as chromosomal abnormalities [59]. Impairment in DNA repair has also been reported with smoking, as the levels of checkpoint kinase 1 (Chk1), which is released in response to DNA damage and causes cell cycle arrest to allow for repair, is decreased with smoking [60]. In addition, increased release of apoptotic spermatozoa with increased SDF has been linked to smoking [61].

Alcohol and Other Lifestyle Risk Factors Excessive alcohol intake can lead to cellular damage via apoptosis, inflammation, OS, and genotoxicity which can lead to DNA strand breaks, including SDF [62]. In one report, non-smoking infertile men who consume daily alcohol were found to have significantly higher SDF levels as measured by TUNEL, when compared to those who did not consume alcohol and did not smoke (25% vs. 16%, $P < 0.05$) [63]. Alcohol has also been reported to negatively affect semen volume, sperm motility and morphology, and male reproductive hormones, with these harmful effects being dependent upon the amount of alcohol ingestion [64]. Elevated SDF levels have also been reported with a sedentary lifestyle, as men who spend more than half of their work time in a seated position were found to have higher SDF compared to those who are sedentary for less than 50% of their work time, which is attributed to higher scrotal temperatures after prolonged sitting [65]. Finally, dietary factors also play a role, as men who consume high amounts of fruits, vegetables, fish, and chicken in their diet were reported to have significantly lower SDF levels than those who mainly eat red meats, sweets, and high-fat foods [66].

Environmental and Occupational Exposures Many different hazardous and noxious materials can also contribute to male infertility by increasing SDF levels. Men are typically exposed to such substances either via their occupation or via environmental exposure. Men who are exposed to ionizing radiation in their jobs were found to have significantly higher SDF levels, which are due to the direct damaging effect of radiation in inducing double-strand DNA breaks [67]. Toxic chemical exposure for long periods of time, such as carbamate and organophosphate pesticides, have also been associated with higher DFI [68]. Other chemicals such as styrene, which is used in manufacturing reinforced plastic, is also a risk factor for elevated SDF [69]. Car painters were found to have significantly higher levels of SDF when compared to men who work in offices (47.7% vs. 14.9%, $P < 0.001$), which may be attributed to the various chemical exposures, leading to OS and DNA damage [70]. Radiofrequency electromagnetic radiation, which is due to cell phones and laptop computers, can also cause DNA strand breaks leading to SDF [71]. Heat stress and scrotal hyperthermia are associated with significantly higher SDF levels [72]. Finally, air pollution is also linked to higher SDF levels [73].

SDF and Further Investigations

Given the many associated causes and risk factors for elevated SDF, infertile men who are found to have elevated SDF may also benefit from additional examinations. Seminal OS is a known contributor for SDF, and therefore men who are at a risk of higher ROS exposure, for example, smokers, may benefit from seminal OS testing methods. These are also described within advanced examinations of the 6th edition WHO laboratory manual for examination and processing of human semen and include luminol, oxidation reduction potential (ORP), and total antioxidant capacity (TAC) tests [74]. Men with leukocytospermia or those with a clinical picture suggestive of genital tract infection may benefit from a semen culture or nucleic acid amplification tests to detect causative microorganisms and diagnose infections. Although varicocele is a clinical diagnosis, a scrotal ultrasound may be performed, particularly if examination is difficult, or to characterize the grade of reflux and confirm the diagnosis [35]. Diabetic men should be assessed for the level of their glycemic control and should be evaluated for other components of the metabolic syndrome, including a lipid profile. Obese men may benefit from a hormonal evaluation, as obesity is known to cause secondary male hypogonadism, which is also associated with impaired male fertility potential [75].

SDF: Non-ART Management

Treating Associated Underlying Etiologies When infertile men are found to have elevated SDF, it is crucial to identify and treat any potential contributing factor. Men with clinical varicocele benefit from varicocele repair, as has been demonstrated by a recent meta-analysis that included 19 studies with over 1000 patients who were infertile and had clinical varicocele and underwent repair [76]. Pooled analysis revealed a significant decrease in SDF after varicocele repair, with a mean difference of -7.23 ($P < 0.00001$). Results of a prospective study on 60 infertile men with clinical varicocele who underwent repair also demonstrated significant improvements in SDF levels, with mean values decreasing from 29.5% to 18.8% ($P < 0.001$), after 3–6 months of surgery [77]. Men with genital tract infections should be treated with the appropriate antibiotics. In a group of infertile men with mycoplasma or chlamydia genital tract infections, antibiotic treatment caused a significant reduction in mean SDF from 37.7% to 24.2% ($P < 0.001$), and 85.7% of the couples were able to conceive after completing the antibiotic course [41]. Obese men must be counseled on the importance of weight loss, as this has been demonstrated to lower SDF. In one study, 105 obese infertile men with were given a 12-week weight loss program consisting of a healthy diet and exercise [78]. After completing the program, significant reductions in SDF were reported. Bariatric surgery has also been proven successful in reducing SDF after weight loss surgery [79]. Furthermore, smokers should be encouraged to quit, men who consume large amounts of alcohol should be counseled to cut down their consumption, and men with known toxic exposure should be educated on their risk and the appropriate personal protection equipment, as well as possible solutions for exposure limitation when feasible.

Antioxidants ROS and OS that may be attributed to various factors as described earlier play a significant role in the accumulation of SDF. It is not surprising that many scientists have investigated the potential benefit of supplying antioxidants to infertile men who have elevated SDF, as a means to counteract the OS contributing to their SDF, lowering their SDF levels, and in turn improving reproductive outcomes. Several clinical trials have investigated supplementing various antioxidants including zinc, vitamins C and E, and docosahexaenoic acid and reported significant reductions in SDF levels compared to no treatment or placebo groups [80–82]. Infertile men with SDF of 15% or more who had failed intracytoplasmic sperm injection (ICSI) were supplemented with vitamin C and E for 2 months and were later able to achieve significantly higher fertilization and implantation rates with a repeat ICSI [83]. More recent studies have also demonstrated the success of various antioxidants in lower SDF, including co-enzyme Q10, n-acetyl-cysteine, and combination antioxidants [84–86]. In general, antioxidant supplementation has shown promising results in managing infertile men with elevated SDF in terms of lowering SDF levels and improving reproductive outcomes, including fertilization rates, pregnancy rates, and live birth rates [87]. However, it is crucial to point out that the controversial aspects of antioxidants for SDF management. Firstly, not all studies have demonstrated improvement in SDF levels or pregnancy outcomes after supplementation, including the recent MOXI trail which included 171 infertile men [88]. A trial by Schisterman et al. actually reported higher SDF levels among the group that received zinc and folic acid for 6 months compared to placebo [89]. Secondly, not all SDF is caused by OS, and supplying antioxidants to men who do not have high ROS may alternatively cause reductive stress to spermatozoa, which can also cause defective sperm maturation, abnormal chromatin integrity, and impaired function [90, 91]. Finally, there is no superior or universally recommended antioxidant regimen, dose, or duration. Different studies have investigated different antioxidants for various durations and have included different populations of infertile men, which has prevented the ability to make solid recommendations [92].

Hormones   A meta-analysis by Santi et al. included six studies that investigated the effect of follicle stimulating hormone (FSH) in reducing SDF in infertile men and reported significant reductions of 4.24% 3 months after treatment [93]. However, the limitations of this meta-analysis are that heterogeneous treatment regimens were used by the different included studies and there was a lack of standardization in SDF measurement among them [94]. Other hormone modulators such as letrozole, an aromatase inhibitor, has also been reported to reduce SDF [95]. Evidence supporting the use of hormonal therapy for management of infertile men with elevated SDF is limited and there are no well-designed clinical trials that allow recommendation of an appropriate hormonal regimen and dose and for an appropriate duration.

SDF and ART Management: Guide ART Choice

Several techniques approaches have been employed aimed at lowering SDF and improving ART outcomes.

Short Abstinence

It has been postulated that prolonged epididymal storage may increase sperm oxidative stress leading to sperm dysfunction and DNA damage. This has prompted investigators to evaluate short abstinence time (1-day abstinence) to reduce sperm DNA fragmentation in whole semen. Although several studies have reported a reduction in sperm DNA fragmentation with short abstinence, this has not been demonstrated in all studies [96]. As such, this strategy has not been accepted universally as a means of improving sperm DNA fragmentation.

Advanced Sperm Processing Techniques

Several specialized sperm sorting techniques have been developed in the hope that they may allow for selection of a highly functional sperm fraction. These techniques have generally been effective in selecting a population of sperm with lower levels of DNA fragmentation than neat semen. However, these techniques require technical expertise, as well as, additional materials and they increase costs. Moreover, they require lengthier sperm incubation. These specialized separation techniques include HA (hyaluronic acid) binding, annexin-V binding, electrophoretic separation, and microfluidic separation.

To date, the application of specialized sperm sorting techniques has not consistently resulted in a significant improvement in ICSI pregnancy rates compared to ICSI with spermatozoa obtained by conventional sperm separation techniques (e.g., density gradient centrifugation and swim-up). A possible explanation as to why these techniques fail to improve pregnancy outcomes is the understanding that most spermatozoa from samples with high sperm DNA fragmentation demonstrate some degree of DNA damage such that the spermatozoa recovered following sperm separation will also possess a measurable degree of DNA damage [97, 98].

Use of Testicular Sperm for ICSI in Men with High Levels of Sperm DNA Fragmentation

The advent of intracytoplasmic sperm injection (ICSI) has revolutionized the management of male factor infertility, and particularly, the treatment of couples with severe male factor infertility. However, it has become evident that ICSI may not overcome significant sperm abnormalities [99]. Moreover, there is some concern that infertile men with abnormal semen parameters could have a sperm genetic defect with a potential adverse impact on ICSI outcomes, including a higher risk of miscarriage [19].

In 2005, Greco et al. reported higher pregnancy rates with ICSI when using testicular rather than ejaculated sperm in couples with sperm DNA damage and observed a lower frequency of sperm showing detectable DNA damage in testicular vs. ejaculated sperm [100]. They hypothesized that the DNA damage in ejaculated sperm begins after spermatozoa are released from Sertoli cells and suggested that the poorer outcome with ejaculated sperm was a result of acquired DNA damage during transit through the epididymis or possibly during ejaculation. In the same year, Suganuma et al. [101] conducted experimental studies using an animal model with abnormal spermatogenesis and incomplete sperm nuclear compaction to test the hypothesis proposed by Greco et al. [100]. They observed that in animals with abnormal spermatogenesis the passage of sperm through the epididymis was associated with a loss of sperm DNA integrity and fertilizing capacity [101]. They proposed that in some men (i.e., those with defective spermatogenesis) the passage of sperm through the epididymis could impair sperm DNA integrity and fertilizing capacity.

The idea that the post-testicular environment or epididymal transit can induce sperm damage has led clinicians to utilize testicular rather than ejaculated sperm for ICSI in men with abnormal spermatogenesis and poor sperm DNA integrity. To date, several prospective and retrospective studies have supported the findings of Greco et al. [83] and have demonstrated higher pregnancy rates with ICSI when using testicular rather than ejaculated sperm in couples with sperm DNA damage [102]. Moreover, several studies have observed a lower mean sperm DNA fragmentation in testicular vs. ejaculated sperm, in men with sperm DNA fragmentation. However, studies on the use of testicular rather than ejaculated sperm in couples with sperm DNA damage are small and non-randomized. As such, the evidence in favor of testicular sperm in these men remains modest. Larger, randomized studies are needed before we can demonstrate a true benefit of testicular rather than ejaculated sperm for ICSI in couples with sperm DNA fragmentation.

Two Case Scenarios

Case 1 A couple presents for fertility evaluation after experiencing three successive miscarriages following spontaneous conception. Neither partner has a child together nor from a previous relationship. The woman is 27-years-old, with no comorbidities, and a completely normal gynecological and hormonal work-up, including all appropriate imaging and karyotype. The man is 28-years-old and has no medical comorbidities. History and physical examination are unremarkable, conventional semen parameters are within normal limits, and laboratory and hormonal work-up are normal. There are no abnormalities on karyotype. He works as a teacher and leads a sedentary lifestyle; he is obese with a BMI of 32 kg/m^2 and is a smoker with 10-pack years.

The American Urological Association/American Society for Reproductive Medicine guidelines recommend that male partners of couples experiencing recurrent pregnancy loss (RPL) be evaluated with SDF testing [25]. A similar recommendation is made by the European Association of Urology (EAU) [103] and the European Society of Human Reproduction and Embryology (ESHRE) [104].

RPL is defined as two or more successive miscarriages and has been associated with elevated SDF. A meta-analysis that included 13 studies with 517 couples experiencing RPL reported a significantly higher rates of SDF among them when compared to 384 fertile couples with a mean difference of 10.7% ($P < 0.0001$) [22]. Tan et al. also reported higher rates of SDF among couples with RPL after spontaneous conception compared to fertile couples with a mean difference of 11.98% ($P < 0.001$) [105].

This man should undergo SDF testing. He should be counseled on his risk factors that contribute to his infertility and potentially elevated SDF and should be encouraged to lose weight, as this has been proven to lower SDF and improve outcomes, and quit smoking. If elevated OS is found, antioxidants may also be supplied to counteract the OS that is conferred by smoking and obesity, and may be contributing to SDF leading to RPL.

Case 2 A 31-year-old man and 29-year-old woman are referred for andrological evaluation after two failures to achieve clinical pregnancy following conventional in vitro fertilization (IVF). The woman was evaluated by her gynecologist and was found to have no obvious underlying cause to explain IVF failure. The man is a radiologist, who has no medical comorbidities and leads a healthy lifestyle. History and physical exam are unremarkable. His basic semen analysis reveals no sperm abnormalities but is remarkable for leukocytospermia. SDF testing was performed using sperm chromatin structure assay (SCSA) and yielded a DFI of 34%, a value interpreted as "elevated" by the performing laboratory.

This man has known factors for his elevated SDF. His occupation as a radiologist puts him at risk due to his exposure to ionizing radiation that can directly induce DNA damage, and the leukocytospermia, which may be attributed to genital tract inflammation or infection, can also lead to SDF via OS. He should be investigated for his leukocytospermia and treated accordingly with antibiotics if infection is found and with antioxidants that can balance the ROS produced by his seminal WBCs.

SDF adversely impacts the outcome of conventional IVF by lowering fertilization rates [106], poor embryo quality [107], lowering implantation rates [108], and lowering clinical pregnancy rates as reported by several meta-analyses. In the meta-analysis by Zini, 1805 IVF cycles from 11 studies were included and pooled analysis revealed significantly lower pregnancy rates after IVF with high sperm DNA damage (OR = 1.7, $P < 0.05$) [109]. The recent meta-analysis by Rabas-Maynou et al. with 15 studies and 3711 IVF cycles yielded similar results of a significantly lower clinical pregnancy with higher SDF (RR = 0.72, $P = 0.02$) [108]. SDF can also lead to miscarriage after IVF [107] and lower live birth rates [108, 110]. Many of the meta-analyses have also investigated the impact of SDF on ICSI outcomes; however, the results are less consistent than those for IVF. Although SDF can affect ICSI and can lead to miscarriage after ICSI, many meta-analyses have revealed no effects of SDF in terms of lowering clinical pregnancy rates [107–109].

For this man with elevated SDF and failed IVF, managing underlying causes should be attempted first and further methods to reduce SDF can be attempted before repeating IVF or ICSI for this couple, including a shorter abstinence period, advanced sperm selection techniques such as magnetic activated cell sorting (MACS), or intracytoplasmic morphologically selected sperm injection (IMSI) which have been shown to lower SDF levels and improve outcomes after assisted reproduction [111]. As a last resort, ICSI with testicular sperm can be used which has less SDF, although evidence behind using this method is of poor quality and puts the patient at the risks of an invasive procedure [112].

Take Home Message

- Tests of sperm DNA damage have helped advance our understanding of sperm chromatin architecture and function and spermatogenesis.
- Studies have shown that sperm DNA fragmentation (SDF) is associated with male infertility.
- SDF is associated with poor reproductive outcomes.
- Correctable clinical and lifestyle factors have been associated with SDF.
- Several approaches have been employed to lower or overcome SDF in preparation for ART.

References

1. Cooper TG, Noonan E, von Eckardstein S, Auger J, Baker HW, Behre HM, Haugen TB, Kruger T, Wang C, Mbizvo MT, Vogelsong KM. World Health Organization reference values for human semen characteristics. Hum Reprod Update. 2010;16(3):231–45.
2. Vinnakota C, Cree L, Peek J, Morbeck DE. Incidence of high sperm DNA fragmentation in a targeted population of subfertile men. Syst Biol Reprod Med. 2019;65(6):451–7.

3. Fernández-Gonzalez R, Moreira PN, Pérez-Crespo M, Sánchez-Martín M, Ramirez MA, Pericuesta E, Bilbao A, Bermejo-Alvarez P, de Dios HJ, de Fonseca FR, Gutiérrez-Adán A. Long-term effects of mouse intracytoplasmic sperm injection with DNA-fragmented sperm on health and behavior of adult offspring. Biol Reprod. 2008;78(4):761–72.

4. Bungum M, Bungum L, Lynch KF, Wedlund L, Humaidan P, Giwercman A. Spermatozoa DNA damage measured by sperm chromatin structure assay (SCSA) and birth characteristics in children conceived by IVF and ICSI. Int J Androl. 2012;35(4):485–90.

5. Ji BT, Shu XO, Linet MS, Zheng W, Wacholder S, Gao YT, Ying DM, Jin F. Paternal cigarette smoking and the risk of childhood cancer among offspring of nonsmoking mothers. J Natl Cancer Inst. 1997;89(3):238–44.

6. Al-Jebari Y, Glimelius I, Berglund Nord C, Cohn-Cedermark G, Ståhl O, Tandstad T, Jensen A, Sagstuen Haugnes H, Daugaard G, Rylander L, Giwercman A. Cancer therapy and risk of congenital malformations in children fathered by men treated for testicular germ-cell cancer: a nationwide register study. PLoS Med. 2019;16(6):e1002816.

7. Zini A, Sigman M. Are tests of sperm DNA damage clinically useful? Pros and cons. J Androl. 2009;30(3):219–29.

8. De Iuliis GN, Thomson LK, Mitchell LA, Finnie JM, Koppers AJ, Hedges A, Nixon B, AitkenRJ. DNA damage in human spermatozoa is highly correlated with the efficiency of chromatin remodeling and the formation of 8-hydroxy-2′-deoxyguanosine, a marker of oxidative stress. Biol Reprod. 2009;81(3):517–24.

9. Erenpreiss J, Bungum M, Spano M, et al. Intra-individual variation in sperm chromatin structure assay parameters in men from infertile couples: clinical implications. Hum Reprod. 2006;21:2061–4.

10. Evenson DP, Jost LK, Baer RK, et al. Individuality of DNA denaturation patterns in human sperm as measured by the sperm chromatin structure assay. Reprod Toxicol. 1991;5:115–25.

11. Neville DM Jr, Bradley DF. Anomalous rotatory dispersion of acridine orange-native deoxyribonucleic acid complexes. Biochim Biophys Acta. 1961;50:397–9.

12. Singh NP, McCoy MT, Tice RR, Schneider EL. A simple technique for quantitation of low levels of DNA damage in individual cells. Exp Cell Res. 1988;175(1):184–91.

13. Speit G, Vasquez M, Hartmann A. The comet assay as an indicator test for germ cell genotoxicity. Mutat Res. 2009;681(1):3–12.

14. Sailer BL, Jost LK, Evenson DP. Mammalian sperm DNA susceptibility to in situ denaturation associated with the presence of DNA strand breaks as measured by the terminal deoxynucleotidyl transferase assay. J Androl. 1995;16(1):80–7.

15. Lewis SE, Agbaje I, Alvarez J. Sperm DNA tests as useful adjuncts to semen analysis. Syst Biol Reprod Med. 2008;54(3):111–25.

16. Ankem MK, Mayer E, Ward WS, et al. Novel assay for determining DNA organization in human spermatozoa: implications for male factor infertility. Urology. 2002;59:575–8.

17. Spano M, Bonde JP, Hjollund HI, Kolstad HA, Cordelli E, Leter G. Sperm chromatin damage impairs human fertility. Fertil Steril. 2000;73:43–50.

18. Sugihara A, Van Avermaete F, Roelant E, Punjabi U, De Neubourg D. The role of sperm DNA fragmentation testing in predicting intra-uterine insemination outcome: a systematic review and meta-analysis. Eur J Obstet Gynecol Reprod Biol. 2020;244:8–15.

19. Simon L, Zini A, Dyachenko A, Ciampi A, Carrell DT. A systematic review and meta-analysis to determine the effect of sperm DNA damage on in vitro fertilization and intracytoplasmic sperm injection outcome. Asian J Androl. 2017;19:80–90.

20. Cissen M, Wely MV, Scholten I, Mansell S, Bruin JP, Mol BW, Braat D, Repping S, Hamer G. Measuring sperm DNA fragmentation and clinical outcomes of medically assisted reproduction: a systematic review and meta-analysis. PLoS ONE. 2016;11(11):e0165125.

21. Zini A, Boman J, Belzile E, Ciampi A. Sperm DNA damage is associated with an increased risk of pregnancy loss after IVF and ICSI: systematic review and meta-analysis. Hum Reprod. 2008;23:2663–8.

22. McQueen DB, Zhang J, Robins JC. Sperm DNA fragmentation and recurrent pregnancy loss: a systematic review and meta-analysis. Fertil Steril. 2019;112(1):54–60.e3. https://doi.org/10.1016/j.fertnstert.2019.03.003. Epub 2019 May 2. PMID: 31056315.

23. Gawecka JE, Boaz S, Kasperson K, Nguyen H, Evenson DP, Ward WS. Luminal fluid of epididymis and vas deferens contributes to sperm chromatin fragmentation. Hum Reprod. 2015;30(12):2725–36.

24. Majzoub A, Agarwal A, Cho CL, Esteves SC. Sperm DNA fragmentation testing: a cross sectional survey on current practices of fertility specialists. Transl Androl Urol. 2017;6(Suppl 4):S710–9.

25. Schlegel PN, Sigman M, Collura B, de Jonge CJ, Eisenberg ML, Lamb DJ, Mulhall JP, Niederberger C, Sandlow JI, Sokol RZ, Spandorfer SD, Tanrikut C, Treadwell JR, Oristaglio JT, Zini A. Diagnosis and treatment of infertility in men: AUA/ASRM guideline part II. J Urol. 2021;205(1):44–51.

26. Agarwal A, Majzoub A, Esteves SC, Ko E, Ramasamy R, Zini A. Clinical utility of sperm DNA fragmentation testing: practice recommendations based on clinical scenarios. Transl Androl Urol. 2016;5(6):935–50.

27. Toriello HV, Meck JM, Professional Practice and Guidelines Committee. Statement on guidance for genetic counseling in advanced paternal age. Genet Med. 2008;10(6):457–60. https://doi.org/10.1097/GIM.0b013e318176fabb. PMID: 18496227; PMCID: PMC3111019.

28. Sharma R, Agarwal A, Rohra VK, Assidi M, Abu-Elmagd M, Turki RF. Effects of increased paternal age on sperm quality, reproductive outcome and associated epigenetic risks to off-spring. Reprod Biol Endocrinol. 2015;13:35. https://doi.org/10.1186/s12958-015-0028-x. PMID: 25928123; PMCID: PMC4455614.

29. Rybar R, Kopecka V, Prinosilova P, Markova P, Rubes J. Male obesity and age in relationship to semen parameters and sperm chromatin integrity. Andrologia. 2011;43(4):286–91. https://doi.org/10.1111/j.1439-0272.2010.01057.x. Epub 2011 Mar 23. PMID: 21486403.

30. Alshahrani S, Agarwal A, Assidi M, Abuzenadah AM, Durairajanayagam D, Ayaz A, Sharma R, Sabanegh E. Infertile men older than 40 years are at higher risk of sperm DNA damage. Reprod Biol Endocrinol. 2014;12:103. https://doi.org/10.1186/1477-7827-12-103. PMID: 25410314; PMCID: PMC4258051.

31. Pino V, Sanz A, Valdés N, Crosby J, Mackenna A. The effects of aging on semen parameters and sperm DNA fragmentation. JBRA Assist Reprod. 2020;24(1):82–6. https://doi.org/10.5935/1518-0557.20190058. PMID: 31692316; PMCID: PMC6993171.

32. Gunes S, Hekim GN, Arslan MA, Asci R. Effects of aging on the male reproductive system. J Assist Reprod Genet. 2016;33(4):441–54. https://doi.org/10.1007/s10815-016-0663-y. Epub 2016 Feb 11. PMID: 26867640; PMCID: PMC4818633.

33. Plastira K, Msaouel P, Angelopoulou R, Zanioti K, Plastiras A, Pothos A, Bolaris S, Paparisteidis N, Mantas D. The effects of age on DNA fragmentation, chromatin packaging and conventional semen parameters in spermatozoa of oligoasthenoteratozoospermic patients. J Assist Reprod Genet. 2007;24(10):437–43. https://doi.org/10.1007/s10815-007-9162-5. Epub 2007 Sep 4. PMID: 17768675; PMCID: PMC3455076.

34. Colasante A, Minasi MG, Scarselli F, Casciani V, Zazzaro V, Ruberti A, Greco P, Varricchio MT, Greco E. The aging male: Relationship between male age, sperm quality and sperm DNA damage in an unselected population of 3124 men attending the fertility centre for the first time. Arch Ital Urol Androl. 2019;90(4):254–9. https://doi.org/10.4081/aiua.2018.4.254. PMID: 30655635.

35. Shah R, Agarwal A, Kavoussi P, Rambhatla A, Saleh R, Cannarella R, et al. Consensus and diversity in the management of varicocele for male infertility: results of a global practice survey and comparison with guidelines and recommendations. World J Men's Health. 2022;41(1):164–97. https://doi.org/10.5534/wjmh.220048. PMID: 35791302.

36. Zhang Y, Zhang W, Wu X, Liu G, Dai Y, Jiang H, Zhang X. Effect of varicocele on sperm DNA damage: A systematic review and meta-analysis. Andrologia. 2022;54(1):e14275. https://doi.org/10.1111/and.14275. Epub 2021 Oct 17. PMID: 34658054.

37. Ni K, Steger K, Yang H, Wang H, Hu K, Zhang T, Chen B. A comprehensive investigation of sperm DNA damage and oxidative stress injury in infertile patients with subclinical, normozoospermic, and astheno/oligozoospermic clinical varicocoele. Andrology. 2016;4(5):816–24. https://doi.org/10.1111/andr.12210. Epub 2016 May 24. PMID: 27218783.

38. Cho CL, Esteves SC, Agarwal A. Novel insights into the pathophysiology of varicocele and its association with reactive oxygen species and sperm DNA fragmentation. Asian J Androl. 2016;18(2):186–93. https://doi.org/10.4103/1008-682X.170441. PMID: 26732105; PMCID: PMC4770484.

39. Sharma R, Gupta S, Agarwal A, Henkel R, Finelli R, Parekh N, et al. Relevance of Leukocytospermia and semen culture and its true place in diagnosing and treating male infertility. World J Men's Health. 2022;40(2):191–207. https://doi.org/10.5534/wjmh.210063. Epub 2021 Jun 9. PMID: 34169683; PMCID: PMC8987138.

40. Lobascio AM, De Felici M, Anibaldi M, Greco P, Minasi MG, Greco E. Involvement of seminal leukocytes, reactive oxygen species, and sperm mitochondrial membrane potential in the DNA damage of the human spermatozoa. Andrology. 2015;3(2):265–70. https://doi.org/10.1111/andr.302. Epub 2015 Jan 19. PMID: 25598385.

41. Gallegos G, Ramos B, Santiso R, Goyanes V, Gosálvez J, Fernández JL. Sperm DNA fragmentation in infertile men with genitourinary infection by Chlamydia trachomatis and Mycoplasma. Fertil Steril. 2008;90(2):328–34. https://doi.org/10.1016/j.fertnstert.2007.06.035. Epub 2007 Oct 22. PMID: 17953955.

42. Eini F, Kutenaei MA, Zareei F, Dastjerdi ZS, Shirzeyli MH, Salehi E. Effect of bacterial infection on sperm quality and DNA fragmentation in subfertile men with Leukocytospermia. BMC Mol Cell Biol. 2021;22(1):42. https://doi.org/10.1186/s12860-021-00380-8. PMID: 34388964; PMCID: PMC8364116.

43. Leisegang K, Sengupta P, Agarwal A, Henkel R. Obesity and male infertility: mechanisms and management. Andrologia. 2021;53(1):e13617. https://doi.org/10.1111/and.13617. Epub 2020 May 12. PMID: 32399992.

44. Dupont C, Faure C, Sermondade N, Boubaya M, Eustache F, Clément P, Briot P, Berthaut I, Levy V, Cedrin-Durnerin I, Benzacken B, Chavatte-Palmer P, Levy R. Obesity leads to higher risk of sperm DNA damage in infertile patients. Asian J Androl. 2013;15(5):622–5. https://doi.org/10.1038/aja.2013.65. Epub 2013 Jun 24. PMID: 23792341; PMCID: PMC3881654.

45. Zhou L, Han L, Liu M, Lu J, Pan S. Impact of metabolic syndrome on sex hormones and reproductive function: a meta-analysis of 2923 cases and 14062 controls. Aging. 2020;13(2):1962–71. https://doi.org/10.18632/aging.202160. Epub 2020 Dec 1. PMID: 33260149; PMCID: PMC7880347.

46. Condorelli RA, La Vignera S, Mongioì LM, Alamo A, Calogero AE. Diabetes mellitus and infertility: different pathophysiological effects in type 1 and type 2 on sperm function. Front Endocrinol. 2018;9:268. https://doi.org/10.3389/fendo.2018.00268. PMID: 29887834; PMCID: PMC5980990.

47. Agbaje IM, McVicar CM, Schock BC, McClure N, Atkinson AB, Rogers D, Lewis SE. Increased concentrations of the oxidative DNA adduct 7,8-dihydro-8-oxo-2--deoxyguanosine in the germ-line of men with type 1 diabetes. Reprod Biomed Online. 2008;16(3):401–9. https://doi.org/10.1016/s1472-6483(10)60602-5.

48. Rama Raju GA, Jaya Prakash G, Murali Krishna K, Madan K, Siva Narayana T, Ravi Krishna CH. Noninsulin-dependent diabetes mellitus: effects on sperm morphological and functional characteristics, nuclear DNA integrity and outcome of assisted reproductive technique. Andrologia. 2012;44(1):490–8. https://doi.org/10.1111/j.1439-0272.2011.01213.x. Epub 2011 Aug 2. PMID: 21806668.

49. Elshal MF, El-Sayed IH, Elsaied MA, El-Masry SA, Kumosani TA. Sperm head defects and disturbances in spermatozoal chromatin and DNA integrities in idiopathic infertile subjects: association with cigarette smoking. Clin Biochem. 2009;42(7-8):589–94. https://doi.org/10.1016/j.clinbiochem.2008.11.012. Epub 2008 Dec 6. PMID: 19094977.

50. Taha EA, Ezz-Aldin AM, Sayed SK, Ghandour NM, Mostafa T. Smoking influence on sperm vitality, DNA fragmentation, reactive oxygen species and zinc in oligoasthenoterato-

zoospermic men with varicocele. Andrologia. 2014;46(6):687–91. https://doi.org/10.1111/and.12136. Epub 2013 Jul 19. PMID: 23866014.

51. Condorelli RA, La Vignera S, Giacone F, Iacoviello L, Vicari E, Mongioi' L, Calogero AE. In vitro effects of nicotine on sperm motility and bio-functional flow cytometry sperm parameters. Int J Immunopathol Pharmacol. 2013;26(3):739–46. https://doi.org/10.1177/039463201302600317. PMID: 24067470.

52. Kumar SB, Chawla B, Bisht S, Yadav RK, Dada R. Tobacco use increases oxidative DNA damage in sperm - possible etiology of childhood cancer. Asian Pac J Cancer Prev. 2015;16(16):6967–72. https://doi.org/10.7314/apjcp.2015.16.16.6967. PMID: 26514476.

53. Shen HM, Chia SE, Ni ZY, New AL, Lee BL, Ong CN. Detection of oxidative DNA damage in human sperm and the association with cigarette smoking. Reprod Toxicol. 1997;11(5):675–80. https://doi.org/10.1016/s0890-6238(97)00032-4. PMID: 9311575.

54. Ranganathan P, Rao KA, Sudan JJ, Balasundaram S. Cadmium effects on sperm morphology and semenogelin with relates to increased ROS in infertile smokers: an in vitro and in silico approach. Reprod Biol. 2018;18(2):189–97. https://doi.org/10.1016/j.repbio.2018.04.003. Epub 2018 May 3. PMID: 29729841.

55. Sipinen V, Laubenthal J, Baumgartner A, Cemeli E, Linschooten JO, Godschalk RW, Van Schooten FJ, Anderson D, Brunborg G. In vitro evaluation of baseline and induced DNA damage in human sperm exposed to benzo[a]pyrene or its metabolite benzo[a]pyrene-7,8-diol-9,10-epoxide, using the comet assay. Mutagenesis. 2010;25(4):417–25. https://doi.org/10.1093/mutage/geq024. Epub 2010 May 20. PMID: 20488941; PMCID: PMC2893308.

56. Saleh RA, Agarwal A, Sharma RK, Nelson DR, Thomas AJ Jr. Effect of cigarette smoking on levels of seminal oxidative stress in infertile men: a prospective study. Fertil Steril. 2002;78(3):491–9. https://doi.org/10.1016/s0015-0282(02)03294-6. PMID: 12215323.

57. Antoniassi MP, Intasqui P, Camargo M, Zylbersztejn DS, Carvalho VM, Cardozo KH, Bertolla RP. Analysis of the functional aspects and seminal plasma proteomic profile of sperm from smokers. BJU Int. 2016;118(5):814–22. https://doi.org/10.1111/bju.13539. Epub 2016 Jun 20.

58. Xu DX, Shen HM, Zhu QX, Chua L, Wang QN, Chia SE, Ong CN. The associations among semen quality, oxidative DNA damage in human spermatozoa and concentrations of cadmium, lead and selenium in seminal plasma. Mutat Res. 2003;534(1-2):155–63. https://doi.org/10.1016/s1383-5718(02)00274-7. PMID: 12504764.

59. Gunes S, Metin Mahmutoglu A, Arslan MA, Henkel R. Smoking-induced genetic and epigenetic alterations in infertile men. Andrologia. 2018;50(9):e13124. https://doi.org/10.1111/and.13124. Epub 2018 Aug 22. PMID: 30132931.

60. Cui X, Jing X, Wu X, Wang Z, Li Q. Potential effect of smoking on semen quality through DNA damage and the downregulation of Chk1 in sperm. Mol Med Rep. 2016;14(1):753–61. https://doi.org/10.3892/mmr.2016.5318. Epub 2016 May 20. PMID: 27221653; PMCID: PMC4918538.

61. Calogero A, Polosa R, Perdichizzi A, Guarino F, La Vignera S, Scarfia A, Fratantonio E, Condorelli R, Bonanno O, Barone N, Burrello N, D'Agata R, Vicari E. Cigarette smoke extract immobilizes human spermatozoa and induces sperm apoptosis. Reprod Biomed Online. 2009;19(4):564–71. https://doi.org/10.1016/j.rbmo.2009.05.004.

62. Finelli R, Mottola F, Agarwal A. Impact of alcohol consumption on male fertility potential: a narrative review. Int J Environ Res Public Health. 2021;19(1):328. https://doi.org/10.3390/ijerph19010328. PMID: 35010587; PMCID: PMC8751073.

63. Aboulmaouahib S, Madkour A, Kaarouch I, Sefrioui O, Saadani B, Copin H, Benkhalifa M, Louanjli N, Cadi R. Impact of alcohol and cigarette smoking consumption in male fertility potential: looks at lipid peroxidation, enzymatic antioxidant activities and sperm DNA damage. Andrologia. 2018;50(3):12926. https://doi.org/10.1111/and.12926. Epub 2017 Nov 21.

64. Durairajanayagam D. Lifestyle causes of male infertility. Arab J Urol. 2018;16(1):10–20. https://doi.org/10.1016/j.aju.2017.12.004. PMID: 29713532; PMCID: PMC5922227.

65. Gill K, Jakubik J, Kups M, Rosiak-Gill A, Kurzawa R, Kurpisz M, Fraczek M, Piasecka M. The impact of sedentary work on sperm nuclear DNA integrity. Folia Histochem

Cytobiol. 2019;57(1):15–22. https://doi.org/10.5603/FHC.a2019.0002. Epub 2019 Mar 14. PMID: 30869154.

66. Jurewicz J, Radwan M, Sobala W, Radwan P, Bochenek M, Hanke W. Dietary patterns and their relationship with semen quality. Am J Mens Health. 2018;12(3):575–83. https://doi.org/10.1177/1557988315627139. Epub 2016 Jan 27. PMID: 26819182; PMCID: PMC5987950.

67. Zhou DD, Hao JL, Guo KM, Lu CW, Liu XD. Sperm quality and DNA damage in men from Jilin Province, China, who are occupationally exposed to ionizing radiation. Genet Mol Res. 2016;15(1):8078. https://doi.org/10.4238/gmr.15018078. PMID: 27050976.

68. Miranda-Contreras L, Gómez-Pérez R, Rojas G, Cruz I, Berrueta L, Salmen S, Colmenares M, Barreto S, Balza A, Zavala L, Morales Y, Molina Y, Valeri L, Contreras CA, Osuna JA. Occupational exposure to organophosphate and carbamate pesticides affects sperm chromatin integrity and reproductive hormone levels among Venezuelan farm workers. J Occup Health. 2013;55(3):195–203. https://doi.org/10.1539/joh.12-0144-fs. Epub 2013 Feb 27. PMID: 23445617.

69. Migliore L, Naccarati A, Zanello A, Scarpato R, Bramanti L, Mariani M. Assessment of sperm DNA integrity in workers exposed to styrene. Hum Reprod. 2002;17(11):2912–8. https://doi.org/10.1093/humrep/17.11.2912. PMID: 12407048.

70. Irnandi DF, Hinting A, Yudiwati R. DNA fragmentation of sperm in automobile painters. Toxicol Ind Health. 2021;37(4):182–8. https://doi.org/10.1177/0748233721989892. Epub 2021 Feb 17. PMID: 33594946.

71. Yadav H, Rai U, Singh R. Radiofrequency radiation: a possible threat to male fertility. Reprod Toxicol. 2021;100:90–100. https://doi.org/10.1016/j.reprotox.2021.01.007. Epub 2021 Jan 23. PMID: 33497741.

72. Fraczek M, Lewandowska A, Budzinska M, Kamieniczna M, Wojnar L, Gill K, Piasecka M, Kups M, Havrylyuk A, Chopyak V, Nakonechnyy J, Nakonechnyy A, Kurpisz M. The role of seminal oxidative stress scavenging system in the pathogenesis of sperm DNA damage in men exposed and not exposed to genital heat stress. Int J Environ Res Public Health. 2022;19(5):2713. https://doi.org/10.3390/ijerph19052713. PMID: 35270405; PMCID: PMC8910598.

73. Bosco L, Notari T, Ruvolo G, Roccheri MC, Martino C, Chiappetta R, Carone D, Lo Bosco G, Carrillo L, Raimondo S, Guglielmino A, Montano L. Sperm DNA fragmentation: an early and reliable marker of air pollution. Environ Toxicol Pharmacol. 2018;58:243–9. https://doi.org/10.1016/j.etap.2018.02.001. Epub 2018 Feb 7.

74. World Health Organization. WHO laboratory manual for the examination and processing of human semen. 6th ed. Geneva: World Health Organization; 2021.

75. Farkouh AN, Zayed AA. An obese 48-year-old man with progressive fatigue and decreased libido. Cleve Clin J Med. 2019;86(5):321–31. https://doi.org/10.3949/ccjm.86a.18097. PMID: 31066666.

76. Lira Neto FT, Roque M, Esteves SC. Effect of varicocelectomy on sperm deoxyribonucleic acid fragmentation rates in infertile men with clinical varicocele: a systematic review and meta-analysis. Fertil Steril. 2021;116(3):696–712. https://doi.org/10.1016/j.fertnstert.2021.04.003. Epub 2021 May 10. PMID: 33985792.

77. Abdelbaki SA, Sabry JH, Al-Adl AM, Sabry HH. The impact of coexisting sperm DNA fragmentation and seminal oxidative stress on the outcome of varicocelectomy in infertile patients: a prospective controlled study. Arab J Urol. 2017;15(2):131–9. https://doi.org/10.1016/j.aju.2017.03.002. PMID: 29071142; PMCID: PMC5653613.

78. Mir J, Franken D, Andrabi SW, Ashraf M, Rao K. Impact of weight loss on sperm DNA integrity in obese men. Andrologia. 2018;50:e12957. https://doi.org/10.1111/and.12957. PMID: 29388233.

79. Wood GJA, Tiseo BC, Paluello DV, de Martin H, Santo MA, Nahas W, Srougi M, Cocuzza M. Bariatric surgery impact on reproductive hormones, semen analysis, and sperm DNA fragmentation in men with severe obesity: prospective study. Obes Surg. 2020;30(12):4840–51. https://doi.org/10.1007/s11695-020-04851-3. Epub 2020 Jul 22. PMID: 32700180.

80. Greco E, Iacobelli M, Rienzi L, Ubaldi F, Ferrero S, Tesarik J. Reduction of the incidence of sperm DNA fragmentation by oral antioxidant treatment. J Androl. 2005;26(3):349–53. https://doi.org/10.2164/jandrol.04146. PMID: 15867002.

81. Omu AE, Al-Azemi MK, Kehinde EO, Anim JT, Oriowo MA, Mathew TC. Indications of the mechanisms involved in improved sperm parameters by zinc therapy. Med Princ Pract. 2008;17(2):108–16. https://doi.org/10.1159/000112963. Epub 2008 Feb 19. PMID: 18287793.

82. Martínez-Soto JC, Domingo JC, Cordobilla B, Nicolás M, Fernández L, Albero P, Gadea J, Landeras J. Dietary supplementation with docosahexaenoic acid (DHA) improves seminal antioxidant status and decreases sperm DNA fragmentation. Syst Biol Reprod Med. 2016;62(6):387–95. https://doi.org/10.1080/19396368.2016.1246623. Epub 2016 Oct 28. PMID: 27792396.

83. Greco E, Romano S, Iacobelli M, Ferrero S, Baroni E, Minasi MG, Ubaldi F, Rienzi L, Tesarik J. ICSI in cases of sperm DNA damage: beneficial effect of oral antioxidant treatment. Hum Reprod. 2005;20(9):2590–4. https://doi.org/10.1093/humrep/dei091. Epub 2005 Jun 2. PMID: 15932912.

84. Alahmar AT, Sengupta P, Dutta S, Calogero AE. Coenzyme Q10, oxidative stress markers, and sperm DNA damage in men with idiopathic oligoasthenoteratospermia. Clin Exp Reprod Med. 2021;48(2):150–5. https://doi.org/10.5653/cerm.2020.04084. Epub 2021 May 25. PMID: 34078008; PMCID: PMC8176152.

85. Jannatifar R, Cheraghi E, Nasr-Esfahani MH, Piroozmanesh H. Association of heat shock protein A2 expression and sperm quality after N-acetyl-cysteine supplementation in astheno-terato-zoospermic infertile men. Andrologia. 2021;53(5):e14024. https://doi.org/10.1111/and.14024. Epub 2021 Mar 4. PMID: 33661545.

86. Ozer C. Antioxidant treatment of increased sperm DNA fragmentation: complex combinations are not more successful. Arch Ital Urol Androl. 2020;92(4):362. https://doi.org/10.4081/aiua.2020.4.362. PMID: 33348968.

87. Majzoub A, Agarwal A. Systematic review of antioxidant types and doses in male infertility: benefits on semen parameters, advanced sperm function, assisted reproduction and live-birth rate. Arab J Urol. 2018;16(1):113–24. https://doi.org/10.1016/j.aju.2017.11.013. PMID: 29713542; PMCID: PMC5922223.

88. Steiner AZ, Hansen KR, Barnhart KT, Cedars MI, Legro RS, Diamond MP, Krawetz SA, Usadi R, Baker VL, Coward RM, Huang H, Wild R, Masson P, Smith JF, Santoro N, Eisenberg E, Zhang H. The effect of antioxidants on male factor infertility: the males, antioxidants, and infertility (MOXI) randomized clinical trial. Fertil Steril. 2020;113(3):552–60. https://doi.org/10.1016/j.fertnstert.2019.11.008. Epub 2020 Feb 25. PMID: 32111479; PMCID: PMC7219515.

89. Schisterman EF, Sjaarda LA, Clemons T, Carrell DT, Perkins NJ, Johnstone E, Lamb D, Chaney K, Van Voorhis BJ, Ryan G, Summers K, Hotaling J, Robins J, Mills JL, Mendola P, Chen Z, DeVilbiss EA, Peterson CM, Mumford SL. Effect of folic acid and zinc supplementation in men on semen quality and live birth among couples undergoing infertility treatment: a randomized clinical trial. JAMA. 2020;323(1):35–48. https://doi.org/10.1001/jama.2019.18714.

90. Rashki Ghaleno L, Alizadeh A, Drevet JR, Shahverdi A, Valojerdi MR. Oxidation of sperm DNA and male infertility. Antioxidants. 2021;10(1):97. https://doi.org/10.3390/antiox10010097. PMID: 33445539; PMCID: PMC7827380.

91. Henkel R, Sandhu IS, Agarwal A. The excessive use of antioxidant therapy: a possible cause of male infertility? Andrologia. 2019;51(1):e13162. https://doi.org/10.1111/and.13162. Epub 2018 Sep 26. PMID: 30259539.

92. Martinez M, Majzoub A. Best laboratory practices and therapeutic interventions to reduce sperm DNA damage. Andrologia. 2021;53(2):e13736. https://doi.org/10.1111/and.13736. Epub 2020 Jul 14. PMID: 32662555.

93. Santi D, Spaggiari G, Simoni M. Sperm DNA fragmentation index as a promising predictive tool for male infertility diagnosis and treatment management - meta-analyses. Reprod

Biomed Online. 2018;37(3):315–26. https://doi.org/10.1016/j.rbmo.2018.06.023. Epub 2018 Jul 10. PMID: 30314886.

94. Muratori M, Baldi E. Effects of FSH on sperm DNA fragmentation: review of clinical studies and possible mechanisms of action. Front Endocrinol. 2018;9:734. https://doi.org/10.3389/fendo.2018.00734. PMID: 30619081; PMCID: PMC6297197.

95. Kooshesh L, Bahmanpour S, Zeighami S, Nasr-Esfahani MH. Effect of letrozole on sperm parameters, chromatin status and ROS level in idiopathic oligo/astheno/teratozoospermia. Reprod Biol Endocrinol. 2020;18(1):47. https://doi.org/10.1186/s12958-020-00591-2. PMID: 32404173; PMCID: PMC7218838.

96. Hanson BM, Aston KI, Jenkins TG, Carrell DT, Hotaling JM. The impact of ejaculatory abstinence on semen analysis parameters: a systematic review. J Assist Reprod Genet. 2018;35(2):213–20.

97. Ramos L, De Boer P, Meuleman EJ, Braat DD, Wetzels AM. Evaluation of ICSI-selected epididymal sperm samples of obstructive azoospermic males by the CKIA system. J Androl. 2004;25(3):406–11.

98. Said TM, Land JA. Effects of advanced selection methods on sperm quality and ART outcome: a systematic review. Hum Reprod Update. 2011;17(6):719–33.

99. Strassburger D, Friedler S, Raziel A, Schachter M, Kasterstein E, Ronel R. Very low sperm count affects the result of intracytoplasmic sperm injection. J Assist Reprod Genet. 2000;17:431–6.

100. Greco E, Scarselli F, Lacobelli M, Rienzi L, Ubaldi F, Ferrero S, Franco G, Anniballo N, Mendoza C, Tesarik J. Efficient treatment of infertility due to sperm DNA damage by ICSI with testicular spermatozoa. Hum Reprod. 2005;20:226–30.

101. Suganuma R, Yanagimachi R, Meistrich ML. Decline in fertility of mouse sperm with abnormal chromatin during epididymal passage as revealed by ICSI. Hum Reprod. 2005;20(11):3101–8.

102. Esteves SC, Roque M, Bradley CK, Garrido N. Reproductive outcomes of testicular versus ejaculated sperm for intracytoplasmic sperm injection among men with high levels of DNA fragmentation in semen: systematic review and meta-analysis. Fertil Steril. 2017;108(3):456–67.

103. Tharakan T, Bettocchi C, Carvalho J, Corona G, Jones TH, Kadioglu A, Salamanca JIM, Serefoglu EC, Verze P, Salonia A, Minhas S, EAU Working Panel on Male Sexual Reproductive Health. European Association of Urology Guidelines Panel on male sexual and reproductive health: a clinical consultation guide on the indications for performing sperm DNA fragmentation testing in men with infertility and testicular sperm extraction in nonazoospermic men. Eur Urol Focus. 2022;8(1):339–50. https://doi.org/10.1016/j.euf.2020.12.017. Epub 2021 Jan 6. PMID: 33422457.

104. Bender Atik R, Christiansen OB, Elson J, Kolte AM, Lewis S, Middeldorp S, Nelen W, Peramo B, Quenby S, Vermeulen N, Goddijn M. ESHRE guideline: recurrent pregnancy loss. Hum Reprod Open. 2018;2018:4. https://doi.org/10.1093/hropen/hoy004. PMID: 31486805; PMCID: PMC6276652.

105. Tan J, Taskin O, Albert A, Bedaiwy MA. Association between sperm DNA fragmentation and idiopathic recurrent pregnancy loss: a systematic review and meta-analysis. Reprod Biomed Online. 2019;38(6):951–60. https://doi.org/10.1016/j.rbmo.2018.12.029. Epub 2018 Dec 22. PMID: 30979611.

106. Li Z, Wang L, Cai J, Huang H. Correlation of sperm DNA damage with IVF and ICSI outcomes: a systematic review and meta-analysis. J Assist Reprod Genet. 2006;23(9-10):367–76. https://doi.org/10.1007/s10815-006-9066-9. Epub 2006 Oct 4. PMID: 17019633; PMCID: PMC3455102.

107. Deng C, Li T, Xie Y, Guo Y, Yang QY, Liang X, Deng CH, Liu GH. Sperm DNA fragmentation index influences assisted reproductive technology outcome: a systematic review and meta-analysis combined with a retrospective cohort study. Andrologia. 2019;51(6):e13263. https://doi.org/10.1111/and.13263. Epub 2019 Mar 5. PMID: 30838696.

108. Ribas-Maynou J, Yeste M, Becerra-Tomás N, Aston KI, James ER, Salas-Huetos A. Clinical implications of sperm DNA damage in IVF and ICSI: updated systematic review and meta-analysis. Biol Rev Camb Philos Soc. 2021;96(4):1284–300. https://doi.org/10.1111/brv.12700. Epub 2021 Mar 1. PMID: 33644978.

109. Zini A. Are sperm chromatin and DNA defects relevant in the clinic? Syst Biol Reprod Med. 2011;57(1-2):78–85. https://doi.org/10.3109/19396368.2010.515704. Epub 2011 Jan 6. PMID: 21208147.

110. Osman A, Alsomait H, Seshadri S, El-Toukhy T, Khalaf Y. The effect of sperm DNA fragmentation on live birth rate after IVF or ICSI: a systematic review and meta-analysis. Reprod Biomed Online. 2015;30(2):120–7. https://doi.org/10.1016/j.rbmo.2014.10.018. Epub 2014 Nov 13. PMID: 25530036.

111. Farkouh A, Salvio G, Kuroda S, Saleh R, Vogiatzi P, Agarwal A. Sperm DNA integrity and male infertility: a narrative review and guide for the reproductive physicians. Transl Androl Urol. 2022;11(7):1023–44. https://doi.org/10.21037/tau-22-149. PMID: 35958895; PMCID: PMC9360512.

112. Agarwal A, Farkouh A, Parekh N, Zini A, Arafa M, Kandil H, et al. Sperm DNA fragmentation: a critical assessment of clinical practice guidelines. World J Men's Health. 2022;40(1):30–7. https://doi.org/10.5534/wjmh.210056. Epub 2021 Apr 21. PMID: 33988000; PMCID: PMC8761233.

Genetic Screening for Sperm Aneuploidy by Fluorescent In Situ Hybridization (FISH) in Severe Cases of Male Infertility

Sezgin Gunes and Nicolás Garrido

Introduction

Infertility is health and social problem affecting 15% of population at reproductive ages, with failure to conceive after 1 year of unprotected intercourse [1, 2].

When the man is not azoospermic then is is difficult to attribute the sole responsibility to the male for this condition, because of the lack of diagnostic tests reliably detecting male or semen characteristics to predict infertility, and because female contribution is also a key factor modulating couple's success. Fertile/infertile condition may change in short periods of time and with different partners.

Nevertheless, among men in reproductive age almost 10% seek medical counseling for infertility related problems [1] and male factor is the cause for 30% of infertility cases while 40% is due to female causes, leaving the last 30% to either a combination of both or unknown reasons [3, 4].

If no sperm is present within the ejaculate, or exists in lower counts, or showing inappropriate physiological or biochemical features not compensable by the oocyte, the result is male infertility.

Spermatogenesis is a complex process requiring precise coordination of the molecular pathways involved [5], and failures involve the creation of incompetent sperm cells unable to trigger a correct fertilization and embryonic development, growth, and implantation leading to a healthy child.

S. Gunes
Department of Medical Biology and Molecular Genetics Subsection, Ondokuz Mayıs University, Samsun, Turkey

N. Garrido (✉)
IVIRMA Global Research Alliance, Valencia, Spain

IVI Foundation, Valencia, Spain
e-mail: nicolas.garrido@ivirma.com

The output of spermatogenesis is the ejaculate, and the way to estimate its fertility potential is through the basic sperm analysis as described on the World Health Organization's (WHO) Manual's criteria [6], by measuring microscopic semen parameters such as concentration, motility, morphology, and viability.

However, it does not provide predictive information on the natural or the assisted reproduction treatment success chances [7]. In fact, about 30% of normozoospermic men are unable to achieve pregnancy [8].

Establishing a threshold to discriminate fertile from infertile ejaculates based on the results of the conventional semen analysis is not possible, since approximately 40% of infertile men have normal parameters [9, 10] making it impossible to make a final diagnosis of infertility based on the classical semen analysis approaches [11].

In any case, male infertility seems to be a multifactorial disorder caused by a wide variety of factors, some impeding conception, while others can be considered as infertility risk factors that may delay it or induce the use of complex assisted reproduction techniques to overcome their physiological limitations.

They include, but are not limited to, chromosomal abnormalities, infections, single gene mutations, varicocele, hormonal disbalances, reproductive tract obstructions [12].

Despite proper diagnostic work-up, given that the detailed knowledge of the process of normal conception is still limited, the cause of infertility is unknown in about half of these cases [12]. Facing that situation, a more detailed physical and clinical examination should be performed [2] probably after using the basic sperm analysis results as a first screening for other underlying infertility causes and also to detect, based on its result, men at risk of having another alteration, such as genetic defects.

When there is no identifiable cause and the results of the semen analysis are normal, patients are categorized as having unexplained male infertility [13] meaning that abnormalities are probably present, but are overlooked by general diagnostic approaches, since the clinical evaluation of male infertility usually does not scrutinize certain aspects and markers of the sperm physiology related to fertility and genetic integrity.

Genetic defects may be in part or completely related to the real cause of infertility in such men. Given that assisted reproductive technology (ART) provides high success rates regardless of the primary infertility cause, this is frequently the medical approach for couples with unexplained infertility, without even identifying the underlying reasons causing the lack of fertility, thus missing the risks evaluation process.

Male infertility can be the end result of a number of genetic disorders, including chromosomal aberrations, monogenic disorders and multifactorial genetic alterations such as epigenetic modifications that influence fertility at both pre- and post-testicular levels, specifically involving the hypothalamic-pituitary axis and overall testicular function, causing spermatogenic defects and altering expression/function of specific genes and areas of critical importance outside the coding regions.

More than 3000 genes are estimated to be involved to some extent in the process of spermatogenesis and male reproductive pathway competence [14] therefore demonstrating that there is a highly intricate genetic interaction resulting in increased heterogeneity in infertility presentations among males [15].

Generally, genetic abnormalities are observed in 13–30% of infertile men [13, 16] with severe presentations of infertility, oligozoospermia or azoospermia, in 20–30% of the cases, whereas 12–40% of infertile men lacking a specific diagnosis are suspected to have a background of genetic association [17–19].

Genetic factors play an important role in the causes of male infertility, including well-accepted genetic causes of human male infertility such as variant karyotypes (e.g., 47, XXY for Klinefelter syndrome) and submicroscopic genomic deletions on the Y chromosome (Yq) [20].

In a study of almost 2000 azoospermic men, 21% were provided with a molecular diagnosis, including 15% with Klinefelter syndrome and 2% with Yq deletions [21], while others were found to have malignancies, obstruction, and endocrine/chronic diseases, leaving for the remaining 46% an "unknown infertility" cause.

However, genetically abnormal spermatozoa, if employed in ART, may generate a wide range of adverse outcomes, from abnormal embryo development that may either cause arrest, fail to implant or result in an increased risk of miscarriage and defects in the offspring [22]. Therefore, it is mandatory to determine the origin of the problem to allow appropriate counseling and management.

The absence of sperm, or the presence of abnormal sperm, in the ejaculate, as well as repeated ART failures may reflect genetic disorders that, unless are specifically characterized, will remain elusive to the etiological evaluation. Most importantly, these may harbor risks not only for reproductive success, but also for the offspring.

Among genetic problems in sperm, aneuploidy is an important cause of early pregnancy loss, offspring cognitive and developmental disorders, and infertility in humans. From 10–30% of all fertilized human eggs exhibit an incorrect number of chromosomes, most being either trisomic or monosomic [23], and embryo aneuploidy has been suggested to be originated either at the stage of germ cell production (due to meiotic errors) or at a post-zygotic level (mitotic missegregation).

Concerning the first, male contribution to meiotic-origin embryo aneuploidies occurs when an aneuploid sperm fertilizes a euploid oocyte, and this may come from cytogenetic abnormalities found on the somatic cells, or only within the germline.

Infertile men frequently show cytogenetic anomalies, and some of them can be detected by karyotype, but those resulting from impaired meiosis are limited to the germ cell line only [24, 25].

The processes of synapsis, recombination, and DNA repair may induce abnormal segregation of homologous chromosomes in meiosis I or sister chromatids in meiosis II and deliver spermatozoa with numerical chromosome abnormalities.

Fluorescence in situ hybridization (FISH) has been used the most to analyze sperm aneuploidies in the past 20 years, and most publications have shown higher incidence of sperm aneuploidies in infertile males compared to the fertile population [26]. Although clinical indications for FISH analysis of sperm are not clearly defined, it has been applied mainly to patients with severely impaired sperm parameters and to couples with a clinical history of recurrent miscarriage (RM) or repeated implantation failure (RIF) [27–32].

In this chapter, we provide an overview of the current clinical indications of FISH in male infertility, along with essential information for healthcare professionals to utilize this test in practice to identify chromosomal abnormalities in sperm. Increasing awareness regarding the use of this tool may help improve the medical management of infertile men and enhance male infertility research.

Chromosomal Content in Sperm, How to Measure It

Spermatogenesis is an organized and productive process in the developing of primordial male germ cells into mature spermatozoa involving proliferation and differentiation via mitosis, meiosis, and spermiogenesis [33]. The first phase is the proliferative process that involves a series of mitotic cell divisions by which the undifferentiated diploid spermatogonial cells (types A and B) called spermatogonia are transformed into primary spermatocytes, which undergo a meiotic process. During the second phase of spermatogenesis, chromosome pairing, crossover, and genetic exchange occur [33–35]. The diploid genome of spermatocyte ($2n$) is reduced to haploid spermatids (n) by two successive cell divisions, meiosis I and II.

Numerical chromosomal aberration of a cell/organism is called aneuploidy which is the leading cause of infertility, pregnancy loss, developmental disorders, and mental retardation of fetuses [23] (Fig. 11.1). Aneuploidies originate from the nondisjunction of sister chromatids and anaphase lagging during meiosis.

Formerly, sperm aneuploidies were detected using conventional karyotype testing. However, nowadays, new methods have been developed, such as a multicolor FISH method for detecting of aneuploidies in sperm nuclei and new sequencing technologies such as next-generation sequencing [36]. The sperm FISH assay is based on identification of multiple chromosomes and or chromosomal segments depends on the spectral properties of chromosomes [37]. Fixation of the epididymal, ejaculated or testicular sperm cells, decondensation, hybridization, post-hybridization, and visualization are five steps of sperm FISH analysis. Briefly, haploid spermatozoal chromosomes are fixed and then decondensate on the slide. After fixation and decondensation, the chromosomes are fluorescently labeled with DNA probes for the specific chromosomes that are analyzed and hybridized. Then, slides are washed and viewed via fluorescent microscopy [38]. Sperm FISH assay gives a relative prediction of the frequency of chromosomal abnormalities in sperm such as disomy, diploidy, and nullisomy. One blue, green, and red signal must be given with reference to chromosome 18, X and Y, respectively, in each normal spermatozoon. In addition, every normal spermatozoon must be differentiated for chromosomes 13 and 21 by giving signals in green and red, respectively. Scoring a large quantity of sperm nuclei is necessary to reach the statistical power for precise quantification of sperm aneuploidy [39]. A study suggested the use of a non-parametric

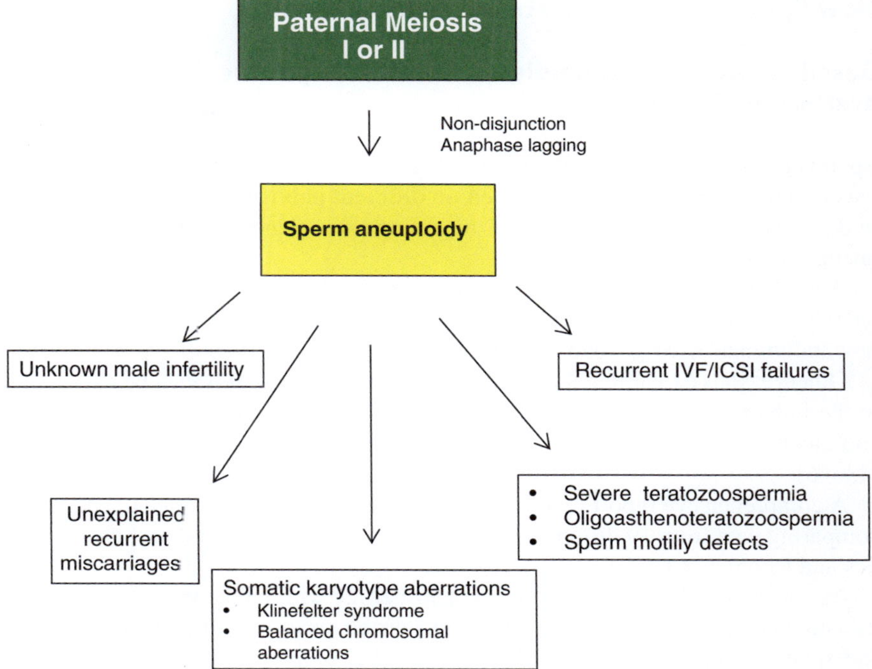

Fig. 11.1 Mechanisms of sperm aneuploidy and their consequences

Wilcoxon Rank Sum test for the statistical evaluation of sperm FISH data, including diploidy, nullisomy, disomy, and a total of 13 chromosomes including 1, 2, 9, 13, 15, 16, 17, 18, 19, 21, 22, X, and Y in human sperm nuclei from 14 fertile men using automatized FISH [40]. Fertile men have been classified as normal or altered regarding the sperm aneuploidy with this approach [40]. Correct assessment of sperm aneuploidy must be performed using standardized evaluation criteria. Indeed, there is no consensus on which statistical analysis of sperm FISH evaluation should be used [38]. The major limitation of the analysis is the laboriousness of the assignment of all chromosomes of spermatozoa. Evaluation of the frequency of clinically relevant chromosomes, including 13, 18, 21, X, and Y is sufficient to reveal the presence of meiotic defects [41]. Branch et al. assessed human sperm aneuploidy rate using semi-automated scoring of triple-probe FISH confocal microscopy and compared their results with manual methods. Their results showed that the method using spectral imaging on a confocal platform is feasible for assessing of sperm numerical chromosomal abnormalities and is comparable to manual methods [42].

How Sperm Ploidy Is Related with Male Fertility

Baseline Sperm Aneuploidies in Normozoospermic and Fertile Controls

Sperm chromosomal aneuploidies normal values have been defined after FISH analysis on normal donors and fertile men on different publications so far, revealing a wide variety of results, mainly regarding prevalence and distribution of aneuploidies.

Several technical reasons can be responsible for these different thresholds, namely, how the protocol is executed, how sample is processed and analyzed, and how individuals used as controls are categorized.

Other reasons explaining these different normality thresholds may be attributable to the influence of external exposures, related to lifestyle factors such as smoking and alcohol, disease and aging, and most importantly, a time-dependent variation [43–46].

A comprehensive report on the topic was published by Gambera and colleagues comparing data from 19 different studies selected on the basis of donor characteristics and techniques [47].

As controls, individuals being normozoospermic with unknown or known fertility, and donors with unknown semen parameters but proven fertility were employed, and sperm aneuploidy rate regarding 13, 18, 21, X, and Y chromosomes investigated, showing a clear variation among them. Quantitative alteration was given as the total frequency of aneuploidies.

Overall information about sperm chromosome autosomal disomy for each chromosome ranged from 0.05% to even 0.14% in normozoospermic and fertile, 0.23% in the normozoospermic group, and 0.09% in already fertile males.

Disomies for chromosomes 13, 18, and 21 have been extensively studied and provide statistically significant background for the interpretation of results. The disomy rate for each chromosome varied only slightly in the three groups and between groups, although chromosome 21 disomy was shown higher in the normozoospermic group, suggesting greater susceptibility to nondisjunction for this chromosome even under normal fertility conditions.

Other studies, for instance, have revealed a high aneuploidy frequency for chromosomes 14, 21, 22, X, and Y [46]. A review of the available literature revealed, interestingly, that only the disomy frequency of 21, X, and Y in reference subjects was increased. This information is highly relevant to establish the normality thresholds enabling us to decide what is abnormal, based on statistically significant differences between the observed rates in controls and in patients analyzed. Important to remark, first, that statistical significance largely depends on the sample size, the total number of sperm analyzed, on the control and the proband, and second, that statistically confirmed differences do not necessarily mean or imply clinically relevant changes.

Then, probably the best approach recommended is to describe each laboratory normality threshold based on own information to establish the normal values, related to clinical relevance.

Sperm Aneuploidies in Infertile Males

Concerning infertile males, there is an overall three-fold increase in the frequency of sperm aneuploidy (around 3%) compared with fertile cases [26, 46, 48] in unexplained infertility, recurrent miscarriage, in vitro fertilization (IVF) failure, and is associated with increased risk of chromosome abnormalities in newborns [26, 49].

Over the last 20 years, a strong correlation between male infertility/subfertility and sperm aneuploidy rates has been confirmed by several authors [50], and infertile males gametes exhibited a significantly higher rate of chromosomal abnormalities compared to the general population [51], and aneuploidy and diploidy frequencies have been directly related to a reduction in the number and progressive motility of sperm [25, 52, 53], high levels of follicle stimulating hormone (FSH), and previous in vitro fertilization (IVF) failures in normozoospermic patients [48].

Sperm Aneuploidies in Low Quality Sperm Samples

Several studies seem to confirm that the incidence of sperm aneuploidy increases proportionally with male factor severity, leading to conclude that in particular cases, paternal contribution to aneuploidy may be more important than that extrapolated from frequencies seen on products of conception and live births [54–57].

Sperm aneuploidy has been associated with severe sperm defects, [58, 59] and more specifically correlated with a relevant reduction in the number and progressive motility [25, 48, 52, 53], as several studies have demonstrated [60, 61], but also morphology, nuclear maturity and DNA fragmentation have been related with significantly high rate of sperm chromosomal defects [62–66].

Among all sperm alterations in the semen analysis, reduced sperm concentration seems to present the stronger association with chromosomal aneuploidies [28, 67, 68], and that may be explained by the already demonstrated correlation between severe quantitative impairment of spermatogenesis and problems with chromosome recombination and segregation during the process of spermatogenesis [48, 69, 70].

Among all, the most frequent nondisjunction happens on chromosomes other than sex chromosomes, given that X and Y are usually presenting only one crossover within the pseudoautosomal region. This may result in triple increase in the rate of disomies observed in chromosomes 13, 18, and 21 in patients with oligoasthenoteratozoospermia (OAT) compared with normozoospermic and fertile controls.

Sex chromosomes seem to be affected in particular in OAT cases, with mean disomy rates increased (mainly for XY disomy) to about 8 times higher than normozoospermic and fertile controls.

We can conclude that men with reduced spermatogenesis exhibit reduced genome-wide recombination directed toward chromosome-specific sperm defects. This may be evident even for each individual alteration within the basic sperm analysis results, concentration, motility, and morphology (particularly high in macrocephalic spermatozoa) in patients otherwise presenting normal karyotype [46, 48, 53, 60, 70–81].

Regarding specific morphologic traits, it was described that sperm with abnormal head morphology showed a frequency of structural chromosomal aberrations of about four times higher compared with those presenting normal morphology [82]. This data was confirmed by others using multicolor FISH analysis with frequency of chromosome 18 disomy approximately eight times higher than in normozoospermic and fertile control, and the same arises for the frequency of disomy for sex chromosomes. In particular, some specific morphological abnormalities are associated with chromosome imbalance, particularly those affecting the sperm head characteristics [83].

In presence of frequent aberrant morphological findings like macrocephalic, multinucleate, globozoospermic and multiflagellate sperm the aneuploidy rate may even rise ten times, as reported by various authors [29, 84–86].

Isolated asthenozoospermia, a rare finding alone, has been reported relevant regarding the presence of aneuploidies in sperm [52, 87, 88] where analyzing a range of chromosomes (1, 4, 8, 12, 13, 18, 21 and sex chromosomes) a noticeable increase on sperm disomy and diploidy rates were detected compared with the controls.

Even more, on particular cases of total asthenozoospermia attributable to anomalies of the flagella, as stump tail syndrome and Kartagener syndrome, or fibrous sheath dysplasia, abnormally high aneuploidy and diploidy rates were found [80, 89, 90].

Increases in sperm aneuploidy are strongly correlated with the severity of infertility, presenting the highest levels of aneuploidy in men with severe OAT and in cases of nonobstructive azoospermia (NOA) where sperm had to be retrieved from the testis [30, 51, 70, 91–94]

Sperm retrieved from epididymis or testicular tissue have a considerably increased risk of presenting aneuploidies [31, 54, 95] in the majority of studies available, including when comparing epididymal vs. ejaculated sperm [30, 31, 92–95].

All these may lead to the creation of embryos with increased rate of chromosomal abnormalities, leading to worse reproductive outcomes, thus requiring the appropriate genetic counseling pre-intracytoplasmic sperm injection (ICSI).

Diploidy of sex chromosomes with a total 24,XY and 24,YY chromosome is the most frequent sperm chromosome aberration of infertile males. Therefore, men with 47,XXY, 47,XYY and mosaics 47,XXY and 47,XYY are candidates for sperm FISH analysis. Hence, men with 47,XXY and 47,XYY karyotypes develop higher sex chromosomes diploidy than men with normal karyotype [96].

The association between age and numerical chromosomal aberrations of human spermatozoa are controversial; several studies showed that structural chromosomal rearrangements are more frequent than aneuploidies in older men [97]. On the hand, sperm analysis from men older than 50 years of age showed significantly higher sperm DNA damage and increased global aneuploidy, and a significantly increased number of embryos with any of trisomies in IVF/ICSI cycles [98].

Studies demonstrated that infertile men with NOA, severe OAT, and severe teratozoospermia are candidates for FISH aneuploidy screening [32, 63, 81]. Additionally, sperm samples retrieved from the testes are suggested to be potential candidates for FISH assay compared to sperm samples retrieved from the epididymis [31, 95]. Finally, men whose female partners are experiencing unexplained recurrent implantation failure (RIF) or recurrent pregnancy loss (RPL) and implantation failure following IVF are reported to get benefit from sperm FISH analysis [40].

Reproductive Outcomes in ART from Men Presenting Sperm Aneuploidies

There is a number of clinical research studies demonstrating a strong correlation between the aneuploidy rate of spermatozoa and ART outcomes, reflected in metrics like implantation, pregnancy, and miscarriage rates after ICSI in OAT males with abnormal FISH results [58, 59]. Additionally, paternally derived de novo chromosome abnormalities in embryos, fetuses, and newborns obtained after ICSI occur in 2–3% of conceptions, that is triple the prevalence of aneuplodies found in natural conceptions [99–101].

This is particularly relevant in cases of ICSI that has also been used in ART even in the absence of a male factor [102].

The main concern of this widespread use of ICSI regards the genetic quality of the embryologist's selected sperm, that bypasses any natural selection process happening in natural conceptions or conventional IVF [103], seemingly causing an approximate three-fold increase in de novo chromosome aberrations in ICSI derived offspring, mimicking the three-fold increase observed in aneuploidy detected in sperm from infertile men [104–106].

Sperm selection based on the observers' interpretation of the right sperm morphology is not always linked with genetic integrity, nor is an indicator of normal genetic constitution [61, 64], thus allowing the possibility of using a genetically incompetent sperm, causing embryo arrest, implantation failure or the transmission of chromosomal abnormalities to offspring.

This seems reinforced by the high aneuploidy rates and recurrent ART failures [56, 107] as well as the abnormally increased levels of aneuploidy in preimplantation embryos and lower pregnancy rates and live births [41, 54, 57, 68, 108, 109].

Embryos from ICSI treatments have higher sex chromosome aneuploidy rates (0.6% versus 0.2%) and autosomal structural alterations (0.4% versus 0.07%) than the general population, as shown in classic studies [105, 110].

Moderate increases in sperm aneuploidy in infertile men have also been postulated to contribute to the higher levels of aneuploid offspring conceived after ICSI [103].

It is well established that sperm aneuploidy is strongly correlated with embryo aneuploidy [108, 111] and also previous IVF failures even in normozoospermic patients [112].

Furthermore, it has been reported that some patients with normal semen parameters may also produce higher sperm aneuploidy levels which could be associated with RPL [113].

Rodrigo et al. evaluated the impact of sperm concentration, motility, morphology, and other indications for sperm FISH analysis on the incidence of numerical sperm abnormalities and also clinical outcome according to the incidence of sperm aneuploidy [114]. Interestingly, not all evidences point to the same direction, and in some cases, almost no effect of sperm aneuploidies on the outcome of ICSI has been reported [63, 115] showing similar fertilization, clinical pregnancy and losses, and, following live births, neonatal malformations.

This could be explained by potential bias toward having comparable results from analyzing only the first embryo transferred (for reproductive outcomes), or due to sperm selection methods applied, although some reports show that classic sperm selection methods do not seem efficient in selecting sperm with the right chromosomal load [116–118].

Another example, hyaluronic acid (HA)–sperm binding, was demonstrated as being able to recover almost 100% of euploid sperm [119], and this has also been reported in a other clinical trial with an overall reduction of miscarriage, thus potentially leading to a higher live birth rate per ICSI performed [120].

Preimplantation Genetic Testing for Aneuploidy (PGT-A) in Patients with Increased Sperm Aneuploidy

The clinical application of PGT-A in patients with increased sperm aneuploidy could lead to increased rates of clinical pregnancies per embryo transfer, reduced rates of miscarriages per pregnancy, lower time to pregnancy, subsequently improved live birth rates and children's health after ART, especially in the case of patients with unexplained RPL or recurrent implantation failure, who are also showing elevated levels of sperm aneuploidy. However, whether PGT-A may improve reproductive outcomes in these patients remains so far unproven, needing further investigation [121–123].

New technologies are being employed, changing from FISH to next-generation sequencing, and from day 3 blastomere biopsy to day 5 trophectoderm biopsy permitting the detection of chromosome mosaicisms and segmental aneuploidies, both of which appear to be common biological phenomena in the early preimplantation embryo [124, 125]. Segmental aneuploidies can be caused by a de novo error in meiosis or through a mitotic error during early gametogenesis. Relevant to the topic is that segmental aneuploidies are not correlated with maternal age and appear to be predominantly mitotic in origin [126].

A study by Rodrigo et al. [114] on couples with female $\leq$37 years old and with abnormal sperm FISH results evaluated PGT-A results from four different groups: (1) conventional IVF/ICSI cycles, in which embryos were selected for transfer on day 5/6 of development by morphological criteria, (2) a group of PGT-A cycles, in which embryos were biopsied in day 3 and 9 chromosomes were screened for aneuploidy by FISH, (3) a group of PGT-A cycles from patients in which 24 chromosomes were screened for aneuploidy in single-cell, day-three embryo biopsies by array comparative genome hybridization (aCGH) or next-generation sequencing (NGS), and (4) a group of PGT-A cycles from patients in which 24 chromosomes were screened for aneuploidy in trophectoderm.

The clinical outcomes were poorer in conventional IVF/ICSI cycles compared to PGT-A cycles, irrespective of the embryo biopsy day and number of chromosomes analyzed, with significant differences in livebirth rate per cycle.

Further research using the new PGT-A methodologies in appropriately designed clinical trials is needed to confirm the real benefit of these procedures for males exhibiting high sperm aneuploidy rates.

Solving Reproductive Problems Linked with Sperm Aneuploidy

Sperm aneuploidy has been found to be associated with paternally transmitted de novo numerical chromosomal aberrations in embryos, fetuses, and newborns conceived after ICSI. These numerical chromosomal abnormalities are 2–3% of ICSI conceptions and are three times higher than natural conceptions [106, 127]. Thus, the evaluation of sperm aneuploidies may be useful in in patient with idiopathic male infertility, structural chromosome rearrangements, Klinefelter syndrome, severe OAT and teratozoospermia, as well as in patients with unexplained or repeated IVF/ICSI RPL failures.

Sperm FISH aneuploidy screening offers a prognostic value as a clinical diagnostic tool to evaluate reproductive potential in infertile men. However, sperm aneuploidy testing has been of limited benefit because of technical difficulties of and/or the cost. High cost of multiple FISH probes and technical difficulties of the test leads to avoidance of the use of sperm aneuploidy testing [128]. In addition, sperm chromosome aneuploidy rate is low among the infertile men. These current problems limit the use of this test as a routine screening tool during male infertility evaluation. However, the assay is used as diagnostic tool in patients with certain pathologies, including severe morphological sperm defects, known structural chromosomal aberrations, unexplained RPL and implantation IVF failure, and increased risk of chromosomal abnormalities in newborns [49, 128]. Aberrations sperm FISH results may create genetic risk for offspring and indicate the necessity of genetic counseling and consideration of options such as preimplantation genetic testing for aneuploidy.

Conclusions

In summary, several male factor conditions linked with reproductive failure, as shown in recurrent miscarriage, RPL, implantation failure, and poor offspring health, could be related to embryo aneuploidy caused by sperm incorrect genetic load. FISH analysis may help in selected group of patients who may benefit from sperm aneuploidy screening such as carriers of chromosome aberrations, OAT, severe teratozoospermia, RM, and unexplained RPL or RIF. The assessment of embryo aneuploidy frequencies by means of FISH has been proposed as a prognostic indicator prior to ART.

Clinical Scenarios

Scenario 1

Couple where female is 34 years old and had experienced three embryo transfers from an IVF program, with both fresh and frozen/thawed embryos, resulting in two miscarriages. Recurrent abortion work-up and studies for the female resulted in normal findings, while sperm analysis shows a diminished sperm count of 12 mill/ml, 20% of motile spermatozoa, and 2.5 ml ejaculate volume. Normal karyotype on both.

Solution: Although not indicated by the total motile sperm count, offering FISH analysis to the couple may bring useful information since repeated failure including several miscarriages has occurred. Risk of having increased sperm aneuploidies exist and applying preimplantation tests to the embryos in future cycles might be advised if a positive result is found.

Scenario 2

Male, 48 years old, two consecutive semen analyzes without spermatozoa present within the ejaculate, normal volume and pH, high FSH, low testicular volume, undergoing TESE.

Solution: FISH is strongly recommended in these cases, if sufficient sperm are found, since the increase of aneuploidy risk is inversely proportional to the testicular production of sperm, mainly below 4–5 mill/ml within the ejaculate. If there is high aneuploidy then PGD-A should be considered.

Take Home Message

- Infertile males present increased risk of chromosomal abnormalities in sperm
- This can be found either in males with normal or abnormal basic semen parameters.

- The risk increases with the decrease on sperm basic analysis results, mainly on reduced counts and extremely abnormal morphology
- These aneuploidies are translated into worse reproductive outcomes
- Little is known about how to treat/avoid these, but applying preimplantation testing on embryos seems the most appropriate current option.

References

1. Esteves SC. A clinical appraisal of the genetic basis in unexplained male infertility. J Hum Reprod Sci. 2013;3:176–82.
2. Practice Committee of the American Society for Reproductive Medicine. Definitions of infertility and recurrent pregnancy loss: a committee opinion. Fertil Steril. 2013;99:63.
3. Vander Borght M, Wyns C. Fertility and infertility: definition and epidemiology. Clin Biochem. 2018;62:2–10.
4. Sharlip ID, Jarow JP, Belker AM, Lipshultz LI, Sigman M, Thomas AJ, Schlegel PN, Howards SS, Nehra A, Damewood MD, et al. Best practice policies for male infertility. Fertil Steril. 2002;77:873–82.
5. Matzuk MM, Lamb DJ. The biology of infertility: research advances and clinical challenges. Nat Med. 2008;14:1197–213.
6. World Health Organization, editor. WHO laboratory manual for the examination and processing of human semen. 6th ed. Geneva: World Health Organization; 2021.
7. Lewis SE. Is sperm evaluation useful in predicting human fertility? Reproduction. 2007;134:31–40.
8. Panner Selvam MK, Agarwal A, Pushparaj PN, Baskaran S, Bendou H. Sperm proteome analysis and identification of fertility-associated biomarkers in unexplained male infertility. Gene. 2019;10:522. https://doi.org/10.3390/genes10070522.
9. Esteves SC, Zini A, Aziz N, Alvarez JG, Sabanegh ES, Agarwal A. Critical appraisal of World Health Organization's new reference values for human semen characteristics and effect on diagnosis and treatment of subfertile men. Urology. 2012;79:16–22.
10. van der Steeg JW, Steures P, Eijkemans MJ, Habbema F, Hompes PG, Kremer JA, van der Leeuw-Harmsen L, Bossuyt PM, Repping S, Silber SJ, et al. Role of semen analysis in subfertile couples. Fertil Steril. 2011;95:1013–9.
11. Rybar R, Markova P, Veznik Z, Faldikova L, Kunetkova M, Zajicova A, Kopecka V, Rubes J. Sperm chromatin integrity in young men with no experiences of infertility and men from idiopathic infertility couples. Andrologia. 2009;41:141–9.
12. Kamel RM. Management of the infertile couple: an evidence-based protocol. Reprod Biol Endocrinol. 2010;8:21–7827.
13. Hamada A, Esteves SC, Nizza M, Agarwal A. Unexplained male infertility: diagnosis and management. Int Braz J Urol. 2012;38:576–94.
14. Neto FT, Bach PV, Najari BB, Li PS, Goldstein M. Genetics of male infertility. Curr Urol Rep. 2016;17:70–6.
15. Lee JD, Kamiguchi Y, Yanagimachi R. Analysis of chromosome constitution of human spermatozoa with normal and aberrant head morphologies after injection into mouse oocytes. Hum Reprod. 1996;11:1942–6.
16. Dohle GR, Halley DJ, Van Hemel JO, van den Ouwel AM, Pieters MH, Weber RF, Govaerts LC. Genetic risk factors in infertile men with severe oligozoospermia and azoospermia. Hum Reprod. 2002;17:13–6.
17. Garrido N, Hervas I. Personalized medicine in infertile men. Urol Clin North Am. 2020;47:245–55.

18. Dong Y, Pan Y, Wang R, Zhang Z, Xi Q, Liu RZ. Copy number variations in spermatogenic failure patients with chromosomal abnormalities and unexplained azoospermia. Genet Mol Res. 2015;14:16041–9.

19. Robay A, Abbasi S, Akil A, El-Bardisi H, Arafa M, Crystal RG, Fakhro KA. A systematic review on the genetics of male infertility in the era of next-generation sequencing. Arab J Urol. 2018;16:53–64.

20. Tuttelmann F, Ruckert C, Ropke A. Disorders of spermatogenesis: perspectives for novel genetic diagnostics after 20 years of unchanged routine. Med Genet. 2018;30:12–20.

21. Tuttelmann F, Werny F, Cooper TG, Kliesch S, Simoni M, Nieschlag E. Clinical experience with azoospermia: aetiology and chances for spermatozoa detection upon biopsy. Int J Androl. 2011;34:291–8.

22. Aitken RJ, Koopman P, Lewis SE. Seeds of concern. Nature. 2004;432:48–52.

23. Hassold T, Hunt P. To err (meiotically) is human: the genesis of human aneuploidy. Nat Rev Genet. 2001;2:280–91.

24. Egozcue J, Templado C, Vidal F, Navarro J, Morer-Fargas F, Marina S. Meiotic studies in a series of 1100 infertile and sterile males. Hum Genet. 1983;65:185–8.

25. Vendrell JM, Garcia F, Veiga A, Calderon G, Egozcue S, Egozcue J, Barri PN. Meiotic abnormalities and spermatogenic parameters in severe oligoasthenozoospermia. Hum Reprod. 1999;14:375–8.

26. Moosani N, Pattinson HA, Carter MD, Cox DM, Rademaker AW, Martin RH. Chromosomal analysis of sperm from men with idiopathic infertility using sperm karyotyping and fluorescence in situ hybridization. Fertil Steril. 1995;64:811–7.

27. Rubio C, Gil-Salom M, Simon C, Vidal F, Rodrigo L, Minguez Y, Remohi J, Pellicer A. Incidence of sperm chromosomal abnormalities in a risk population: relationship with sperm quality and ICSI outcome. Hum Reprod. 2001;16:2084–92.

28. Martin RH, Rademaker AW, Greene C, Ko E, Hoang T, Barclay L, Chernos J. A comparison of the frequency of sperm chromosome abnormalities in men with mild, moderate, and severe oligozoospermia. Biol Reprod. 2003;69:535–9.

29. Mateu E, Rodrigo L, Prados N, Gil-Salom M, Remohi J, Pellicer A, Rubio C. High incidence of chromosomal abnormalities in large-headed and multiple-tailed spermatozoa. J Androl. 2006;27:6–10.

30. Levron J, Aviram-Goldring A, Madgar I, Raviv G, Barkai G, Dor J. Sperm chromosome abnormalities in men with severe male factor infertility who are undergoing in vitro fertilization with intracytoplasmic sperm injection. Fertil Steril. 2001;76:479–84.

31. Rodrigo L, Rubio C, Mateu E, Simon C, Remohi J, Pellicer A, Gil-Salom M. Analysis of chromosomal abnormalities in testicular and epididymal spermatozoa from azoospermic ICSI patients by fluorescence in-situ hybridization. Hum Reprod. 2004;19:118–23.

32. Sarrate Z, Vidal F, Blanco J. Role of sperm fluorescent in situ hybridization studies in infertile patients: indications, study approach, and clinical relevance. Fertil Steril. 2010;93:1892–902.

33. Gunes S, Al-Sadaan M, Agarwal A. Spermatogenesis, DNA damage and DNA repair mechanisms in male infertility. Reprod Biomed Online. 2015;31:309–19.

34. Clermont Y. Kinetics of spermatogenesis in mammals: seminiferous epithelium cycle and spermatogonial renewal. Physiol Rev. 1972;52:198–236.

35. Neto FTL, Flannigan R, Goldstein M. Regulation of human spermatogenesis. Adv Exp Med Biol. 2021;1288:255–86.

36. Colaco S, Sakkas D. Paternal factors contributing to embryo quality. J Assist Reprod Genet. 2018;35:1953–68.

37. Liyanage M, Coleman A, Du Manoir S, Veldman T, McCormack S, Dickson RB, Barlow C, Wynshaw-Boris A, Janz S, Wienberg J, Ferguson-Smith MA, Schrock E, Ried T. Multicolour spectral karyotyping of mouse chromosomes. Nat Genet. 1996;14:312–5.

38. Sarrate Z, Anton E. Fluorescence in situ hybridization (fish) protocol in human sperm. J Vis Exp. 2009;31:1405.

39. Levsky JM, Singer RH. Fluorescence in situ hybridization: past, present and future. J Cell Sci. 2003;116:2833–8.

40. Garcia-Mengual E, Trivino JC, Saez-Cuevas A, Bataller J, Ruiz-Jorro M, Vendrell X. Male infertility: establishing sperm aneuploidy thresholds in the laboratory. J Assist Reprod Genet. 2019;36:371–81.
41. Sanchez-Castro M, Jimenez-Macedo AR, Sandalinas M, Blanco J. Prognostic value of sperm fluorescence in situ hybridization analysis over PGD. Hum Reprod. 2009;24:1516–21.
42. Branch F, Nguyen G, Porter N, Young HA, Martenies SE, Mccray N, Deloid G, Popratiloff A, Perry MJ. Semi-automated scoring of triple-probe fish in human sperm using confocal microscopy. Cytometry. 2017;91:859–66.
43. Bosch M, Rajmil O, Martinez-Pasarell O, Egozcue J, Templado C. Linear increase of diploidy in human sperm with age: a four-colour FISH study. Eur J Hum Genet. 2001;9:533–8.
44. Bosch M, Rajmil O, Egozcue J, Templado C. Linear increase of structural and numerical chromosome 9 abnormalities in human sperm regarding age. Eur J Hum Genet. 2003;11:754–9.
45. Naccarati A, Zanello A, Landi S, Consigli R, Migliore L. Sperm-FISH analysis and human monitoring: a study on workers occupationally exposed to styrene. Mutat Res. 2003;537:131–40.
46. Templado C, Bosch M, Benet J. Frequency and distribution of chromosome abnormalities in human spermatozoa. Cytogenet Genome Res. 2005;111:199–205.
47. Gambera L, Morgante G, Serafini F, et al. Human sperm aneuploidy: FISH analysis in fertile and infertile men. Expert Rev Obstet Gynecol. 2011;6:609–27.
48. Sarrate Z, Blanco J, Anton E, Egozcue S, Egozcue J, Vidal F. FISH studies of chromosome abnormalities in germ cells and its relevance in reproductive counseling. Asian J Androl. 2005;7:227–36.
49. Tempest HG, Martin RH. Cytogenetic risks in chromosomally normal infertile men. Curr Opin Obstet Gynecol. 2009;21:223–7.
50. Burrello N, Arcidiacono G, Vicari E, Asero P, Di Benedetto D, De Palma A, Romeo R, D'Agata R, Calogero AE. Morphologically normal spermatozoa of patients with secretory oligo-astheno-teratozoospermia have an increased aneuploidy rate. Hum Reprod. 2004;19:2298–302.
51. Egozcue J, Blanco J, Anton E, Egozcue S, Sarrate Z, Vidal F. Genetic analysis of sperm and implications of severe male infertility–a review. Placenta. 2003;24:62–5.
52. Collodel G, Capitani S, Baccetti B, Pammolli A, Moretti E. Sperm aneuploidies and low progressive motility. Hum Reprod. 2007;22:1893–8.
53. Vegetti W, Van Assche E, Frias A, Verheyen G, Bianchi MM, Bonduelle M, Liebaers I, Van Steirteghem A. Correlation between semen parameters and sperm aneuploidy rates investigated by fluorescence in-situ hybridization in infertile men. Hum Reprod. 2000;15:351–65.
54. Gianaroli L, Magli MC, Cavallini G, Crippa A, Nadalini M, Bernardini L, Menchini Fabris GF, Voliani S, Ferraretti AP. Frequency of aneuploidy in sperm from patients with extremely severe male factor infertility. Hum Reprod. 2005;20:2140–52.
55. Harton GL, Tempest HG. Chromosomal disorders and male infertility. Asian J Androl. 2012;14:32–9.
56. Kahraman S, Findikli N, Biricik A, Oncu N, Ogur C, Sertyel S, Karlikaya G, Karagozoglu H, Saglam Y. Preliminary FISH studies on spermatozoa and embryos in patients with variable degrees of teratozoospermia and a history of poor prognosis. Reprod Biomed Online. 2006;12:752–61.
57. Magli MC, Gianaroli L, Ferraretti AP, Gordts S, Fredericks V, Crippa A. Paternal contribution to aneuploidy in preimplantation embryos. Reprod Biomed Online. 2009;18:536–42.
58. Martinez G, Gillois P, Le Mitouard M, Borye R, Esquerre-Lamare C, Satre V, Bujan L, Hennebicq S. FISH and tips: a large scale analysis of automated versus manual scoring for sperm aneuploidy detection. Basic Clin Androl. 2013;23:13–4190.
59. Molina O, Sarrate Z, Vidal F, Blanco J. FISH on sperm: spot-counting to stop counting? Not yet. Fertil Steril. 2009;92:1474–80.
60. Ushijima C, Kumasako Y, Kihaile PE, Hirotsuru K, Utsunomiya T. Analysis of chromosomal abnormalities in human spermatozoa using multi-colour fluorescence in-situ hybridization. Hum Reprod. 2000;15:1107–11.

61. Celik-Ozenci C, Jakab A, Kovacs T, Catalanotti J, Demir R, Bray-Ward P, Ward D, Huszar G. Sperm selection for ICSI: shape properties do not predict the absence or presence of numerical chromosomal aberrations. Hum Reprod. 2004;19:2052–9.

62. Bernardini L, Borini A, Preti S, Conte N, Flamigni C, Capitanio GL, Venturini PL. Study of aneuploidy in normal and abnormal germ cells from semen of fertile and infertile men. Hum Reprod. 1998;13:3406–13.

63. Calogero AE, De Palma A, Grazioso C, Barone N, Burrello N, Palermo I, Gulisano A, Pafumi C, D'Agata R. High sperm aneuploidy rate in unselected infertile patients and its relationship with intracytoplasmic sperm injection outcome. Hum Reprod. 2001;16:1433–9.

64. Ryu HM, Lin WW, Lamb DJ, Chuang W, Lipshultz LI, Bischoff FZ. Increased chromosome X, Y, and 18 nondisjunction in sperm from infertile patients that were identified as normal by strict morphology: implication for intracytoplasmic sperm injection. Fertil Steril. 2001;76:879–83.

65. Carrell DT, Emery BR, Wilcox AL, Campbell B, Erickson L, Hatasaka HH, Jones KP, Peterson CM. Sperm chromosome aneuploidy as related to male factor infertility and some ultrastructure defects. Arch Androl. 2004;50:181–5.

66. Kovanci E, Kovacs T, Moretti E, Vigue L, Bray-Ward P, Ward DC, Huszar G. FISH assessment of aneuploidy frequencies in mature and immature human spermatozoa classified by the absence or presence of cytoplasmic retention. Hum Reprod. 2001;16:1209–17.

67. Ohashi Y, Miharu N, Honda H, Samura O, Ohama K. High frequency of XY disomy in spermatozoa of severe oligozoospermic men. Hum Reprod. 2001;16:703–8.

68. Nagvenkar P, Zaveri K, Hinduja I. Comparison of the sperm aneuploidy rate in severe oligozoospermic and oligozoospermic men and its relation to intracytoplasmic sperm injection outcome. Fertil Steril. 2005;84:925–31.

69. Egozcue J, Sarrate Z, Codina-Pascual M, Egozcue S, Oliver-Bonet M, Blanco J, Navarro J, Benet J, Vidal F. Meiotic abnormalities in infertile males. Cytogenet Genome Res. 2005;111:337–42.

70. Miharu N. Chromosome abnormalities in sperm from infertile men with normal somatic karyotypes: oligozoospermia. Cytogenet Genome Res. 2005;111:347–51.

71. Bernardini L, Martini E, Geraedts JP, Hopman AH, Lanteri S, Conte N, Capitanio GL. Comparison of gonosomal aneuploidy in spermatozoa of normal fertile men and those with severe male factor detected by in-situ hybridization. Mol Hum Reprod. 1997;3:431–8.

72. Lahdetie J, Saari N, Ajosenpaa-Saari M, Mykkanen J. Incidence of aneuploid spermatozoa among infertile men studied by multicolor fluorescence in situ hybridization. Am J Med Genet. 1997;71:115–21.

73. McInnes B, Rademaker A, Greene CA, Ko E, Barclay L, Martin RH. Abnormalities for chromosomes 13 and 21 detected in spermatozoa from infertile men. Hum Reprod. 1998;13:2787–90.

74. Storeng RT, Plachot M, Theophile D, Mandelbaum J, Belaisch-Allart J, Vekemans M. Incidence of sex chromosome abnormalities in spermatozoa from patients entering an IVF or ICSI protocol. Acta Obstet Gynecol Scand. 1998;77:191–7.

75. Pang MG, Hoegerman SF, Cuticchia AJ, Moon SY, Doncel GF, Acosta AA, Kearns WG. Detection of aneuploidy for chromosomes 4, 6, 7, 8, 9, 10, 11, 12, 13, 17, 18, 21, X and Y by fluorescence in-situ hybridization in spermatozoa from nine patients with oligoasthenoteratozoospermia undergoing intracytoplasmic sperm injection. Hum Reprod. 1999;14:1266–73.

76. Calogero AE, De Palma A, Grazioso C, Barone N, Romeo R, Rappazzo G, D'Agata R. Aneuploidy rate in spermatozoa of selected men with abnormal semen parameters. Hum Reprod. 2001;16:1172–9.

77. Rives N, Mousset-Simeon N, Sibert L, Duchesne V, Mace L, Milazzo JP, Mazurier S, Mace B. Chromosome abnormalities of spermatozoa. Gynecol Obstet Fertil. 2004;32:771–8.

78. Brahem S, Elghezal H, Ghedir H, Landolsi H, Amara A, Ibala S, Gribaa M, Saad A, Mehdi M. Cytogenetic and molecular aspects of absolute teratozoospermia: comparison between polymorphic and monomorphic forms. Urology. 2011;78:1313–9.

79. Brahem S, Mehdi M, Elghezal H, Saad A. Study of aneuploidy rate and sperm DNA fragmentation in large-headed, multiple-tailed spermatozoa. Andrologia. 2012;44:130–5.
80. Moretti E, Collodel G. Three cases of genetic defects affecting sperm tail: a FISH study. J Submicrosc Cytol Pathol. 2006;38:137–41.
81. Mehdi M, Gmidene A, Brahem S, Guerin JF, Elghezal H, Saad A. Aneuploidy rate in spermatozoa of selected men with severe teratozoospermia. Andrologia. 2012;44(Suppl 1):139–43.
82. Lee SR, Lee TH, Song SH, Kim DS, Choi KH, Lee JH, Kim DK. Update on genetic screening and treatment for infertile men with genetic disorders in the era of assisted reproductive technology. Clin Exp Reprod Med. 2021;48:283–94.
83. Sun F, Ko E, Martin RH. Is there a relationship between sperm chromosome abnormalities and sperm morphology? Reprod Biol Endocrinol. 2006;4:1–7827.
84. Carrell DT, Emery BR, Liu L. Characterization of aneuploidy rates, protamine levels, ultrastructure, and functional ability of round-headed sperm from two siblings and implications for intracytoplasmic sperm injection. Fertil Steril. 1999;71:511–6.
85. Carrell DT, Wilcox AL, Udoff LC, Thorp C, Campbell B. Chromosome 15 aneuploidy in the sperm and conceptus of a sibling with variable familial expression of round-headed sperm syndrome. Fertil Steril. 2001;76:1258–60.
86. Moretti E, Collodel G, Scapigliati G, Cosci I, Sartini B, Baccetti B. 'Round head' sperm defect. Ultrastructural and meiotic segregation study. J Submicrosc Cytol Pathol. 2005;37:297–303.
87. Aran B, Blanco J, Vidal F, Vendrell JM, Egozcue S, Barri PN, Egozcue J, Veiga A. Screening for abnormalities of chromosomes X, Y, and 18 and for diploidy in spermatozoa from infertile men participating in an in vitro fertilization-intracytoplasmic sperm injection program. Fertil Steril. 1999;72:696–701.
88. Bernardini LM, Calogero AE, Bottazzi C, Lanteri S, Venturini PL, Burrello N, De Palma A, Conte N, Ragni N. Low total normal motile count values are associated with increased sperm disomy and diploidy rates in infertile patients. Int J Androl. 2005;28:328–36.
89. Baccetti B, Collodel G, Gambera L, Moretti E, Serafini F, Piomboni P. Fluorescence in situ hybridization and molecular studies in infertile men with dysplasia of the fibrous sheath. Fertil Steril. 2005;84:123–9.
90. Rives N, Mousset-Simeon N, Mazurier S, Mace B. Primary flagellar abnormality is associated with an increased rate of spermatozoa aneuploidy. J Androl. 2005;26:61–9.
91. Vidal F, Blanco J, Egozcue J. Chromosomal abnormalities in sperm. Mol Cell Endocrinol. 2001;183(1):51–4.
92. Bernardini L, Gianaroli L, Fortini D, Conte N, Magli C, Cavani S, Gaggero G, Tindiglia C, Ragni N, Venturini PL. Frequency of hyper-, hypohaploidy and diploidy in ejaculate, epididymal and testicular germ cells of infertile patients. Hum Reprod. 2000;15:2165–72.
93. Burrello N, Calogero AE, De Palma A, Grazioso C, Torrisi C, Barone N, Pafumi C, D'Agata R, Vicari E. Chromosome analysis of epididymal and testicular spermatozoa in patients with azoospermia. Eur J Hum Genet. 2002;10:362–6.
94. Mateizel I, Verheyen G, Van Assche E, Tournaye H, Liebaers I, Van Steirteghem A. FISH analysis of chromosome X, Y and 18 abnormalities in testicular sperm from azoospermic patients. Hum Reprod. 2002;17:2249–57.
95. Palermo GD, Colombero LT, Hariprashad JJ, Schlegel PN, Rosenwaks Z. Chromosome analysis of epididymal and testicular sperm in azoospermic patients undergoing ICSI. Hum Reprod. 2002;17:570–5.
96. Caseiro AL, Regalo A, Pereira E, Esteves T, Fernandes F, Carvalho J. Implication of sperm chromosomal abnormalities in recurrent abortion and multiple implantation failure. Reprod Biomed Online. 2015;31:481–5.
97. Gunes S, Hekim GN, Arslan MA, Asci R. Effects of aging on the male reproductive system. J Assist Reprod Genet. 2016;33:441–54.
98. Garcia-Ferreyra J, Luna D, Villegas L, Romero R, Zavala P, Hilario R, Duenas-Chacon J. High aneuploidy rates observed in embryos derived from donated oocytes are related to male aging and high percentages of sperm DNA fragmentation. Clin Med Insights Reprod Health. 2015;9:21–7.

99. Netten H, Young IT, van Vliet LJ, Tanke HJ, Vroljik H, Sloos WC. FISH and chips: automation of fluorescent dot counting in interphase cell nuclei. Cytometry. 1997;28:1–10.
100. Perry MJ, Chen X, Lu X. Automated scoring of multiprobe FISH in human spermatozoa. Cytometry A. 2007;71:968–72.
101. Perry MJ, Chen X, McAuliffe ME, Maity A, Deloid GM. Semi-automated scoring of triple-probe FISH in human sperm: methods and further validation. Cytometry A. 2011;79:661–6.
102. Boulet SL, Mehta A, Kissin DM, Warner L, Kawwass JF, Jamieson DJ. Trends in use of and reproductive outcomes associated with intracytoplasmic sperm injection. JAMA. 2015;313:255–63.
103. Griffin DK, Hyland P, Tempest HG, Homa ST. Safety issues in assisted reproduction technology: should men undergoing ICSI be screened for chromosome abnormalities in their sperm? Hum Reprod. 2003;18:229–35.
104. Aboulghar H, Aboulghar M, Mansour R, Serour G, Amin Y, Al-Inany H. A prospective controlled study of karyotyping for 430 consecutive babies conceived through intracytoplasmic sperm injection. Fertil Steril. 2001;76:249–53.
105. Bonduelle M, Aytoz A, Van Assche E, Devroey P, Liebaers I, Van Steghem A. Incidence of chromosomal aberrations in children born after assisted reproduction through intracytoplasmic sperm injection. Hum Reprod. 1998;13:781–2.
106. Van Steirteghem A, Bonduelle M, Devroey P, Liebaers I. Follow-up of children born after ICSI. Hum Reprod Update. 2002;8:111–6.
107. Petit FM, Frydman N, Benkhalifa M, Le Du A, Aboura A, Fanchin R, Frydman R, Tachdjian G. Could sperm aneuploidy rate determination be used as a predictive test before intracytoplasmic sperm injection? J Androl. 2005;26:235–41.
108. Rodrigo L, Peinado V, Mateu E, Remohi J, Pellicer A, Simon C, Gil-Salom M, Rubio C. Impact of different patterns of sperm chromosomal abnormalities on the chromosomal constitution of preimplantation embryos. Fertil Steril. 2010;94:1380–6.
109. Coates A, Hesla JS, Hurliman A, Coate B, Holmes E, Matthews R, Mounts EL, Turner KJ, Thornhill AR, Griffin DK. Use of suboptimal sperm increases the risk of aneuploidy of the sex chromosomes in preimplantation blastocyst embryos. Fertil Steril. 2015;104:866–72.
110. Veld PA, Weber RF, Los FJ, den Hollander N, Dhont M, Pieters MH, Van Hemel JO. Two cases of Robertsonian translocations in oligozoospermic males and their consequences for pregnancies induced by intracytoplasmic sperm injection. Hum Reprod. 1997;12:1642–4.
111. Sills ES, Li X, Frederick JL, Khoury CD, Potter DA. Determining parental origin of embryo aneuploidy: analysis of genetic error observed in 305 embryos derived from anonymous donor oocyte IVF cycles. Mol Cytogenet. 2014;7:68. eCollection 2014.
112. Blanco J, Anton E, Sarrate Navas Z, Vidal Dominguez F. Diagnóstico genético del varón infértil: hibridación "in situ" fluorescente en espermatozoides. Folia Clín Obstetr Ginecol. 2006;59:54–9.
113. Ramasamy R, Scovell JM, Kovac JR, Cook PJ, Lamb DJ, Lipshultz LI. Fluorescence in situ hybridization detects increased sperm aneuploidy in men with recurrent pregnancy loss. Fertil Steril. 2015;103:906–909.e1.
114. Rodrigo L. Sperm genetic abnormalities and their contribution to embryo aneuploidy miscarriage. Best Pract Res Clin Endocrinol Metab. 2020;34:101477.
115. Colombero LT, Hariprashad JJ, Tsai MC, Rosenwaks Z, Palermo GD. Incidence of sperm aneuploidy in relation to semen characteristics and assisted reproductive outcome. Fertil Steril. 1999;72:90–6.
116. Samura O, Miharu N, He H, Okamoto E, Ohama K. Assessment of sex chromosome ratio and aneuploidy rate in motile spermatozoa selected by three different methods. Hum Reprod. 1997;12:2437–42.
117. Pfeffer J, Pang MG, Hoegerman SF, Osgood CJ, Stacey MW, Mayer J, Oehninger S, Kearns WG. Aneuploidy frequencies in semen fractions from ten oligoasthenoteratozoospermic patients donating sperm for intracytoplasmic sperm injection. Fertil Steril. 1999;72:472–8.

118. Van Dyk Q, Lanzendorf S, Kolm P, Hodgen GD, Mahony MC. Incidence of aneuploid spermatozoa from subfertile men: selected with motility versus hemizona-bound. Hum Reprod. 2000;15:1529–36.
119. Huszar G, Jakab A, Sakkas D, Ozenci CC, Cayli S, Delpiano E, Ozkavukcu S. Fertility testing and ICSI sperm selection by hyaluronic acid binding: clinical and genetic aspects. Reprod Biomed Online. 2007;14:650–63.
120. Miller D, Pavitt S, Sharma V, Forbes G, Hooper R, Bhattacharya S, Kirkman-Brown J, Coomarasamy A, Lewis S, Cutting R, Brison D, Pacey A, West R, Brian K, Griffin D, Khalaf Y. Physiological, hyaluronan-selected intracytoplasmic sperm injection for infertility treatment (HABSelect): a parallel, two-group, randomised trial. Lancet. 2019;393(10170):416–22.
121. Rubio C, Buendia P, Rodrigo L, Mercader A, Mateu E, Peinado V, Delgado A, Milan M, Mir P, Simon C, et al. Prognostic factors for preimplantation genetic screening in repeated pregnancy loss. Reprod Biomed Online. 2009;18:687–93.
122. Murugappan G, Shahine LK, Perfetto CO, Hickok LR, Lathi RB. Intent to treat analysis of in vitro fertilization and preimplantation genetic screening versus expectant management in patients with recurrent pregnancy loss. Hum Reprod. 2016;31:1668–74.
123. Esquerre-Lamare C, Walschaerts M, Chansel Debordeaux L, Moreau J, Bretelle F, Isus F, Karsenty G, Monteil L, Perrin J, Papaxanthos-Roche A, et al. Sperm aneuploidy and DNA fragmentation in unexplained recurrent pregnancy loss: a multicenter case-control study. Basic Clin Androl. 2018;28:4–6.
124. Fragouli E, Katz-Jaffe M, Alfarawati S, Stevens J, Colls P, Goodall NN, Tormasi S, Gutierrez-Mateo C, Prates R, Schoolcraft WB, et al. Comprehensive chromosome screening of polar bodies and blastocysts from couples experiencing repeated implantation failure. Fertil Steril. 2010;94:875–87.
125. Babariya D, Fragouli E, Alfarawati S, Spath K, Wells D. The incidence and origin of segmental aneuploidy in human oocytes and preimplantation embryos. Hum Reprod. 2017;32:2549–60.
126. Vera-Rodriguez M, Michel CE, Mercader A, Bladon AJ, Rodrigo L, Kokocinski F, Mateu E, Al-Asmar N, Blesa D, Simon C, et al. Distribution patterns of segmental aneuploidies in human blastocysts identified by next-generation sequencing. Fertil Steril. 2016;105:1047–55.
127. Bonduelle M, Ponjaert I, Steirteghem AV, et al. Developmental outcome at 2 years of age for children born after ICSI compared with children born after IVF. Hum Reprod. 2002;18:342–50.
128. Hotaling J, Carrell DT. Clinical genetic testing for male factor infertility: current applications and future directions. Andrology. 2014;2:339–50.

Part IV

Advanced Examinations in Clinical Practice

Assessment of Seminal Oxidative Stress

Pallav Sengupta, Sulagna Dutta, and Ramadan Saleh

Introduction

Oxidative stress (OS) is a disequilibrium between the generation of reactive oxygen species (ROS) and the capacity of the cellular antioxidant system to counteract them [1]. ROS, which are highly reactive molecular entities, are typically the outcome of standard metabolic activities within cells and have the potential to induce detrimental effects on lipids, proteins, and nucleic acids. When the creation of ROS surpasses the cellular antioxidant defenses, it results in OS. This state has been associated with numerous pathologies, including male infertility [2, 3].

Male infertility significantly affects a considerable number of couples attempting to achieve pregnancy, with the cause remaining unidentified in roughly 30–40% of instances [4]. Increasing evidence indicates that OS within the male reproductive system is a critical component in the pathophysiology of infertility [1]. The balance between the production of ROS and the antioxidant defense systems is fundamental for normal sperm functionality, encompassing aspects such as sperm motility, capacitation, and DNA integrity. Disruptions favoring excessive ROS production may culminate in compromised sperm functionality, reduction in sperm count, and escalation of DNA damage, ultimately leading to infertility [5, 6]. Given the importance of seminal OS in male infertility, the most recent version of the World Health

P. Sengupta
Global Andrology Forum, Moreland Hills, OH, USA

College of Medicine, Gulf Medical University, Ajman, UAE

School of Medicine, Avalon University, Willemstad, Curaçao

S. Dutta
Global Andrology Forum, Moreland Hills, OH, USA

R. Saleh (✉)
Dermatology, Venereology, & Andrology, Sohag University, Sohag, Egypt

A. Agarwal et al. (eds.), *Human Semen Analysis*,
https://doi.org/10.1007/978-3-031-55337-0_12

Organization (WHO) manual of semen analysis has incorporated the evaluation of seminal OS as an "Advanced test of semen" [7]. This acknowledgment underscores the growing awareness of the deleterious impact of OS on male reproductive health and underlines the importance of examining this aspect in the appraisal of semen quality.

The objective of this chapter is to provide a comprehensive summary of the appraisal of seminal OS within the framework of male infertility. The diverse techniques utilized for quantifying OS in seminal fluid will be reviewed, encompassing the evaluation of ROS concentrations, lipid peroxidation, antioxidant potential, and oxidative DNA damage. Additionally, we will delve into the clinical implications of seminal OS assessment, such as its prognostic capacity concerning fertility outcomes and its potential as a treatment objective in managing male infertility. Through the critical analysis of existing knowledge and studies in this area, this chapter strives to enhance the comprehension of the significance of seminal OS in male infertility and deliver essential perspectives for clinical protocols and prospective research pathways.

Pathophysiology of Seminal Reactive Oxygen Species (ROS)

The origin of seminal ROS pertains to the fundamental mechanisms and processes responsible for the genesis and influence of ROS in seminal fluid [8]. ROS, representing highly reactive molecular entities with oxygen atoms, include examples like superoxide anion ($O_2^{\cdot-}$), hydrogen peroxide (H_2O_2), and hydroxyl radical ($\cdot OH$). Under standard physiological circumstances, the production of ROS occurs in controlled amounts. Nonetheless, in instances where an escalation in ROS production is coupled with a malfunction in the antioxidant defense mechanisms, the phenomenon known as OS may ensue. This situation amplifies the adverse effects on spermatogenesis and the overall health of the male reproductive system, potentially undermining fertility [3, 5].

Various factors play a crucial role in the genesis of ROS in seminal plasma [1]. Such determinants encompass leukocyte invasion within the reproductive system, infection, inflammation, exposure to xenobiotic toxins, along with lifestyle attributes like tobacco usage and ethanol intake. Moreover, spermatozoa themselves are integral to the ROS synthesis via enzymatic processes inherent to the sperm, particularly localized in the mitochondria [1, 5].

The deleterious consequences of heightened ROS levels on sperm functionality are complex and varied. ROS have the capacity to inflict direct harm on spermatozoa by inducing lipid peroxidation in the spermatozoal membrane, subsequently resulting in compromised membrane stability and a decline in sperm motility [5]. These phenomena may further precipitate the deterioration of DNA integrity, characterized by single- and double-strand DNA breaks, alterations in nucleobases, and the synthesis of covalent bonds among nucleotides, potentially jeopardizing sperm chromatin integrity and escalating the probability of genetic aberrations in progeny. Additionally, ROS can interfere with sperm capacitation, a multifaceted biological process pivotal for the sperm to gain fertilizing potential [1, 5]. ROS have the ability to modulate intracellular signaling cascades, obstruct ion transportation, and influence protein phosphorylation, thereby obstructing capacitation. An excess of ROS can also disturb the engagement between the sperm and oocyte by impeding the acrosomal reaction, a critical physiological process necessary for sperm to penetrate the oocyte [5, 6].

In order to counteract the detrimental impact of ROS, an array of both enzymatic and non-enzymatic antioxidants are contained within seminal plasma. These include, but are not restricted to, catalase, superoxide dismutase, glutathione peroxidase, and vitamins C and E. The primary function of these antioxidants is to neutralize ROS via a process known as scavenging, thereby thwarting potential oxidative harm to the spermatozoa. However, an imbalance in the equilibrium between ROS production and the antioxidative defensive mechanism could precipitate OS, which has been identified as a potential contributor to male infertility [6, 9]. Hence, the seminal ROS play a pivotal role in the pathophysiology underpinning male infertility. Overproduction of ROS and impaired antioxidant defenses could culminate in OS, leading to compromised sperm function, DNA damage, and decreased fertility. Comprehending the pathophysiological mechanisms associated with seminal ROS could offer valuable information for the creation of therapeutic strategies intended to alleviate OS [2, 5].

Physiological Role of ROS in Male Reproductive System

ROS have been recognized as pivotal players in a broad spectrum of biological processes, notably, male reproduction. While the pathophysiological implications of ROS in male infertility have been well-documented, the nuanced roles of ROS in maintaining the physiological balance necessary for successful male reproduction have also begun to emerge [6].

Spermatozoa are unique in their dual role of conveying paternal genetic information while simultaneously acting as vehicles of biochemical mediators, including ROS. However, the relationship between ROS and male reproductive function is rather paradoxical and subject to fine-tuning. Minimal to intermediate quantities of ROS are indispensable for key reproductive mechanisms such as sperm capacitation and hyperactivation, acrosomal reaction, and ultimately, fertilization [1, 6]. However, excess ROS can precipitate OS, negatively impacting spermatozoa morphology and functionality, potentially resulting in male infertility. From a molecular perspective, ROS, a collection of chemically active molecules originating from oxygen, possess the ability to alter cellular constituents like lipids, proteins, and DNA [10]. Within the sperm cell, ROS regulate several physiological processes. Primarily, ROS activate multiple signaling pathways involved in sperm maturation. They modulate intracellular concentrations of cyclic adenosine monophosphate (cAMP), a crucial regulator of sperm motility, leading to sperm capacitation, a prerequisite for successful fertilization [6].

ROS also facilitates the fusion of the sperm acrosome with the zona pellucida of oocyte, necessary for successful fertilization. Additionally, ROS contribute to sperm hyperactivation, characterized by vigorous flagellar movement, enabling the sperm to penetrate the oocyte [11]. Furthermore, ROS, in controlled concentrations, assist in chromatin condensation during spermiogenesis—a critical step in the transformation of spermatids into mature, motile spermatozoa. They also partake in the regulation of the redox potential within the reproductive tract, thereby influencing the overall reproductive homeostasis [12].

Pathological Role of ROS

Excessive ROS can inflict oxidative damage on sperm DNA, result in lipid peroxidation, and oxidize proteins, thereby affecting sperm integrity and functions, ultimately inducing male infertility. Causes of excess seminal ROS production include varicocele, genital tract inflammation/infection, lifestyle factors among others.

Varicocele

Varicoceles represent one of the prevalent causes of male infertility, implicated in approximately 40% of cases [13]. As varicocele formation is essentially a state of increased OS in the testicular milieu, ROS plays a crucial role in varicocele-induced male infertility [8]. In the pathophysiology of varicoceles, increased venous pressure and resultant hyperthermia can lead to hypoxia and subsequent ROS overproduction. The elevated ROS levels then instigate OS by outweighing the capacity of the testicular antioxidant system [3, 8]. The varicocele-induced OS culminates in the deterioration of sperm parameters, compromising sperm motility, morphology, and concentration, thereby instigating male infertility [13].

One major casualty of ROS overproduction is sperm DNA fragmentation (SDF), as the susceptibility of spermatozoa to OS is particularly high, primarily due to their deficient antioxidative defense mechanisms and the significant presence of polyunsaturated fatty acids in their plasma membrane. OS can inflict DNA fragmentation in sperm, significantly diminishing the DNA integrity and causing apoptosis of spermatozoa [14]. This oxidative DNA damage poses a severe threat to male fertility, as it not only diminishes the fertilizing capability of sperm but also jeopardizes the subsequent embryo development and the health of the offspring. Moreover, ROS can impinge upon sperm function by oxidizing lipids in the sperm plasma membrane, altering its fluidity and integrity, and impairing the sperm capacitation and acrosome reaction (Fig. 12.1). Furthermore, the elevated OS in varicocele cases has been associated with mitochondrial dysfunction in spermatozoa. As mitochondria are significant ROS producers, their dysfunction exacerbates ROS production, creating a vicious cycle of OS. Damaged mitochondria can also impair the production of adenosine triphosphate (ATP), crucial for sperm motility, hence contributing to asthenozoospermia [15].

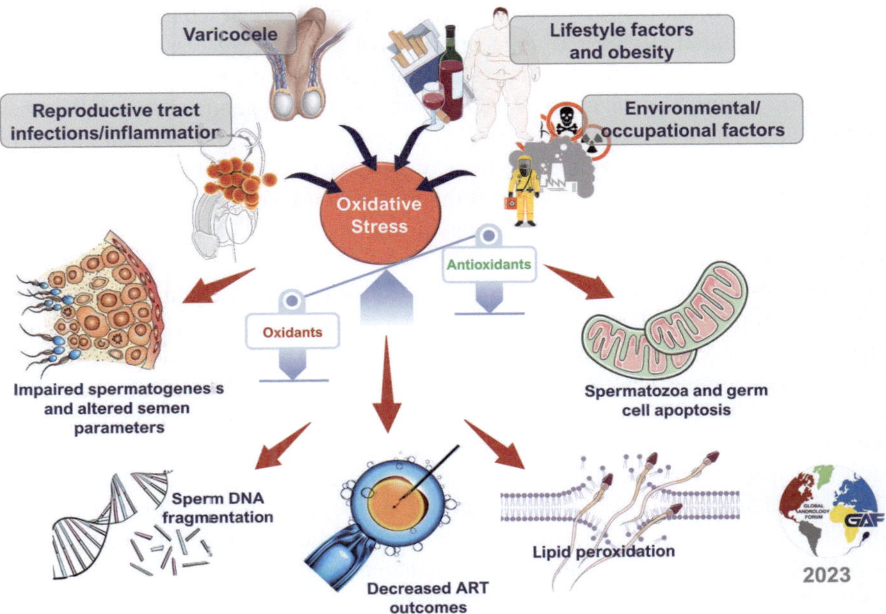

Fig. 12.1 Causes and consequences of oxidative stress in male reproduction. Oxidative stress (OS), resulting from an imbalance between reactive oxygen species production and antioxidant defense mechanisms, can arise from various factors such as environmental toxins, lifestyle factors, reproductive tract inflammation/infections and varicocele. In male reproductive system, OS induces sperm DNA damage, lipid peroxidation, and protein oxidation, leading to impaired sperm motility, morphology abnormalities, and reduced fertilization capacity

Thus, the influence of ROS on male infertility in patients with varicocele is diverse and significant [5], and consequently, the regulation of OS and ROS may provide a potent strategy for addressing varicocele-related male infertility [13]. As our understanding of the mechanisms of ROS production and the role of antioxidant system in the testicular environment deepens, targeted therapies can be developed [16].

Genital Tract Inflammation/Infection

Bacterial organisms, notably genital mycoplasmas encompassing species such as *Ureaplasma urealyticum* and *Mycoplasma hominis*, are prevalent invaders of the reproductive pathways [17]. Urethritis, prostatitis, and, in some cases, orchitis can be caused by either *Ureaplasma urealyticum* or *Mycoplasma hominis*. Ureaplasmas have been confirmed to cause non-gonococcal, non-chlamydial, urethritis in males [18]. Despite substantial research evidence, it appears that *Ureaplasma urealyticum* and *Mycoplasma hominis* do not significantly impact the quality of spermatozoa. However, it has been empirically observed that exposure to *M. hominis* can negatively influence spermatozoan motility, morphological characteristics, and fecundity potential. Enhanced concentrations of granulocyte elastase in seminal plasma act as verifying factors and signals of male genitourinary tract infections. The World Health Organization (WHO) reports that silent genitourinary inflammations are present in approximately 20–30% of infertile males [19, 20]. Alterations in the attributes of spermatozoa, indications of apoptosis, an overabundance of leukocytes in semen due to inflammation of the male reproductive system, and the generation of harmful ROS linked to pathogenic agents, collectively serve as potential contributors to male infertility [21].

The primary sources of ROS encompass immature sperm containing excessive residual cytoplasm and high levels of seminal leukocytes [22, 23]. It is worth noting that the presence of low concentration of leukocytes is a normal occurrence in semen, even among healthy fertile men without any genital tract infection [24]. However, while leukocytes play a crucial role in the immune system, an increase in their numbers may not be favorable in certain aspects, signifying an abnormal condition in specific regions of the body. Consequently, close monitoring is necessary. The identification of a substantial quantity of leukocytes in a semen sample poses a problem, as it indicates a potential infection in the reproductive tract. If left untreated, this can further compromise testicular function and sperm production. Notwithstanding their indispensable function in physiological processes, leukocytes generate a substantial quantity of ROS, with production rates estimated to be 1000-fold higher in relation to ROS [25], particularly during immunological vigilance and phagocytic activities, encompassing the removal of aberrant spermatozoa [25, 26]. However, there is an increased presence of leukocytes in seminal fluid, surpassing the norm by approximately 20–30% in males grappling with infertility. This escalation culminates in a marked amplification of ROS production, often correlated with genitourinary infections, inflammatory responses, and cellular defense mechanisms [9, 27]. The diversity of leukocyte populations in seminal fluid is contingent upon individual variability and the nature of the infection. Polymorphonuclear (PMN) granulocytes constitute the predominant class of leukocytes, accounting for 50–60% of the total leukocyte population in semen. In contrast, macrophages and lymphocytes represent 20–30% and 2–5% of the leukocyte population, respectively. It is notable that granulocytes primarily originate from the prostate gland and seminal vesicles, whereas the epididymis and rete testis are principally implicated in the genesis of other white blood cell types [23, 28].

In assessing the concentrations of leukocytes in seminal fluid among fertile and infertile males, it is observed that the count of white blood cells is generally lower in fertile individuals. However, due to the substantial overlap in leukocyte concentrations between these two groups, it becomes challenging to utilize seminal leucocyte levels as a diagnostic marker for male infertility [28]. The WHO, in its updated Laboratory Manual for Human Semen Analysis, has endorsed [29] a clinical threshold of 1×10^6 leucocytes/mL of semen. However, various studies [30, 31] have raised concerns regarding the appropriateness of this threshold, considering it to be excessively high. Certain scholars have posited that even elevated levels of leukocytes may not adversely impact male fertility [32], and might even promote the initiation of acrosome reactions [33]. Barraud-Lange et al. [34] observed that concentrations of leukocytes below the 1×10^6/mL threshold correlated with enhanced fertilization rates and pregnancy outcomes. However, contemporary research has not definitively demonstrated a negative effect of elevated leukocyte concentrations on sperm function [35, 36].

Clinical observations of asthenozoospermia and azoospermia suggest a correlation between male genital tract infections, inflammation, and the deleterious impact of leukocytospermia on sperm function and structural integrity [37, 38]. In contrast, within established ART clinics, leukocytes have not been observed to exert a detrimental impact on fertilization or pregnancy rates [39, 40]. The effects of leukocytospermia may vary among individuals. In the context of bacterial infections, activated leukocytes have been reported to exert more harmful effects in patients with fertility impairments [41]. These activated leukocytes infiltrate the infected organs, releasing substantial quantities of ROS which can induce infertility through OS [42]. Further investigations are imperative to elucidate the relationship between leukocyte levels and the fertility potential in males.

Lifestyle Factors

Several lifestyle factors can precipitate or exacerbate OS and thereby influence male fertility. Cigarette smoking is a known risk factor, inducing OS through a dual mechanism. First, the combustion products of tobacco are rich in free radicals, which directly contribute to the oxidative load. Second, several toxins in cigarette smoke impair the natural antioxidant systems of the body, leading to an imbalance favoring ROS [43]. Excessive alcohol consumption is another key player in this context. Metabolism of ethanol in the liver generates acetaldehyde and ROS as by-products. Chronic heavy drinking can lead to a systemic state of OS, which can cause testicular damage and impaired spermatogenesis, contributing to male infertility [43]. Poor dietary habits, such as a diet rich in saturated fats and low in antioxidants, can also induce OS. A diet deficient in antioxidants, like vitamins C and E, or selenium and zinc, impairs the body's ability to neutralize ROS. Simultaneously, a high intake of processed and fried foods, which are rich in trans fats, can stimulate endogenous ROS production, adding to the oxidative load. Physical inactivity and obesity are interrelated lifestyle factors that enhance OS. Obesity promotes a pro-inflammatory state, which is often accompanied by OS. In turn, this can result in sperm DNA damage and impaired fertility. On the other hand, regular physical activity promotes antioxidant defense mechanisms. However, over-exercise without proper recovery can also generate ROS, underlining the need for a balanced approach to physical activity [43]. Environmental factors like exposure to pollutants and toxins can induce OS by introducing exogenous free radicals and disrupting endogenous antioxidant systems. Occupational exposure to heavy metals, pesticides, and industrial chemicals has been linked to decreased sperm quality and infertility [44].

Thus, numerous lifestyle factors playing a role in the genesis of OS and male infertility (Fig. 12.1). These factors, often modifiable, offer promising avenues for intervention to prevent or mitigate OS-induced male infertility [43, 44]. Lifestyle modification, including smoking cessation, moderating alcohol consumption, adopting a balanced diet rich in antioxidants, and maintaining a healthy weight through regular, balanced physical activity, can be instrumental in managing OS and improving male fertility. Further research is warranted to fully elucidate these relationships and their therapeutic potential [43].

Male Oxidative Stress Infertility (MOSI)

Despite remarkable progress in the realm of male reproductive health, the issue of idiopathic male infertility—a state where altered semen characteristics in males exist without a discernible cause, and where there is an absence of female factor infertility- continues to pose considerable diagnostic and management challenges [4]. It is explained how growing scientific evidence indicate that OS has an autonomous role in the genesis of male infertility, as observed in 30–80% of infertile men with augmented levels of seminal ROS [45].

Agarwal et al. [46] had introduced the term male oxidative stress infertility (MOSI) to describe infertile men who exhibit abnormal semen parameters and OS, a group that includes many who were previously classified under idiopathic male infertility. This pioneering article also emphasized that oxidation–reduction potential (ORP), which encompasses the levels of both oxidizing and reducing agents (antioxidants), could serve as a practical clinical biomarker for the categorization of MOSI [46, 47]. The precision in categorization aid treatment strategies for OS, such as the administration of antioxidants, which previously lacked strong evidence-based foundation and carried risk of complications [46]. Employing a simple, reproducible, and economical test to measure OS might provide a rationale for delivering antioxidant therapy, thereby mitigating the danger of antioxidant overdose [48]. The increasing recognition and comprehension of MOSI as a distinct category of male infertility offer opportunities for future research to foster the formulation of therapy based on evidence that directly target its root cause.

Correlation Between Seminal OS and Semen Parameters

Correlation with Basic Sperm Parameters

Body of evidence underscores the significance of OS in the pathophysiology of male infertility, with a special focus on its correlation with basic sperm parameters—sperm concentration, motility, and morphology. An inverse relationship has been documented between OS and sperm concentration, owing to the cytotoxic effects of ROS. High ROS levels are known to interfere with spermatogenesis, potentially leading to a decline in sperm production. Increased OS can disrupt the delicate equilibrium of germ cells, compromising their function and consequently diminishing sperm concentration [49]. Sperm motility, a key determinant of male fertility, is crucial for successful fertilization, as it enables sperm to traverse the female reproductive tract. Elevated ROS levels can inflict lipid peroxidation, causing cellular damage that impairs sperm motility. ROS can interfere with the energy metabolism of sperm, impinging on their ability to move efficiently. Sperm morphology is another vital parameter of sperm quality. Abnormal sperm morphology is often associated with reduced fertility potential [50]. ROS can initiate peroxidative damage to the sperm membrane, altering its architecture, and negatively affecting the acrosomal reaction necessary for fertilization [14, 51].

A study by Homa et al. [52] compared ROS levels in semen across three distinct cohorts: Group 1, normal semen parameters without leukocytospermia; Group 2, abnormal semen parameters without leukocytospermia; and Group 3, any semen parameters with leukocytospermia. As expected, the most elevated ROS levels were observed in Group 3 subjects. Nevertheless, Group 2 displayed significantly increased ROS levels in comparison to Group 1 subjects, implying a negative correlation between ROS and standard semen parameters. Agarwal et al. [53] similarly studied semen parameters and ROS levels in the ejaculates of infertile men and confirmed fertile men. Infertile men exhibited notably higher ROS levels compared to fertile controls, with significant positive correlations found between ROS levels and sperm concentration and motility across all men, infertile men, and fertile controls. Another investigation revealed seminal malondialdehyde (MDA), nitric oxide (NO), zinc, and TAC levels in infertile and fertile men, with infertile men showing significantly elevated MDA and NO and significantly decreased zinc and TAC. Negative correlations were observed between sperm concentration, motility, and morphology and MDA and NO levels, while positive correlations were found with zinc and TAC levels.

A study by Venkatesh et al. [54] explored the relationship between various sperm morphological abnormalities and seminal OS in infertile and fertile men. Infertile men exhibited a median ROS level up to 124-fold higher compared to fertile men. Among the morphological anomalies, a significantly increased percentage of sperm with cytoplasmic droplets was identified in infertile men, possibly attributable to the raised ROS levels in their semen samples. Another study confirmed an adverse effect of OS on acrosomal structures, demonstrating a significant positive correlation between acrosomal anomalies and MDA values [55].

Correlation Between Seminal OS and Sperm DNA Fragmentation (SDF)

The integrity of sperm DNA is a crucial factor in male fertility. Over recent years, an association has been suggested between seminal OS and SDF [14]. A significant number of studies have underlined this correlation, providing a novel insight into the etiology of male infertility [56, 57]. Emerging research implicates seminal OS as a key driver of SDF, indicating the potential utility of SDF testing in male infertility diagnosis [58]. Iommiello et al. [51] identified a notable positive association between OS, as evaluated by oxiSperm® (Halotech DNA, SL, Madrid, Spain), and DNA fragmentation index, assessed via sperm chromatin structure assay (SCSA®; SCSA Diagnostics, Volga, SD). A separate investigation highlighted a greater prevalence of spermatozoa DNA fragmentation in infertile males relative to fertile counterparts, alongside a meaningful positive relationship between SDF and seminal MDA levels [57]. A study evaluated the impact of seminal ORP and SDF (gauged through sperm chromatin dispersion) on sperm morphology aberrations in both fertile and infertile populations [53]. In the latter study, both ORP and SDF were correlated positively with sperm head defects and negatively with normal sperm morphology in infertile men. Additionally, an inverse relationship was noted between ORP, SDF, and the prevalence of normal sperm morphology (both $P <$ 0.001) [56]. Elevated SDF levels have been associated with reduced fertilization rates, poor embryo quality, lower pregnancy rates, and a higher risk of early pregnancy loss. An increasing body of evidence points to a robust correlation between seminal OS and SDF [10]. Infertile men with high SDF levels also exhibited increased markers of OS, signifying an underlying link between these two parameters [56]. Experimental models have demonstrated that exogenously induced OS leads to an increase in SDF, thereby directly substantiating this association [59, 60]. Furthermore, interventional studies have shown that the reduction of seminal OS through antioxidant therapy leads to a decrease in SDF, improving the overall fertility outcomes [61–63]. These studies provide compelling evidence for a positive correlation between seminal OS and SDF.

The link between OS and SDF is hypothesized to be mediated via oxidative DNA damage mechanism (Fig. 12.1). Excessive ROS can inflict base modifications, strand breaks, and chromatin crosslinks, resulting in the SDF [10, 14]. However, the precise molecular pathways underlying this link require further investigation.

Correlation Between Seminal OS and Assisted Reproductive Technique Outcomes

Impact on the Outcome of Intrauterine Insemination

Intrauterine insemination (IUI) is a widely employed fertility treatment, used especially in cases of unexplained infertility or male factor infertility [64]. High ROS levels negatively influence sperm parameters such as motility, morphology, and concentration, which are crucial for successful IUI [65]. The sperm preparation techniques used in IUI might further increase ROS production, especially during the centrifugation process [66]. Additionally, high ROS levels might cause DNA fragmentation in sperm, which is associated with a decrease in fertilization rates, impaired embryonic development, and increased miscarriage rates [14]. Furthermore, seminal OS may potentially affect female reproductive tract function and embryonic development. Experimental evidence suggests that ROS can induce an inflammatory response in the female reproductive tract, which could be deleterious to sperm transit, oocyte fertilization, and embryo implantation. ROS can also trigger DNA damage in the oocyte, potentially impacting embryonic development and the pregnancy outcome [57]. Novel diagnostic tools for accurate ROS measurement and customized antioxidant supplementation based on individual OS profiles might pave the way for improved IUI outcomes in the future.

Impact on the Outcome of In Vitro Fertilization/Intracytoplasmic Sperm Injection (IVF/ICSI)

The impact of seminal OS on the outcome of in vitro fertilization (IVF) and intracytoplasmic sperm injection (ICSI) has emerged as a prominent area of research in recent years [68].

A negative correlation has been found between elevated levels of seminal OS and the success rates of IVF/ICSI [68]. It appears that ROS-induced damage can compromise the sperm's fertilizing capacity, thus, adversely affecting embryo development and implantation rates following IVF/ICSI. In particular, SDF, a direct consequence of OS, has been significantly associated with lower rates of fertilization, poor embryo quality, and higher incidences of early pregnancy loss after IVF and ICSI procedures [68]. Given that both IVF and ICSI depend heavily on the integrity of the sperm genome for the initiation and sustenance of a successful pregnancy, these observations underline the importance of OS as a critical determinant of treatment outcome [69]. Similarly, lipid peroxidation, triggered by excessive ROS, can destabilize the integrity of the sperm membrane. This can lead to a decrease in sperm motility and hamper the acrosome reaction, two crucial prerequisites for successful fertilization [5, 6]. It is noteworthy that ICSI, which bypasses the need for natural sperm-oocyte fusion, might be less impacted by these changes compared to IVF. Nevertheless, even in ICSI, the overall sperm quality still influences the embryo development post-fertilization.

Further exacerbating the issue, it is worth noting that ARTs themselves might amplify OS due to sperm manipulation and exposure to light and temperature fluctuations [69]. Consequently, understanding the contribution of OS to sperm function and IVF/ICSI outcomes has practical implications for the refinement of these procedures. Although mitigating seminal OS remains a challenge, several strategies are under investigation [68]. Antioxidant supplementation, for example, has shown promise in improving semen parameters and the outcomes of IVF/ICSI. However, well-designed randomized controlled trials are required to conclusively establish the efficacy and optimal dosage of such interventions [16]. Therefore, seminal OS represents a significant hurdle to the success of IVF/ICSI (Fig. 12.1). It has the potential to inflict multifaceted damage on sperm cells, thus negatively affecting key outcomes of assisted reproduction. As such, routine screening for OS markers in semen analysis could aid in providing personalized care and optimizing ART outcomes.

Methods of Seminal OS Testing

Assessing elevated levels of ROS in males is a logical investigative step of male factor infertility. However, certain obstacles such as the inconvenience and cost associated with ROS screening, coupled with the absence of a universally acknowledged effective analytical method, limit the inclusion of ROS measurements as a crucial part of male fertility evaluations, notwithstanding its substantial significance. Till current, in excess of 30 different assays for ROS and OS measurement in the semen of infertile men are reported in the scientific literature [8].

Standard Semen Analysis

The standard evaluation of semen parameters (sperm count, morphology, and motility) provides clinicians with an indirect measure of seminal OS, with asthenozoospermia potentially serving as the most accurate OS indicator [70]. An increase in the viscosity of seminal plasma corresponds to an augmentation in seminal plasma malondialdehyde (MDA) levels and a decline in antioxidant status within the seminal plasma [70]. Additionally, infection by *Ureaplasma urealyticum* in semen has been correlated with an increased seminal plasma viscosity and excessive ROS generation [70]. The identification of an excessive number of round cells could denote the existence of leukocytospermia, a recognized source of excessive ROS production, as indicated earlier. However, to exclude the possibility of these round cells being immature spermatozoa, supplemental tests such as the peroxidase test, seminal elastase determination, or cluster of differentiation 45 (CD45, a cell surface-expressed transmembrane glycoprotein) antibody staining should be conducted. Aberrant sperm morphology and the presence of cytoplasmic droplets are distinctive attributes of abnormal spermatozoa, leading to unregulated ROS generation. Lastly, compromised sperm membrane integrity, which can be evaluated through the hypo-osmotic swelling test (HOST), has been associated with the existence of OS [8].

Evaluation of ROS via Chemiluminescence

Primarily, the assessment of ROS in seminal fluid is executed through the chemiluminescence assay (Fig. 12.2). This methodology necessitates the use of a luminometer and a chemiluminescent agent such as luminal (5-amino-2,3-dihydro-1,4-phthalazinedione; Sigma-Aldrich, St. Louis, MO). Segments of liquefied semen are subjected to centrifugation at 300 g for a duration of 7 min. Subsequently, the seminal plasma, divided into aliquots, is frozen at $-20\ ^{\circ}\mathrm{C}$ in anticipation of assessing total antioxidant capacities. The pellet is cleansed with PBS (pH 7.4), and 400-μL aliquots of 2×10^6 sperm/mL are reconstituted in the washing solution for basal ROS level examination. A volume of 10 mL of 5-mM luminol in 400 mL of PBS serves as the negative control. Luminol (5-mM stock in dimethyl sulphoxide) is

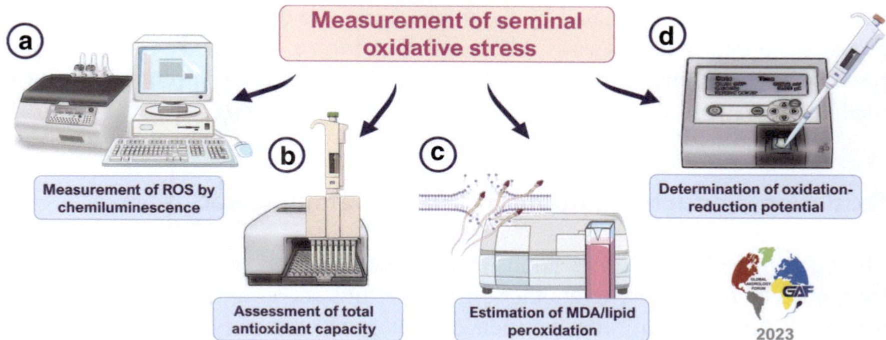

Fig. 12.2 Different methods of measurement of seminal oxidative stress. The comparative summary showcases (**a**) The method of chemiluminescence accurately identifies the presence of reactive oxygen species (ROS) in seminal plasma, (**b**) the evaluation of total antioxidant capacity (TAC) measures the combined strength of antioxidant defenses present in the semen sample, (**c**) the analysis of lipid peroxidation measures the oxidative damage to lipids, which has implications for the integrity of the sperm membrane, and (**d**) the MiOXSYS analyzer is used to gauge the oxidation-reduction potential (ORP), which serves as an indicator of the equilibrium between oxidizing agents and antioxidants. While each technique provides distinct information, MiOXSYS delivers a more holistic understanding of the oxidative state within semen

introduced into the blend to function as a probe, and the test tubes are placed within the luminometer for 15 min to quantify ROS concentrations. Luminol is capable of detecting both extracellular and intracellular ROS. The free radicals contained within the semen sample interact with luminal to generate a light signal, which is transduced into an electric (photon) signal by the luminometer. The enumeration of the free radicals produced is expressed in relative light units/s/10^6 sperm. In washed sperm suspensions, normal ROS concentrations span between 0.10 and 1.03×10^6 counted photons/min/20×10^6 sperm [71].

Quantifying Total Antioxidant Capacity (TAC)

For measurement of the TAC within seminal plasma, luminol is also employed. This measurement is standardized against "Trolox," a water-soluble analogue of vitamin E. The outcomes are represented as a ROS-TAC score, signifying the aggregated antioxidant activities invoked by all constituents, inclusive of vitamins, lipids, and proteins [71].

Lipid Peroxidation (LPO) Markers

Accumulation of lipid peroxides within spermatozoa results in diverse degradation products such as malondialdehyde (MDA), acrolein (2-propenal), hydroxynonenal, and isoprostanes. These can be quantified as markers of OS [72]. Among these,

MDA quantification, mediated by the thiobarbituric acid (TBA) assay, is the most prevalent approach. In this assay, MDA and TBA form a 1:2 adduct, a colored compound whose concentration can be evaluated by fluorometric or spectrophotometric methods [8, 72].

Oxidation–Reduction Potential (ORP) in Seminal Fluid

The ORP provides a quantification of the capacity of electrons to be transferred from one chemical entity to another [73]. ORP thus serves as an aggregate metric for the dynamic equilibrium between oxidizing and reducing agents, offering a comprehensive assessment of OS (Fig. 12.2). Recent advancements in technology have introduced a galvanostatic approach for assessing the movement of electrons, a tool that has found applications in evaluating alterations in OS following traumatic incidents or extreme physical exertion [74].

MiOXSYS Analyzer

Concurrent OS assessment and standard semen analysis are performed to discern the etiology underlying substandard semen quality and male infertility. The MiOXSYS analyzer (Male Infertility Oxidative System; Aytu BioScience), an ultra-high impedance electrometer, gauges the ORP levels in a semen sample by quantifying the electron transfer between antioxidants and oxidants [75]. The ORP measurement through the MiOXSYS technique, in contrast to other methods, does not demand specialized personnel training or specific sample processing. Additionally, it examines ORP in a minuscule quantity of either fresh or frozen specimens (30 µl) in less than 4 min, yielding consistent outcomes for up to 120 min post semen sample collection [75]. Thus, freezing the specimen is advocated if evaluation is not feasible within 120 min post-liquefaction.

Alternative Probes and Analyzers

ORP sensors, functioning analogously to pH sensors, measure solution ORP via redox potential disparity between a working electrode and a gold or platinum reference electrode. Sensorex Inc has devised a range of sensors for specific applications withstanding temperatures up to 100 °C. These sensors interface wirelessly with Android devices, enabling data storage and retrieval. Certain sensors concurrently detect ORP, temperature, pH, and additional water parameters including dissolved oxygen, conductivity, salinity, ammonium, nitrate, and chloride. In healthcare, analyzer selection is contingent on sample type, with smaller electrodes utilized for reduced sample volumes. Thermo Scientific Orion analyzers, for instance, were employed for ORP measurement in cell cultures [76], while the RedoxSYS Diagnostic System, predecessor to MiOXSYS, was used for ORP determination in human blood plasma [77, 78].

Future Prospects of Seminal OS Testing

The 6th edition of the WHO manual of human semen analysis classified seminal OS test as an emerging technology, and provided a brief description of ORP as a promising assay for seminal OS assessment [7]. Several studies highlighted the diagnostic significance of ORP testing in the context of male infertility [76, 77]. More recently, results of seminal ORP test have been significantly correlated with ICSI outcomes [78]. Thus, seminal OS analysis demonstrates considerable potential in the management of infertility. In fact, the diagnostic significance of seminal OS testing in routine infertility investigations cannot be overstated. Elevated levels of ROS in seminal fluid can detrimentally impact sperm function, which commonly contributes to male infertility. Accurate assessment of OS levels through seminal OS testing aids in the identification of men who may be causally linked to infertility, thus enabling targeted interventions.

In the domain of male infertility prognosis, seminal OS analysis occupies a paramount position. Oxidative stress is implicated in a myriad of sperm anomalies, such as DNA fragmentation and impaired motility. Comprehension of OS levels illuminates the severity and etiological factors of male infertility, equipping medical professionals to deliver precise prognostic information, thus enabling couples to make informed decisions. Seminal OS assessment becomes indispensable in devising treatment strategies for couples experiencing infertility and monitoring the responses to treatments. Individualized therapeutic interventions, such as antioxidant supplementation or lifestyle alterations, can be proposed based on the data derived from seminal OS analysis. This personalized methodology amplifies the possibility of ameliorating sperm quality and functionality. Moreover, tracking changes in seminal OS levels during treatment provision can furnish empirical evidence of the efficacy of the intervention, permitting prompt modifications to the treatment regimen if deemed necessary. In summary, the seminal OS assessment is an invaluable diagnostic and prognostic instrument for infertility. By paving the way for bespoke treatment plans and providing ongoing monitoring, OS testing may enhance the reproductive outcomes of infertile couples. Robust data on reliable cutoff values of seminal OS are warranted for the test to be incorporated in routine infertility workup.

References

1. Agarwal A, Sengupta P. Oxidative stress and its association with male infertility. In: Male infertility: contemporary clinical approaches, andrology, ART and antioxidants. Cham: Springer; 2020. p. 57–68.
2. Saleh RA. Oxidative stress and male infertility: from research bench to clinical practice. J Androl. 2002;23(6):737–52.
3. Makker K, Agarwal A, Sharma R. Oxidative stress & male infertility. Indian J Med Res. 2009;129(4):357–67.
4. Agarwal A, Mulgund A, Hamada A, Chyatte MR. A unique view on male infertility around the globe. Reprod Biol Endocrinol. 2015;13(1):1–9.

5. Agarwal A, Leisegang K, Sengupta P. Oxidative stress in pathologies of male reproductive disorders. In: Pathology. Amsterdam: Elsevier; 2020. p. 15–27.

6. Dutta S, Henkel R, Sengupta P, Agarwal A. Physiological role of ROS in sperm function. In: Male infertility: contemporary clinical approaches, andrology, ART and antioxidants. Cham: Springer; 2020. p. 337–45.

7. World Health Organization. WHO laboratory manual for the examination and processing of human semen. Geneva: World Health Organization; 2021.

8. Agarwal A, Virk G, Ong C, Du Plessis SS. Effect of oxidative stress on male reproduction. World J Mens Health. 2014;32(1):1–17.

9. Izuka E, Menuba I, Sengupta P, Dutta S, Nwagha U. Antioxidants, anti-inflammatory drugs and antibiotics in the treatment of reproductive tract infections and their association with male infertility. Chem Biol Lett. 2020;7(2):156–65.

10. Agarwal A, Majzoub A, Baskaran S, Selvam MKP, Cho CL, Henkel R, et al. Sperm DNA fragmentation: a new guideline for clinicians. World J Mens Health. 2020;38(4):412.

11. Gunes S, Sengupta P, Henkel R, Alguraigari A, Sinigaglia MM, Kayal M, et al. Microtubular dysfunction and male infertility. World J Mens Health. 2020;38(1):9–23.

12. Sengupta P, Arafa M, Elbardisi H. Hormonal regulation of spermatogenesis. In: Molecular signaling in spermatogenesis and male infertility. CRC Press: Boca Raton; 2019. p. 41–9.

13. Agarwal A, Finelli R, Durairajanayagam D, Leisegang K, Henkel R, Salvio G, et al. Comprehensive analysis of global research on human varicocele: a scientometric approach. World J Mens Health. 2022;40(4):636.

14. Panner Selvam MK, Sengupta P, Agarwal A. Sperm DNA fragmentation and male infertility. In: Genetics of male infertility: a case-based guide for clinicians. Cham: Springer; 2020. p. 155–72.

15. Sengupta P, Durairajanayagam D, Agarwal A. Fuel/energy sources of spermatozoa. In: Male infertility: contemporary clinical approaches, andrology, ART and antioxidants. Cham: Springer; 2020. p. 323–35.

16. Agarwal A, Finelli R, Selvam MKP, Leisegang K, Majzoub A, Tadros N, et al. A global survey of reproductive specialists to determine the clinical utility of oxidative stress testing and antioxidant use in male infertility. World J Mens Health. 2021;39(3):470.

17. Andrade-Rocha FT. Ureaplasma urealyticum and Mycoplasma hominis in men attending for routine semen analysis. Urol Int. 2003;71(4):377–81.

18. Taylor-Robinson D. Infections due to species of mycoplasma and ureaplasma: an update. Clin Infect Dis. 1996;23:671–82.

19. Zorn B, Virant-klun I, Vidmar G, Sešek-Briški A, Kolbezen M, Meden-vrtovec H. Seminal elastase-inhibitor complex, a marker of genital tract inflammation, and negative IVF outcome measures: role for a silent inflammation? Int J Androl. 2004;27(6):368–74.

20. Rowe P, Comhaire F, Hargreave T, Mahmoud A. Objective criteria for diagnostic categories in the standardized management of male infertility: male accessory gland infection (MAGI). In: WHO manual for the standardized investigation, diagnosis and management of the infertile male. Geneva: World Health Organization; 2000. p. 52–4.

21. Dutta S, Sengupta P, Slama P, Roychoudhury S. Oxidative stress, testicular inflammatory pathways, and male reproduction. Int J Mol Sci. 2021;22(18):10043.

22. Dutta S, Majzoub A, Agarwal A. Oxidative stress and sperm function: a systematic review on evaluation and management. Arab J Urol. 2019;17(2):87–97.

23. Sengupta P. Current trends of male reproductive health disorders and the changing semen quality. Int J Prev Med. 2014;5(1):1.

24. Wallach EE, Wolff H. The biologic significance of white blood cells in semen. Fertil Steril. 1995;63(6):1143–57.

25. Ford W, Whittington K, Williams A. Reactive oxygen species in human sperm suspensions: production by leukocytes and the generation of NADPH to protect sperm against their effects. Int J Androl. 1997;20:44–9.

26. Plante M, de Lamirande E, Gagnon C. Reactive oxygen species released by activated neutrophils, but not by deficient spermatozoa, are sufficient to affect normal sperm motility. Fertil Steril. 1994;62(2):387–93.
27. Irez T, Bicer S, Sahin S, Dutta S, Sengupta P. Cytokines and adipokines in the regulation of spermatogenesis and semen quality. Chem Biol Lett. 2020;7(2):131–9.
28. de Lamirande E, Gagnon C. Capacitation-associated production of superoxide anion by human spermatozoa. Free Radic Biol Med. 1995;18(3):487–95.
29. World Health Organization. WHO laboratory manual for the examination and processing of human semen. Geneva: World Health Organization; 2010.
30. Sharma RK, Pasqualotto FF, Nelson DR, Agarwal A. Relationship between seminal white blood cell counts and oxidative stress in men treated at an infertility clinic. J Androl. 2001;22(4):575–83.
31. Punab M, Lõivukene K, Kermes K, Mändar R. The limit of leucocytospermia from the microbiological viewpoint. Andrologia. 2003;35(5):271–8.
32. Yanushpolsky EH, Politch JA, Hill JA, Anderson DJ. Is leukocytospermia clinically relevant? Fertil Steril. 1996;66(5):822–5.
33. Kaleli S, Öçer F, Irez T, Budak E, Aksu MF. Does leukocytospermia associate with poor semen parameters and sperm functions in male infertility? The role of different seminal leukocyte concentrations. Eur J Obstet Gynecol Reprod Biol. 2000;89(2):185–91.
34. Barraud-Lange V, Pont J-C, Ziyyat A, Pocate K, Sifer C, Cedrin-Durnerin I, et al. Seminal leukocytes are good Samaritans for spermatozoa. Fertil Steril. 2011;96(6):1315–9.
35. Sandoval JS, Raburn D, Muasher S. Leukocytospermia: overview of diagnosis, implications, and management of a controversial finding. Middle East Fertil Soc J. 2013;18(3):129–34.
36. Fraczek M, Hryhorowicz M, Gill K, Zarzycka M, Gaczarzewicz D, Jedrzejczak P, et al. The effect of bacteriospermia and leukocytospermia on conventional and nonconventional semen parameters in healthy young normozoospermic males. J Reprod Immunol. 2016;118:18–27.
37. Dohle G, Colpi G, Hargreave T, Papp G, Jungwirth A, Weidner W, et al. EAU guidelines on male infertility. Eur Urol. 2005;48(5):703–11.
38. Lackner JE, Herwig R, Schmidbauer J, Schatzl G, Kratzik C, Marberger M. Correlation of leukocytospermia with clinical infection and the positive effect of antiinflammatory treatment on semen quality. Fertil Steril. 2006;86(3):601–5.
39. Cavagna M, Oliveira JBA, Petersen CG, Mauri AL, Silva LF, Massaro FC, et al. The influence of leukocytospermia on the outcomes of assisted reproductive technology. Reprod Biol Endocrinol. 2012;10(1):44.
40. Ricci G, Granzotto M, Luppi S, Giolo E, Martinelli M, Zito G, et al. Effect of seminal leukocytes on in vitro fertilization and intracytoplasmic sperm injection outcomes. Fertil Steril. 2015;104(1):87–93.
41. Moretti E, Capitani S, Figura N, Pammolli A, Federico MG, Giannerini V, et al. The presence of bacteria species in semen and sperm quality. J Assist Reprod Genet. 2009;26(1):47.
42. Martínez P, Proverbio F, Camejo MI. Sperm lipid peroxidation and pro-inflammatory cytokines. Asian J Androl. 2007;9(1):102–7.
43. Durairajanayagam D. Lifestyle causes of male infertility. Arab J Urol. 2018;16(1):10–20.
44. Sengupta P. Environmental and occupational exposure of metals and their role in male reproductive functions. Drug Chem Toxicol. 2013;36(3):353–68.
45. Agarwal A, Majzoub A, Parekh N, Henkel R. A schematic overview of the current status of male infertility practice. World J Mens Health. 2020;38(3):308.
46. Agarwal A, Parekh N, Selvam MKP, Henkel R, Shah R, Homa ST, et al. Male oxidative stress infertility (MOSI): proposed terminology and clinical practice guidelines for management of idiopathic male infertility. World J Mens Health. 2019;37(3):296–312.
47. Arafa M, Agarwal A, Majzoub A, Panner Selvam MK, Baskaran S, Henkel R, et al. Efficacy of antioxidant supplementation on conventional and advanced sperm function tests in patients with idiopathic male infertility. Antioxidants. 2020;9(3):219.
48. Panner Selvam MK, Finelli R, Agarwal A, Henkel R. Evaluation of seminal oxidation–reduction potential in male infertility. Andrologia. 2021;53(2):e13610.

49. Sengupta P, Dutta S, Krajewska-Kulak E. The disappearing sperms: analysis of reports published between 1980 and 2015. Am J Mens Health. 2017;11(4):1279–304.
50. Guthrie H, Welch G. Effects of reactive oxygen species on sperm function. Theriogenology. 2012;78(8):1700–8.
51. Iommiello VM, Albani E, Di Rosa A, Marras A, Menduni F, Morreale G, et al. Ejaculate oxidative stress is related with sperm DNA fragmentation and round cells. Int J Endocrinol. 2015;2015:321901.
52. Homa ST, Vessey W, Perez-Miranda A, Riyait T, Agarwal A. Reactive oxygen species (ROS) in human semen: determination of a reference range. J Assist Reprod Genet. 2015;32:757–64.
53. Agarwal A, Sharma RK, Sharma R, Assidi M, Abuzenadah AM, Alshahrani S, et al. Characterizing semen parameters and their association with reactive oxygen species in infertile men. Reprod Biol Endocrinol. 2014;12(1):1–9.
54. Venkatesh S, Singh G, Gupta NP, Kumar R, Deecaraman M, Dada R. Correlation of sperm morphology and oxidative stress in infertile men. Iran J Reprod Med. 2009;7(1):29–34.
55. El-Taieb MA, Ali MA, Nada EA. Oxidative stress and acrosomal morphology: a cause of infertility in patients with normal semen parameters. Middle East Fertil Soc J. 2015;20(2):79–85.
56. Majzoub A, Arafa M, Mahdi M, Agarwal A, Al Said S, Al-Emadi I, et al. Oxidation–reduction potential and sperm DNA fragmentation, and their associations with sperm morphological anomalies amongst fertile and infertile men. Arab J Urol. 2018;16(1):87–95.
57. Dorostghoal M, Kazeminejad S, Shahbazian N, Pourmehdi M, Jabbari A. Oxidative stress status and sperm DNA fragmentation in fertile and infertile men. Andrologia. 2017;49(10):e12762.
58. El-Sakka AI. Routine assessment of sperm DNA fragmentation in clinical practice: commentary and perspective. Transl Androl Urol. 2017;6(4):640.
59. Kumar TR, Doreswamy K, Shrilatha B. Oxidative stress associated DNA damage in testis of mice: induction of abnormal sperms and effects on fertility. Mutat Res. 2002;513(1-2):103–11.
60. La Maestra S, De Flora S, Micale RT. Effect of cigarette smoke on DNA damage, oxidative stress, and morphological alterations in mouse testis and spermatozoa. Int J Hyg Environ Health. 2015;218(1):117–22.
61. Greco E, Iacobelli M, Rienzi L, Ubaldi F, Ferrero S, Tesarik J. Reduction of the incidence of sperm DNA fragmentation by oral antioxidant treatment. J Androl. 2005;26(3):349–53.
62. Martínez-Soto JC, Domingo JC, Cordobilla B, Nicolás M, Fernández L, Albero P, et al. Dietary supplementation with docosahexaenoic acid (DHA) improves seminal antioxidant status and decreases sperm DNA fragmentation. Syst Biol Reprod Med. 2016;62(6):387–95.
63. Abad C, Amengual M, Gosálvez J, Coward K, Hannaoui N, Benet J, et al. Effects of oral antioxidant treatment upon the dynamics of human sperm DNA fragmentation and subpopulations of sperm with highly degraded DNA. Andrologia. 2013;45(3):211–6.
64. Sengupta P, Roychoudhury S, Nath M, Dutta S. Oxidative stress and idiopathic male infertility. In: Oxidative stress and toxicity in reproductive biology and medicine: a comprehensive update on male infertility, vol. 1. Cham: Springer; 2022. p. 181–204.
65. Sikka SC. Andrology lab corner: role of oxidative stress and antioxidants in andrology and assisted reproductive technology. J Androl. 2004;25(1):5–18.
66. Henkel RR, Schill W-B. Sperm preparation for ART. Reprod Biol Endocrinol. 2003;1(1):1–22.
67. Sengupta P, Dutta S, Alahmar AT. Reproductive tract infection, inflammation and male infertility. Chem Biol Lett. 2020;7(2):75–84.
68. Ribas-Maynou J, Yeste M, Salas-Huetos A. The relationship between sperm oxidative stress alterations and IVF/ICSI outcomes: a systematic review from nonhuman mammals. Biology. 2020;9(7):178.
69. Gupta S, Sekhon L, Kim Y, Agarwal A. The role of oxidative stress and antioxidants in assisted reproduction. Curr Womens Health Rev. 2010;6:227–38.
70. Aydemir B, Onaran I, Kiziler AR, Alici B, Akyolcu MC. The influence of oxidative damage on viscosity of seminal fluid in infertile men. J Androl. 2008;29(1):41–6.
71. Agarwal A, Majzoub A. Laboratory tests for oxidative stress. Indian J Urol. 2017;33(3):199.
72. Aitken RJ. Free radicals, lipid peroxidation and sperm function. Reprod Fertil Dev. 1995;7(4):659–68.

73. McCord JM. The evolution of free radicals and oxidative stress. Am J Med. 2000;108(8):652–9.
74. Rael LT, Bar-Or R, Mains CW, Slone DS, Levy AS, Bar-Or D. Plasma oxidation-reduction potential and protein oxidation in traumatic brain injury. J Neurotrauma. 2009;26(8):1203–11.
75. Agarwal A, Sharma R, Roychoudhury S, Du Plessis S, Sabanegh E. MiOXSYS: a novel method of measuring oxidation reduction potential in semen and seminal plasma. Fertil Steril. 2016;106(3):566–73.
76. Pluschkell SB, Flickinger MC. Improved methods for investigating the external redox potential in hybridoma cell culture. Cytotechnology. 1995;19(1):11–26.
77. Polson D, Villalba N, Freeman K. Optimization of a diagnostic platform for oxidation–reduction potential (ORP) measurement in human plasma. Red Rep. 2018;23(1):125–9.
78. Stagos D, Goutzourelas N, Bar-Or D, Ntontou A-M, Bella E, Becker AT, et al. Application of a new oxidation-reduction potential assessment method in strenuous exercise-induced oxidative stress. Red Rep. 2015;20(4):154–62.

Acrosome Reaction

13

Fahmi Bahar and Tan V. Le

Introduction

Semen analysis is the first step in the evaluation of male fertility. However, conventional semen parameters are insufficient to assess spermatozoa's capacity for in vivo or in vitro fertilization (IVF). Therefore, a thorough investigation of sub-microscopic factors that support the sperm's fertilization capacity is required. Deoxyribonucleic acid (DNA) fragmentation, capacitation, hyperactivation, and acrosome response were among these factors [1–3].

Acrosome reaction is included in the section on advanced examinations of the sixth edition of the WHO laboratory manual for semen examination [4]. The spermatozoa's acrosome, which has a hat-like form, plays a crucial role in fertilization. The fusing of two human gamete cell nuclei begins with an AR in the pellucid zone of the oocyte. The effects of the AR on male fertility or infertility, as well as potential therapies to alter AR to support impregnation will be discussed in detail in this chapter.

F. Bahar (✉)
Siloam Sriwijaya Palembang Hospital, Palembang, Indonesia

Global Andrology Forum (GAF), Moreland Hills, OH, USA

Faculty of Medicine, Muhammadiyah Palembang University, Palembang, Indonesia

T. V. Le
Department of Andrology, Binh Dan Hospital, Da Nang, Vietnam

Department of Andrology and Urology, Pham Ngoc Thach University of Medicine, Ho Chi Minh City, Vietnam

Global Andrology Forum (GAF), Moreland Hills, OH, USA

Physiology of Acrosome Reaction

The acrosome covers two-thirds of the front of the spermatozoa's head like a cap over the nucleus. Additionally, spermatozoan morphology typically shows vacuoles in the head either minor or large. Big vacuoles in the head of spermatozoa are believed to be responsible for the spermatozoa's subpar acrosome reactivity [5].

The acrosome includes several enzymes, including protease, hyaluronidase, glycosidase, and acrosin (which is exclusively found in the sperm of mammals). The two enzymes having the greatest impact on spermatozoa fertilizing ability are hyaluronidase and acrosin (serin proteinase acrosin) [6]. For penetration to take place, both enzymes operated by untangling proteins protecting the oocyte's shell.

The renin-angiotensin system (RAS) has an important component called angiotensin-converting enzyme (ACE), which is another enzyme that contributes to the activation process and AR of the human sperm cell. Testicular ACE (tACE) and somatic ACE (sACE) are the two types of ACE with the same coding. While the second is a component of the seminal plasma, the first is a part of the germinal cells. The tACE isoform is the more critical component for spermatozoa motility, capacitation, and acrosome response. The oocyte fertilization by spermatozoa was negatively impacted by a drop in tACE level [1]. Additionally, the cleavage and embryo quality following fertilization were affected by this enzyme [3].

The renin-angiotensin system is important for spermatozoa function. Renin has been discovered in the testis, epididymis, and seminal plasma. It affects the AR through the (Pro)Renin Receptor (PRR), which is situated in the post-acrosome area of the spermatozoa head (and along the tail). Low sperm motility, inability to form blastocytes, and poor embryo quality are all effects of high PRR level in seminal fluid [3]. This is assumed to be caused by its impact on spermatozoa's capacitation and acrosome response.

An essential requirement for fertilization is spermatozoa with an intact acrosome that contains acrosin, proacrosin, and hyaluronidase and can undergo the acrosome response phase. Spermatozoa need the zona pellucida 3 (ZP3) protein to attach to the pellucid zone of the oocyte when they encounter it. The spermatozoa head-encircling acrosome membrane then undergoes a response known as the AR (Fig. 13.1). The sperm membrane contains the Izumo1 protein, which interacts with its partner, Juno, a receptor in the oocyte, to promote the union of two gamete cells [7–10]. The fertilization process's most significant high point is this step.

An excellent method for identifying male infertility, particularly in unexplained infertility, is the examination of acrosome function. Acrosome activity on human sperm cells has been assessed using various techniques, including western blotting, spectrophotometry, radioimmunoassay (RIA), fluorometry, and substrate assay. Currently, three techniques were utilized to study the acrosome response on human spermatozoa: fluorescent labels, dyes for bright-field microscopy (DBM), and transmission electron microscopy (TEM) [6]. Since AR occurs naturally in the female reproductive system (in vivo), a chemical is used to elicit the reaction to study it. Commonly utilized compounds included progesterone, calcium ionophore, and protein from ZP [4, 6].

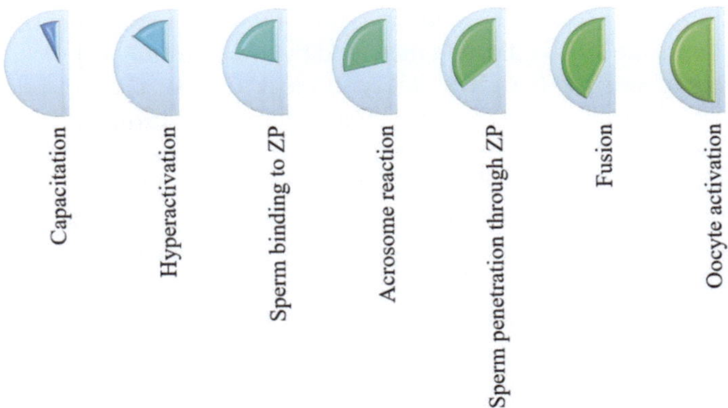

Fig. 13.1 Schematic process when sperm meets oocyte

AR and Diagnosis of Fertility and Infertility

The acrosome response must occur just before the spermatozoa and oocyte come into contact. Acrosome response that happens prematurely will prevent fertilization by preventing spermatozoa from recognizing the pellucid zone. On the other hand, if the acrosome response and spermatozoa activation both fail, there would not be gamete fusion since the spermatozoa would not be able to enter the oocyte [11]. The seminal plasma plays a crucial role in delaying premature acrosome response till the spermatozoa enter the female reproductive system [12].

Oxidative stress, which results from an imbalance between antioxidants and free radicals (ROS), is a condition that frequently harms spermatozoa. This component affects sperm's microscopic characteristics (motility, normal morphology, and concentration) as well as their essential function in fertilizing the oocyte. Oxidative stress can have an impact on the acrosome response phase of fertilization. However, for excellent sperm function, such as capacitation and AR, ROS is required in sufficient amounts [13–16].

Melatonin was introduced to the sperm preparation procedure in sperm that had undergone oxidative stress damage and were intended to undergo IVF/ICSI. This may help the sperm function and acrosome response [16, 17]. Including pinus massoniana bark extract (PMBE) in the cryopreservation procedure may improve the capacity of sperm to fertilize oocytes [17].

A perfect pH level is necessary for the catalytic and acrosome reaction, which include Catsper channels. The seminal fluid's pH level is 7.2, which is thought to be the ideal level for producing acceptable sperm parameters and ensuring that the sperm act well during fertilization [18, 19].

Inositol acts as a mediator to enhance the intracellular amount of calcium in the Catsper channel. Myo-inositol group, a complex vitamin B, is a type of inositol frequently present in the body. The percentage of spermatozoa that exhibit an acrosome response, sperm concentration, motility, total sperm count, and serum inhibin B levels are all significantly increased by myo-inositol [11].

Catsper inhibitor HC-056456's ability to block Catsper channel prior, during, and following capacitation was demonstrated during in vitro and in vivo experiments, as it stopped calcium from entering the cell, and blocked the AR. This chemical was considered as a non-hormonal form of birth control [20].

Mutation (deletion) of SLO3, a potassium channel subfamily that contributes to the shape and function of sperm, may seriously harm spermatozoa morphology and impair motility. An inspection of the ultra-microscopic structure showed a hypoplastic acrosome and damaged mitochondrial sheath [21]. In this instance, ICSI may help the couple become parents.

Numerous proteins were believed to have a role in the spermatogenesis process from a genetic perspective. One of these is the chromosome 6 gene for the Parkinson's disease protein (PARK7). The PARK7 protein was found between the surface and middle of the sperm head and was the main component in charge of binding to the oocyte during fertilization. Higher PARK7-level sperm showed improved capacitation [22].

The genetic anomaly known as globozoospermia, which is characterized by a circular sperm head and no acrosome, affects the acrosome response. This situation is responsible for around 0.1% of male infertility and is caused by a mutation in one of these three genes—DPY19L2, PICK1, and SPATA16. ICSI is required but due to its low fertilization rate (related to deficiency of phospholipase C zeta), addition of calcium ionophore should be considered to activate the oocyte [5, 23].

AR and Etiological Diagnosis of Male Reproductive Functions and Dysfunctions

Mechanism of AR Inducer

The AR may be created artificially by using test yolk buffer, albumin addition, follicular fluid, calcium ionophore, ZP, a lengthy incubation duration, a low incubation temperature, and hypertonic medium (in vitro). Since the AR capability of sperm corresponds with the success of IVF, it can be employed as a sperm function test. Hypothermia, calcium ionophore, and progesterone are the three most often employed AR inducers [24]. These techniques are described below:

Low Temperature Low temperature promotes AR. The sperm suspensions are given two distinct treatments after swim up: (1) The control group is incubated for 24 h at room temperature and then for an additional 3 h at 37 °C; (2) The experimental low temperature group is incubated for 24 h at 4 °C and then for an additional 3 h at 37 °C. After the experiment, slides containing spermatozoa are created to ascertain the spermatozoa's acrosome status. With an overall AR <13% and an induction AR <7.5% links with few fertilized oocytes, this approach correlates well with IVF [24].

Calcium Ionophore Make a stock solution of the calcium ionophore A23187 [9.55 × 10^{-3}M in 100% dimethyl sulfoxide (DMSO)] and keep it at room temperature. Thirty minutes before stimulating the AR, the solution is made by diluting the frozen ionophore stock solution 1:10 in modified human tubular fluid. To produce a concentration of 10 uM ionophore (0.1% v/v DMSO), add an aliquot of the working solution to the sample. The same treatment procedures are used to treat the control samples concurrently, with the exception that just 0.1% DMSO without an ionophore is used. Men who are infertile exhibit a significant decrease in spermatozoa with AR. Male infertility is indicated by a difference in percentage of 5% [24].

Progesterone Sperm are prepared in Biggers, Whitter, and Whittingham's medium (BWW, pH 7.2; Genmed Scientifics Inc., USA) and incubated for 3 h at 37 °C and 0.5% CO_2 (sperm viability >95% after hatching). Progesterone (P4) (P4; final concentration 40 uM) is blended with aliquots of capacitated sperm. In the end, P4-induced AR needs to be higher than 24% and significantly associated with high IVF success rates [24].

The Etiology of Male Reproductive Dysfunctions due to Acrosomal Defects

Male fertility can be hampered by certain illnesses and conditions, particularly those that affect the acrosome (Table 13.1).

Obese Due to altered circulation levels of sperm cholesterol content and estradiol (E2), men with obesity have defective sperm AR, reduced responsiveness to P-AR and higher spontaneous acrosome reaction (sAR). There is a significant relationship between sAR and waist size, weight, and BMI. Spermatozoa from obese individuals

Table 13.1 Summary of causes impairing acrosome reaction

Causes	Result	Reference
Obesity	Sperm from 13 obese men had a higher sAR than those from 19 normal men (17.9% vs. 8.3%), which resulted in a reduced P-AR reactivity as determined by P-AR challenge parameters (3.5% vs 17.6%)	[25]
Varicocele	There are substantial correlations between mitochondrial health and sperm fertility in men with varicocele, which leads to AR dysfunction	[26, 27]
Chronic prostatitis	Men with chronic prostatitis had a markedly higher proportion of spermatozoa with sAR ($P = 0.0472$ and $P = 0.0011$, respectively) and a lower level of AR inducibility ($P = 0.0036$ and $P = 0.0088$, respectively)	[28, 29]
Leukemia	Acute myeloid leukemia (AML) reduces male fertility potential and the number of offspring (in animal studies) while altering sperm parameters and increasing spontaneous AR	[30]

had a significantly higher spontaneous degree of AR than those from normal individuals when the ability of sperm to undergo AR was tested. Furthermore, in a mixed cohort study of overweight individuals, the response to P4 was reduced in obese spermatozoa compared to normal males; this is regarded as an indicator of the inducible response to P-AR. These two features of spermatozoa of obese men may combine to reduce the ability of spermatozoa to fertilize in this metabolic disorder [25].

Varicocele When men are checked for infertility, varicocele is the most common cause discovered [26].

Acrosin activity, AR capacity, and chromatin integrity were all put at risk by the breakdown of sperm mitochondrial membrane potential (MMP). Additionally, human spermatozoa lost adenosine triphosphate (ATP) and their ability to produce ROS as a result of sperm MMP collapse, which may explain why MMP dissipation is dangerous for these critical sperm reproductive capability markers [27].

Zhang et al. offered epidemiological proof of the intimate connections between acrosin activity and mitochondrial function. It showed that MMP dissipation might result in considerable reductions in acrosin activity and AR capability as well as increases in DNA fragmentation index (DFI). These changes were associated by higher levels of ROS generation and lower ATP concentrations [27].

Chronic Prostatitis The total antioxidant capacity (TAC) of seminal plasma, which is a function of chemicals secreted by the prostate, is much lower in individuals with chronic prostatitis. On the one hand, a decreased zinc content in seminal plasma was substantially related with chronic prostatitis [28]. The plasma membrane may get damaged due to oxidative stress, affecting how well it functions. This hypothesis is supported by the finding by Ichikawa et al. that seminal ROS levels are negatively correlated with acrosomal function. Finally, the results of this investigation demonstrated that regardless of whether the disease is inflammatory (NIH IIIA) or non-inflammatory, acrosomal activity was significantly compromised in those with chronic prostatitis (NIH IIIB) [31, 32]. As potential causes of this dysfunction, it is important to look at the negative effects of ROS and the decreased overall antioxidative capacity of the seminal vesicles in people with chronic prostatitis. The pathophysiology of genital tract inflammations impacting sperm activity, fertilization, and pregnancy heavily depends on the balance between sperm ROS generation and antioxidant capacity [32].

Both the NIH IIIA and NIH IIIB patient groups' spontaneous AR and the inducibility of AR, are significantly impacted by prostatitis [31].

Leukemia One of the most prevalent cancers among young individuals is leukemia. Anticancer treatment with intense chemotherapy or radiation, has been shown to have negative effects on the reproductive system, resulting in oligospermia or azoospermia in a significant proportion of patients, and this may be irreversible in some [33]. The outcome supported past research showing that sperm parameters are decreased by AML disease. Male infertility can be caused by AML alone, and chemotherapy will make the condition worse [30]. Future treatments for male infertility in cancer patients may be developed as a result of better understanding of how AML and chemotherapy function.

AR and Planning of Further Investigations

Several methods, including optical and electron microscopy, indirect immunofluorescence employing polyclonal and monoclonal antibodies, and labeling with fluorescein-binding lectin, have been proposed to identify intact acrosomes from acrosome-reacted human sperm (Fig. 13.2) [24].

Direct Tests

Transmission electron microscopy is not an easy way to assess AR. The fact that it requires expensive equipment and trained staff for preparation and analysis limits its usage in clinical practice and research, despite the fact that it is thought to be the most accurate approach for identifying AR. Transmission electron microscopy is a time-consuming approach that only assesses a small number of cells [24].

Indirect Tests

For AR, numerous indirect tests are employed. These are the tests which are most often performed and can be based on various histochemical staining techniques with a light microscopy. These include immunofluorescence microscopy or flow cytometry, or by the triplicate staining method or fluorescently tagged antibodies and lectins [24].

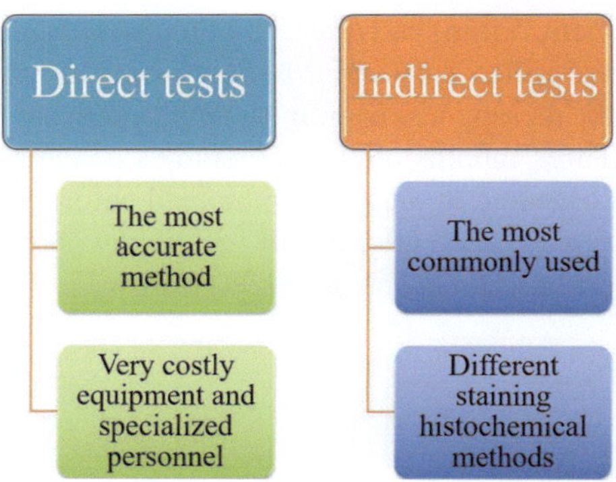

Fig. 13.2 Acrosome reaction tests

AR and Non-ART Management: Treatment and Response Monitoring

The results of the induced AR are more relevant since the acrosome response to ionophore challenge (ARIC) can discriminate between spontaneous and induced AR. To induce AR, a wide range of stimuli have been used, with various degrees of success. The potential for fertilization of a sample can be determined through ARIC testing. The ARIC test has been utilized to assess couples undergoing IVF because it was shown that a low proportion of naturally occurring spontaneous AR was associated with lower fertilization rates [29].

$$\text{ARIC score} = \left(\%iAR - \%sAR \right)$$

$\%iAR$ percentage of induced acrosome reaction, $\% sAR$ percentage of spontaneous AR.

The normal value [34, 35]:

$$\text{ARIC} = 15\%$$

Abnormal sperm function: ARIC 10–15%, %ARIC >20% suggest occurrence premature AR.

With excellent specificity (80.6%) and sensitivity (63.2%), an individual prediction for at least 60% of fertilization was made possible using ARIC and sperm morphology [29]. There are various non-ART therapies for AR available right now.

Atorvastatin and Cholesterol-Lowering Therapy

In capacitating settings, capacitation and AR were tested to gauge spermatozoa's capacity for fertilization. Treatment with atorvastatin had no impact on the percentage of spermatozoa or the P-Tyr levels of the P110 and P80 protein markers of capacitation. The level of P-Tyr did, however, appear to trend to rise both during therapy and three months following atorvastatin discontinuation. The cholesterol-lowering therapy had a tendency to reduce the percentage of spermatozoa with spontaneous acrosome reaction (16.1 ± 3.0% during vs. 26.1 ± 7.8% prior to treatment, 5 min) and after 3 h of incubation under capacitating conditions (28.3 ± 7.4% vs. 36.1 ± 8.5% prior to atorvastatin intake). This pattern persisted 3 months after the therapy was over. It became significant for the AR percentage after three months. Three months after the therapy's conclusion, this pattern was still present. When compared to the results obtained before the atorvastatin treatment, the AR percentage acquired after 3 h of incubation under capacitating conditions became significant ($12.3 \pm 2.0\%$, $p < 0.05$) [36].

Dietary Supplementation with Calcium

Cellular and molecular processes including sperm motility, chemotaxis, capacitation, and acrosome responses are all regulated by calcium. It has been demonstrated that dietary calcium can aid infertility. Calcium is involved in hormone regulation, oocyte maturation, and uterine receptivity, potentially benefiting reproductive health. While more research is needed for a comprehensive understanding, consulting healthcare professionals before making dietary changes is essential. As a result, it is necessary to look into the function of calcium and its levels in human sperm with idiopathic anomalies [37].

Role of Zinc in Male Infertility

The idea that actin polymerization during sperm capacitation is necessary for preventing sAR is supported by the fact that adding 5–10 uM Zn^{2+} to bovine sperm encourages actin polymerization and reduces the sAR rate. The integrity of the sperm acrosome is probably threatened in sperm with high sAR. As a result, improving sperm acrosome integrity while taking dietary supplements of Zn^{2+} supports Zn^{2+}'s role in preventing sAR. These therapies are supported only by small studies, thus to address this problem, future research should demand more reliable study designs [38].

AR and ART Management: Guide ART Choice

Progesterone-Induced Sperm AR Rate and the Fertilization In Vitro

Although there was no significant correlation between the AR rate of the progesterone group and the rates of fertilization or the development of high-quality embryos ($r = 0.053$, $P > 0.01$), the progesterone group's AR rate was statistically greater than the control group's ($15.6 \pm 5.88\%$ versus $9.66 \pm 5.771\%$, $P < 0.05$). Additionally, there was no correlation between normal sperm morphology and the quantity of tripronuclear (3PN) zygotes ($r = 0.029$, $P > 0.01$), rate of production of 3PN zygotes ($r = 0.20$, $P > 0.01$), rate of development of 3PN embryos ($r = 0.406$, $P > 0.01$), rate of fertilization ($r = 0.148$, $P > 0.01$), or rate of progesterone-induced AR progesterone can significantly enhance AR in vitro, although this may not be a decent indication of the rate of fertilization. In vitro fertilization rate may not be accurately predicted by progesterone levels, and the morphology of the sperm may not represent the rate of 3PN fertilization. To completely comprehend the association between progesterone-induced AR and fertilization rate, as well as the relationship between typical sperm morphology and 3PN fertilization rate, a broader patient group must be studied [39].

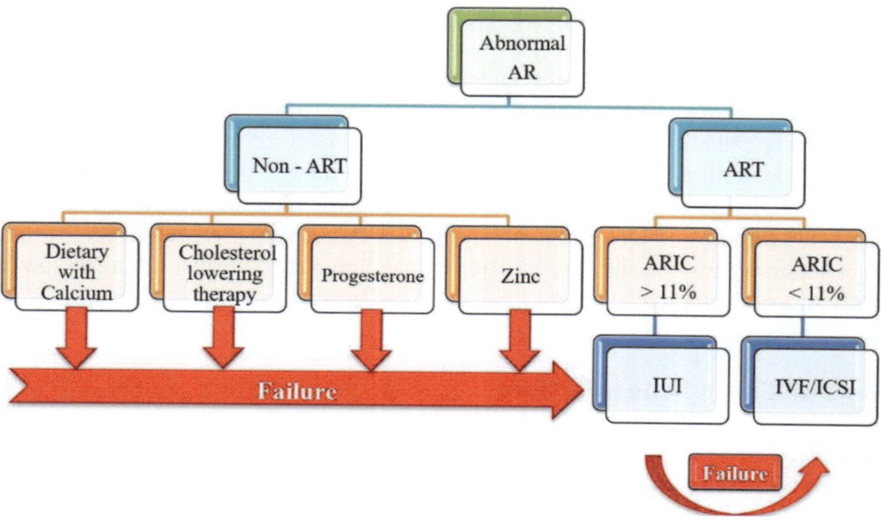

Fig. 13.3 Summary for management of acrosome reaction and ART

For the purpose of diagnosing male factor infertility and treating patients in IVF/ICSI procedures, AR monitoring was added to routine sperm analysis. Regular sperm testing and AR monitoring may support clinical diagnosis and treatment of these patients (Fig. 13.3) [24].

For predicting total fertilization failure and pregnancy in IVF, the ROC curves' calculated AR threshold values were 21% and 26%, respectively. They were the only independent predictors from the conventional semen study. Additionally, when ARIC scores fell below 11%, no pregnancies were achieved by IUI [40].

Two Clinical Scenarios

In the first case, a 36-year-old woman and 32-year-old man have been attempting to conceive for the past 3 years. Despite having frequent and regular sex, they have never gotten pregnant. They look for assistance from an infertility expert. The doctor diagnosed unexplained infertility after doing a number of tests and exams. The lady had a regular menstruation, and the man's semen analysis from three different tests was consistently normal. Nothing else pointed to another reason of infertility. The AR tests were then requested and they were directed to an andrologist. The findings revealed that the ARIC was 10%, much below the expected range. The doctor advised the pair to get ICSI treatment because failing sperm fertilization in IVF is possible with faulty AR. In the first oocyte collection cycle, the couple consented to ICSI treatment. Eight oocytes were harvested and injected with ICSI; six of them were fertilized with two pronuclei, yielding five high-quality embryos. On day three, a single embryo was implanted; the lady conceived and gave birth to a male

39 weeks later. Five more embryos that belonged to the couple are still stored in the freezer.

In the second case, a young couple (a 28-year-old male and a 27-year-old woman) has been attempting to conceive for the past 2 years. The female partner was in good health, had regular periods, and was physically fit. Despite having frequent and regular sex, the couple has never become pregnant. They consult an infertility expert, who does a number of tests and exams. For the female spouse, everything was good; there was no sign of an infertility-related issue. According to the WHO guidelines, the male partner's semen assay revealed 3.3 mL of semen, 60 million sperm/mL of semen, 65% overall motility, 49% progressive motility, and 2% normal sperm morphology. In order to determine if the sperm had the typical capacity to penetrate the ZP in IVF circumstances, the doctor next ordered the AR tests. According to test findings, ARIC was just 10%. The doctor once more suggested the couple think about ICSI therapy in light of these test findings. But during the first oocyte harvest cycle, the patient persisted on undergoing IVF therapy. Subsequently 14 oocytes were retrieved and inseminated for this procedure; however, despite all oocytes being mature and morphologically normal, none of them fertilized. The couple chose to employ ICSI for the second IVF round after the previous cycle's underwhelming outcome. In this procedure, a total of ten mature oocytes were used; nine of them were fertilized, and eight healthy embryos were produced. After the initial transfer of a single embryo on day three, the couple subsequently became pregnant. A baby girl was born at 37 weeks' gestation. Seven more embryos are still in storage and will be used in the future.

Take Home Messages
- To forecast spermatozoa's capacity to fertilize an oocyte, semen analysis alone is insufficient. This is because semen analysis solely refers to the physical assessment of spermatozoa outside of the human body. On the contrary, spermatozoa in the female reproductive system will go through a number of steps, including capacitation, hyperactivation, AR, binding to ZP, fusion, and activation of the oocyte.
- The acrosome is a region that surrounds the nucleus of the sperm head and occupies the front two-thirds of the spermatozoa. The "meeting" of spermatozoa with the oocyte sheath is caused by the acrosome (pellucid zone).
- Normozoospermia alone from semen analysis does not secure pregnancy, hence in unexplained male infertility (UMI) situations, an acrosome test may be the solution. If ARIC <11%, the couple can be advised to have IVF/ICSI despite both of them being found normal during preliminary screening.
- The evaluation of AR using TEM is the most accurate but it requires expensive equipment and trained professionals. In contrast, indirect tests such as immunofluorescence and flow cytometry may be selected as a less expensive option.
- First line therapy for aberrant AR may include lifestyle changes, varicocelectomy, weight loss, treatment of infections of prostate and seminal vesicles, and supplementation with zinc or calcium. If pregnancy is still not achieved, ART may be explored.

References

1. Pencheva M, Keskinova D, Rashev P, Koeva Y, Atanassova N. Localization and distribution of testicular angiotensin I converting enzyme (ACE) in neck and mid-piece of spermatozoa from infertile men in relation to sperm motility. Cell. 2021;10(12):3572. Available from: http://www.pubmedcentral.nih.gov/articlerender.fcgi?artid=PMC8700477.

2. Jairajpuri ZS, Rana S, Ali MA, Pujani M, Jetley S. Patterns of semen analysis: experiences of a laboratory catering to semi urban population of Delhi. Bangladesh J Med Sci. 2017;16(2):314–9. Available from: https://www.banglajol.info/index.php/BJMS/article/view/31944.

3. Gianzo M, Urizar-Arenaza I, Muñoa-Hoyos I, Larreategui Z, Garrido N, Irazusta J, et al. (Pro) renin receptor is present in human sperm and it adversely affects sperm fertility ability. Int J Mol Sci. 2021;22(6):3215. Available from: https://www.mdpi.com/1422-0067/22/6/3215.

4. WHO, editor. WHO laboratory manual for the examination and processing of human semen. 6th ed. Geneva: WHO; 2021. Available from: https://www.who.int/publications/i/item/9789240030787.

5. De Vos A, Polyzos NP, Verheyen G, Tournaye H. Intracytoplasmic morphologically selected sperm injection (IMSI): a critical and evidence-based review. Basic Clin Androl. 2013;23(1):10. https://doi.org/10.1186/2051-4190-23-10.

6. Xu F, Guo G, Zhu W, Fan L. Human sperm acrosome function assays are predictive of fertilization rate in vitro: a retrospective cohort study and meta-analysis. Reprod Biol Endocrinol. 2018;16(1):81. https://doi.org/10.1186/s12958-018-0398-y.

7. Gonzalez SN, Sulzyk V, Weigel Muñoz M, Cuasnicu PS. Cysteine-rich secretory proteins (CRISP) are key players in mammalian fertilization and fertility. Front Cell Dev Biol. 2021;9(December):1–13. https://doi.org/10.3389/fcell.2021.800351/full.

8. Gupta SK. Human zona pellucida glycoproteins: binding characteristics with human spermatozoa and induction of acrosome reaction. Front Cell Dev Biol. 2021;9(February):1–13. https://doi.org/10.3389/fcell.2021.619868/full.

9. Zafar MI, Lu S, Li H. Sperm-oocyte interplay: an overview of spermatozoon's role in oocyte activation and current perspectives in diagnosis and fertility treatment. Cell Biosci. 2021;11(1):4. https://doi.org/10.1186/s13578-020-00520-1.

10. Cannarella R, Condorelli RA, Mongioì LM, La Vignera S, Calogero AE. Molecular biology of spermatogenesis: novel targets of apparently idiopathic male infertility. Int J Mol Sci. 2020;21(5):1728. Available from: https://www.mdpi.com/1422-0067/21/5/1728.

11. Calogero AE, Gullo G, La Vignera S, Condorelli RA, Vaiarelli A. Myoinositol improves sperm parameters and serum reproductive hormones in patients with idiopathic infertility: a prospective double-blind randomized placebo-controlled study. Andrology. 2015;3(3):491–5. https://doi.org/10.1111/andr.12025.

12. Luddi A, Governini L, Wilmskötter D, Gudermann T, Boekhoff I, Piomboni P. Taste receptors: new players in sperm biology. Int J Mol Sci. 2019;20(4):967. Available from: http://www.mdpi.com/1422-0067/20/4/967.

13. Dutta S, Majzoub A, Agarwal A. Oxidative stress and sperm function: a systematic review on evaluation and management. Arab J Urol. 2019;17(2):87–97. https://doi.org/10.1080/2090598X.2019.1599624.

14. Ribas-Maynou J, Yeste M. Oxidative stress in male infertility: causes, effects in assisted reproductive techniques, and protective support of antioxidants. Biology. 2020;9(4):77. Available from: https://www.mdpi.com/2079-7737/9/4/77.

15. Gualtieri R, Kalthur G, Barbato V, Longobardi S, Di Rella F, Adiga SK, et al. Sperm oxidative stress during in vitro manipulation and its effects on sperm function and embryo development. Antioxidants. 2021;10(7):1025. Available from: https://www.mdpi.com/2076-3921/10/7/1025.

16. Minucci S, Venditti M. New insight on the in vitro effects of melatonin in preserving human sperm quality. Int J Mol Sci. 2022;23(9):5128. Available from: https://www.mdpi.com/1422-0067/23/9/5128.

17. Li Y, Zhang T, Jia Y, Yang H, Liu W, Pan J, et al. Supplementation of cryoprotectant with Pinus massoniana bark extract improves human sperm vitality and fertility potential. Andrology. 2021;9(2):700–19. https://doi.org/10.1111/andr.12945.

18. Sun X, Zhu Y, Wang L, Liu H, Ling Y, Li Z, et al. The Catsper channel and its roles in male fertility: a systematic review. Reprod Biol Endocrinol. 2017;15(1):65. https://doi.org/10.1186/s12958-017-0281-2.
19. Mishra AK, Kumar A, Swain DK, Yadav S, Nigam R. Insights into pH regulatory mechanisms in mediating spermatozoa functions. Vet World. 2018;11(6):852–8. Available from: http://www.veterinaryworld.org/Vol.11/June-2018/19.html.
20. Curci L, Carvajal G, Sulzyk V, Gonzalez SN, Cuasnicú PS. Pharmacological inactivation of CatSper blocks sperm fertilizing ability independently of the capacitation status of the cells: implications for non-hormonal contraception. Front Cell Dev Biol. 2021;9(July):1–13. https://doi.org/10.3389/fcell.2021.686461/full.
21. Lv M, Liu C, Ma C, Yu H, Shao Z, Gao Y, et al. Homozygous mutation in SLO3 leads to severe asthenoteratozoospermia due to acrosome hypoplasia and mitochondrial sheath malformations. Reprod Biol Endocrinol. 2022;20(1):5. https://doi.org/10.1186/s12958-021-00880-4.
22. Recuero S, Delgado-Bermúdez A, Mateo-Otero Y, Garcia-Bonavila E, Llavanera M, Yeste M. Parkinson disease protein 7 (PARK7) is related to the ability of mammalian sperm to undergo in vitro capacitation. Int J Mol Sci. 2021;22(19):10804. Available from: https://www.mdpi.com/1422-0067/22/19/10804.
23. Aitken RJ, Baker MA. The role of genetics and oxidative stress in the etiology of male infertility—a unifying hypothesis? Front Endocrinol. 2020;11(September):1–22. https://doi.org/10.3389/fendo.2020.581838/full.
24. Sanchez R, Zambrano F, Uribe P. Manual of sperm function testing in human assisted reproduction. In: Agarwal A, Henkel R, Majzoub A, editors. Manual of sperm function testing in human assisted reproduction. 1st ed. Cambridge: Cambridge University Press; 2021. p. 72–80.
25. Samavat J, Natali I, Degl'Innocenti S, Filimberti E, Cantini G, Di Franco A, et al. Acrosome reaction is impaired in spermatozoa of obese men: a preliminary study. Fertil Steril. 2014;102(5):1274–81. https://doi.org/10.1016/j.fertnstert.2014.07.1248.
26. Poli G, Fabi C, Sugoni C, Bellet MM, Costantini C, Luca G, et al. The role of NLRP3 inflammasome activation and oxidative stress in varicocele-mediated male hypofertility. Int J Mol Sci. 2022;23(9):5233. Available from: https://www.mdpi.com/1422-0067/23/9/5233.
27. Zhang G, Yang W, Zou P, Jiang F, Zeng Y, Chen Q, et al. Mitochondrial functionality modifies human sperm acrosin activity, acrosome reaction capability and chromatin integrity. Hum Reprod. 2019;34(1):3–11. Available from: https://academic.oup.com/humrep/article/34/1/3/5181595.
28. Condorelli RA, Russo GI, Calogero AE, Morgia G, La Vignera S. Chronic prostatitis and its detrimental impact on sperm parameters: a systematic review and meta-analysis. J Endocrinol Investig. 2017;40(11):1209–18. https://doi.org/10.1007/s40618-017-0684-0.
29. Tello-Mora P, Hernández-Cadena L, Pedraza J, López-Bayghen E, Quintanilla-Vega B. Acrosome reaction and chromatin integrity as additional parameters of semen analysis to predict fertilization and blastocyst rates. Reprod Biol Endocrinol. 2018;16(1):102. https://doi.org/10.1186/s12958-018-0408-0.
30. Michailov Y, Lunenfeld E, Kapilushnik J, Friedler S, Meese E, Huleihel M. Acute myeloid leukemia affects mouse sperm parameters, spontaneous acrosome reaction, and fertility capacity. Int J Mol Sci. 2019;20(1):219. Available from: https://www.mdpi.com/1422-0067/20/1/219.
31. Henkel R, Ludwig M, Schuppe H-C, Diemer T, Schill W-B, Weidner W. Chronic pelvic pain syndrome/chronic prostatitis affect the acrosome reaction in human spermatozoa. World J Urol. 2006;24(1):39–44. https://doi.org/10.1007/s00345-005-0038-y.
32. Ichikawa T, Oeda T, Ohmori T, Schill W. Reactive oxygen species influence the acrosome reaction but not acrosin activity in human spermatozoa. Int J Androl. 1999;22(1):37–42. https://doi.org/10.1007/s40618-017-0684-0.
33. Tournaye H, Goossens E, Verheyen G, Frederickx V, De Block G, Devroey P, et al. Preserving the reproductive potential of men and boys with cancer: current concepts and future prospects. Hum Reprod Update. 2004;10(6):525–32. Available from: http://academic.oup.com/humupd/article/10/6/525/626465/Preserving-the-reproductive-potential-of-men-and.
34. Oehninger S, Franken DR, Ombelet W. Sperm functional tests. Fertil Steril. 2014;102(6):1528–33. https://doi.org/10.1016/j.fertnstert.2014.09.044.

35. Bastiaan HS, Menkveld R, Oehninger S, Franken DR. Zona pellucida induced acrosome reaction, sperm morphology, and sperm-zona binding assessments among subfertile men. J Assist Reprod Genet. 2002;19(7):329–34. Available from: http://www.ncbi.nlm.nih.gov/pubmed/12168733.

36. Pons-Rejraji H, Brugnon F, Sion B, Maqdasy S, Gouby G, Pereira B, et al. Evaluation of atorvastatin efficacy and toxicity on spermatozoa, accessory glands and gonadal hormones of healthy men: a pilot prospective clinical trial. Reprod Biol Endocrinol. 2014;12(1):65. https://doi.org/10.1186/1477-7827-12-65.

37. Shah SMH, Ali S, Zubair M, Jamil H, Ahmad N. Effect of supplementation of feed with Flaxseed (Linumusitatisimum) oil on libido and semen quality of Nilli-Ravi buffalo bulls. J Anim Sci Technol. 2016;58(1):25. https://doi.org/10.1186/s40781-016-0107-3.

38. Allouche-Fitoussi D, Breitbart H. The role of zinc in male fertility. Int J Mol Sci. 2020;21(20):7796. Available from: https://www.mdpi.com/1422-0067/21/20/7796.

39. Jiang T, Qin Y, Ye T, Wang Y, Pan J, Zhu Y, et al. Correlation analysis of the progesterone-induced sperm acrosome reaction rate and the fertilisation rate in vitro. Andrologia. 2014;47(8):945–50. https://doi.org/10.1111/and.12361.

40. Katsuki T, Hara T, Ueda K, Tanaka J, Ohama K. Prediction of outcomes of assisted reproduction treatment using the calcium ionophore-induced acrosome reaction. Hum Reprod. 2005;20(2):469–75. Available from: http://academic.oup.com/humrep/article/20/2/469/603306/Prediction-of-outcomes-of-assisted-reproduction.

Sperm Chromatin Condensation

14

Hussein Kandil [iD], Pallav Sengupta [iD],
and Ramadan Saleh [iD]

Introduction

Basic semen analysis is known for its modest capability as a tool for fertility evaluation and hence many infertile males can still present with normal conventional semen parameters [1]. This fact indicates the need for a more profound analysis within the genetic aspects, directing the focus toward the sperm nucleus. It has been demonstrated that nuclear chromatin condensation and stability are essential for sperm maturity and hence, its normal function [2]. Disturbance of the stability of the sperm chromatin is associated with lower fertilization in assisted reproduction [3]. However, there is lack of robust data to suggest routine use of sperm chromatin condensation (SCC) testing in the infertility practice. Therefore, Editors of the latest 6th edition of the World Health Organization (WHO) manual of human semen analysis considered the assessment of SCC as an advanced test of semen [4]. This indicates the need for new studies to investigate the clinical utility of this test in the infertility practice. Indeed, this step should include determining accurate cutoff values that can reliably differentiate between normal and abnormal sperm chromatin. This chapter aims to discuss the physiology of SCC and the impact of sperm chromatin abnormalities on natural and assisted reproduction. Additionally, we

H. Kandil
Fakih IVF Fertility Center, Abu Dhabi, UAE

Global Andrology Forum (GAF), Cleveland, OH, USA

P. Sengupta
Global Andrology Forum (GAF), Cleveland, OH, USA

College of Medicine, Gulf Medical University, Ajman, UAE

R. Saleh (✉)
Dermatology, Venereology, & Andrology, Sohag University, Sohag, Egypt

© The Author(s), under exclusive license to Springer Nature Switzerland AG 2024

A. Agarwal et al. (eds.), *Human Semen Analysis*,
https://doi.org/10.1007/978-3-031-55337-0_14

summarize the current methods for SCC testing and highlight their potential role in the management of infertile couples.

Physiology of Sperm Chromatin Condensation

Sperm chromatin condensation is an intricate physiological process that plays an essential role in ensuring the structural integrity of sperm DNA, which is a crucial factor for effective fertilization [5]. The complexity of this procedure reflects the evolutionary importance of encoding genetic data in a way that conserves its integrity, while also enabling the efficient transfer of genetic information to offspring [6]. Throughout the maturation phase of spermatozoa, the initially relaxed chromatin undergoes a series of molecular modifications to reach an extremely compact state. This metamorphosis entails a mixture of transcriptional shifts, structural adjustments, nucleosomal reductions, and ultimately, protamination [6]. Protamination stands out as a key step in chromatin condensation.

As spermatozoa mature, their passage from the proximal to distal segments of the epididymis signifies progressive phases of chromatin condensation, indicating a systematic procedure of nuclear reconfiguration [7]. Protamines are central to this condensation strategy [8]. These arginine-dense proteins supplant histones, resulting in the genesis of a tightly-packed chromatin framework. The act of protamination is propelled by the oxidation of cysteine-thiol groups, leading to the creation of disulfide linkages [8]. This oxidative process is amplified by nicotinamide adenine dinucleotide phosphate oxidation, highlighting the vital nature of this chemical route in upholding chromatin stability [9–11]. Moreover, the interplay between sperm DNA and protamines culminates in the emergence of a distinct toroidal architecture, described as doughnut loops [12]. This structural layout arises from the disulfide connections established among protamines and is reinforced by the potent binding tendency exhibited by arginine and cysteine residues in protamines to DNA [13–15]. The abundance of arginine in protamines imparts a positive charge, enhancing DNA binding. Simultaneously, involvement of cysteine in disulfide bond formation is vital for the rigorous compaction of chromatin [8].

The molecular mechanisms governing SCC are not only a testament to biological integrity but also vital for reproductive functions. The functionality of mature sperm is closely associated with the structural integrity of its DNA [13]. Thus, deviations in chromatin packaging processes can lead to sperm exhibiting deficient chromatin condensation. As the primary function of sperm is the fertilization of oocyte, it is clear that proper SCC is essential for successful fertilization and, consequently, reproductive outcome [16].

Pathogenesis of Abnormal Sperm Chromatin Condensation

The mechanism(s) by which SCC abnormalities takes place is not clear, but environmental toxicants, including endocrine disrupting chemicals (EDCs) may play a role. It is conceivable that EDCs impact steroidogenesis by interacting with normal hormonal homeostasis. Endocrine disrupting chemicals may exert a hormonal agonistic or antagonistic action through interference with the hormonal binding to androgen or estrogen receptors [17]. Additionally, EDCs can cause oxidative stress (OS) affecting steroidogenesis, germinal epithelium differentiation and alter testicular and epididymal structures, and ultimately impair sperm quality and sperm chromatin integrity. It has been suggested that exposure to EDCs during embryo development may have negative consequences on reproductive function and semen quality in the adult life [18]. This may be attributed to the damage of Sertoli and Leydig cell function due to decrease of androgen action.

Human exposure to EDCs such as polychlorinated biphenyls was found to negatively impact the sperm chromatin integrity of adult European males [19]. Similarly, higher incidence of chromatin defective spermatozoa was observed in young South African males professionally exposed to dichlorodiphenyltrichloroethane [20]. It may also be speculated that SCC abnormalities could be attributed to factors known to cause high sperm DNA fragmentation (SDF) as both conditions have several aspects in common. Risk factors and causes of high SDF include smoking [21], male genital tract infections [22], metabolic syndrome [23–25], and varicocele [26, 27].

Genetic anomalies in PRM1 and PRM2 can result in inadequate or disproportionate protamine synthesis, a prominent factor in compromised chromatin assembly [28]. Enzymes implicated in protamine remodeling, namely histone acetyltransferases and histone deacetylases, play crucial roles in chromatin reconfiguration [29]. A disparity in their functionality can impede the histone-to-protamine conversion [30]. Additionally, an overabundance of reactive oxygen species (ROS) has the potential to harm DNA and obstruct proteins vital for chromatin condensation [31]. While a mild ROS presence is essential for optimal sperm function, excessive ROS generation or insufficient neutralization jeopardizes chromatin stability [32, 33].

Potential Etiologies, Risk Factors, and Implications of Sperm Chromatin Abnormalities

Lifestyle determinants, such as tobacco use, alcohol intake, dietary patterns, and obesity, can also influence SCC, either directly or via promoting OS [34]. Both cigarette smoking and heightened alcohol consumption have links to perturbations in sperm DNA quality. Tobacco constituents can stimulate OS and DNA impairment [35, 36]. In parallel, chronic alcohol ingestion might disrupt the equilibrium between deacetylation and acetylation processes, pivotal for chromatin remodeling [37]. A diet lacking antioxidants amplifies the vulnerability of sperm to oxidative injuries,

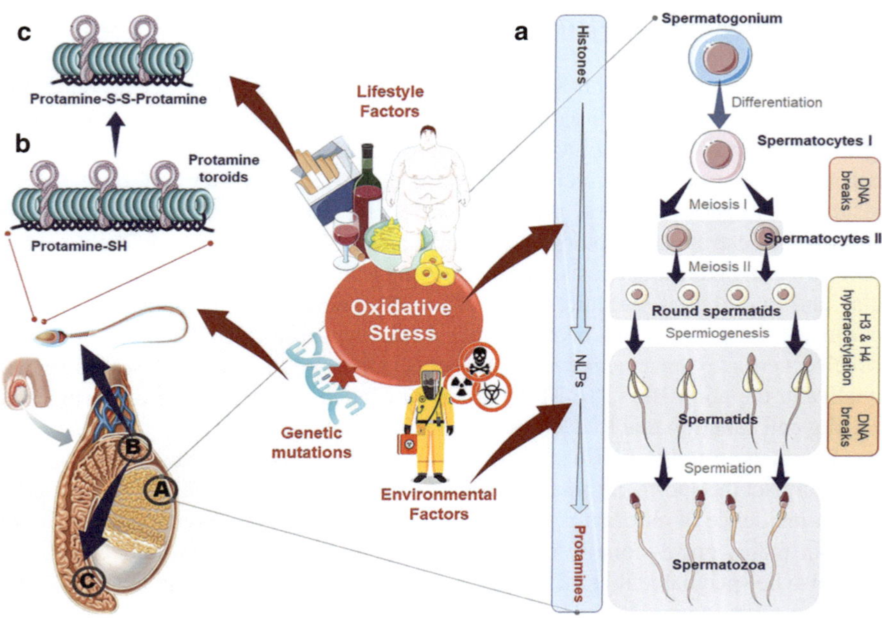

Fig. 14.1 Etiopathogenesis of dysregulation of sperm chromatin integrity. Physiological factors, genetic mutations of regulatory proteins, lifestyle and environmental factors, and oxidative stress affecting protamination of sperm chromatin (**a**), as well as chromatin compaction in its various stages in caput (**b**) and cauda epididymis (**c**)

thereby degrading chromatin caliber. On the other hand, diets abundant in antioxidants, including vitamins C and E, can provide a defensive effect [34]. A surge in body mass index may also be associated with elevated SDF, possibly stemming from amplified ROS synthesis [38] (Fig. 14.1).

Sperm chromatin integrity is not only essential for normal sperm function, but also for the integrity of the developing embryo, with evidence that poor SCC is linked to miscarriages and poor assisted reproductive technique (ART) outcome [39]. Additionally, abnormal SCC has been correlated with DNA impairment in the sperm [40]. This finding has been demonstrated in studies that used protamine deficiency as indicator of chromatin abnormalities with SDF [41, 42] all of which translates a poor fertilization outcome [43]. A study by Sadek et al. demonstrated that SCC was significantly higher in varicocele patients when compared to fertile males with evidence of improvement following varicocele repair [44]. Causes of chromatin disruption are numerous, including genital tract inflammatory condition which was shown to compromise DNA integrity especially when seminal leukocyte count surpasses 0.5 million/ml [45]. Furthermore, the absence of leukocytes does not preclude inflammatory process [46]. Malignancies and their therapies can be associated with a degree of chromatin disruption and epigenetic changes that may exist up to 2 years following the cancer treatment [47]. Another cause of chromatin disruption is hazardous exposure, whether at the environmental or occupational level, which can either directly affect sperm DNA or indirectly through increasing the influx of ROS, which if persist can result in permanent epigenetic changes [48]. Sperm cryopreservation can be associated with alteration in chromatin integrity [49]. A study compared liquid nitrogen freezing of sperm and computerized program freezing and demonstrated a significantly higher SDF occurring with liquid nitrogen [50]. Moreover, Duty et al. noted that rapid freezing through immersion of the semen sample directly into liquid nitrogen without using a cryopreservative showed the highest correlation to fresh semen sample ($R = 0.88$) when SDF was assessed using comet assay [51].

Methods of Sperm Chromatin Condensation Testing

Sperm chromatin structural defects can be associated with sperm DNA strand breaks and/or abnormal nucleoprotein content [18]. Different techniques are available for assessment of SDF such as terminal deoxynucleotidyl transferase mediated dUTP Nick End Labeling assay, sperm chromatin structure assay, sperm chromatin dispersion [4]. These tests are detailed in a separate chapter on "sperm DNA fragmentation." On the other hand, abnormalities of nucleoprotein content can be evaluated by dyes that bind to histones such as aniline blue (AB) or chromomycin A_3 (CMA3) [4], Toludine blue (TB) stain [52] (Table 14.1) or by Raman spectroscopy [43].

Assessing chromatin integrity is usually performed following the staining by either fluorescent or non-fluorescent stains to the sperm sample, this is followed by assessment either through manual observation, which could be associated with variability in test results, or more reliable automated methods as with flowcytometry

Table 14.1 Different sperm chromatin integrity testing

Method	Principle	Assessment parameter(s)	Advantages	Limitations
Toluidine blue staining	It is a metachromatic dye, binding more densely to DNA regions with defects	Intensity and location of staining; DNA maturity and integrity	Simple, inexpensive	Subjective interpretation of staining intensity and location
Aniline blue staining	Differentiates between lysine-rich histones and arginine/serine-rich protamines in the sperm nucleus	Staining intensity; histone-rich vs. protamine-rich areas	Relatively simple and cheap	Subjective interpretation. Not as precise as other assays
Chromomycin A3	Binds specifically to guanosine-cytosine rich regions where protamines are deficient	Fluorescence intensity; protamine deficiency areas	More specific than aniline blue	Requires a fluorescence microscope. Can be expensive

[53, 54] which is performed after applying different stains as acridine orange and propidium iodide and is capable of accurately assessing 10,000 cells in a short time interval [55, 56]. Existing methods assessing SCC may result in functional changes that render the sample not suitable for use e.g., acidic aniline blue; furthermore, these tools are incapable of evaluating the fertilizing capability of the viable sperm [43].

Aniline Blue

Acidic aniline blue (AAB) stain is used to differentiate between histones and protamines based on their respective different chemical composition. Acidic aniline blue tends to interact with lysine present in the nuclear histones and results in blue staining, unlike protamine which is less abundant in lysine and hence will not react with the AB [57]. A negative correlation exists between sperm chromatin integrity with results of AAB staining [58]. Moreover, AAB harbors a good predictability in regard to in vitro fertilization (IVF) outcome [59].

Toluidine Blue

Another method is using TB stain, which is a metachromatic dye highly attracted to acidic entities including nucleic acids [52], hence it has the ability to assess the intensity of chromatin abnormality [60]. Despite being affordable and simple, both AAB and TB are subject to variability in the dye preparation and limitation in the allocated number of cells [61].

Chromomycin A3

Chromomycin A3 (CMA3) is also used in assessing sperm chromatin through its competitive binding with protamine to the DNA [54] and demonstrating abnormal protamination when the population of CMA3 stained sperm are high, with a sensitivity and specificity in determining IVF success of 73% and 75%, respectively [62].

Raman Spectroscopy

Raman spectroscopy is another tool that has been studied in the assessment of chromatin condensation. Raman spectroscopy is a non-invasive and label-free spectroscopic tool, assessing the interaction between light (in-elastic scattering) and the different chemical bonds and has the ability to identify SDF and chromatin condensation abnormalities as efficiently as the currently available staining methods [43].

Management of Abnormal Sperm Chromatin Condensation

A major restraint in managing abnormal SCC lies in the insufficiency of holistic data. While certain interventions have demonstrated potential in improving sperm chromatin quality, a detailed understanding on SCC remains at the forefront of scientific analysis. Emphasis has been placed on the potential benefits of regulating environmental exposures as a means to sustain sperm chromatin integrity and reduce SCC discrepancies [19, 63]. Environmental pollutants, especially EDCs, are implicated in instigating sperm chromatin abnormalities and DNA fragmentation [64, 65]. The precise mechanisms through which EDCs induce such insults are still under investigation, but some research has illuminated potential mitigative approaches. Specifically, OS has been reported as the key regulator, elicited by these pollutants significantly contributes to SCC anomalies [31, 66]. Hence, the role of antioxidants has become increasingly prominent. These compounds possess the inherent capability to quench ROS, thereby reducing OS, a recognized inducer of SCC anomalies and SDF [67]. Vitamin C has shown efficacy in promoting sperm chromatin structural integrity. Studies have indicated that vitamin C supplementation supports sperm chromatin maturation [68, 69]. Combining vitamin C with ellagic acid also manifested protective properties against environmental pollutant-induced damage and improved seminal parameters [70]. Most notably, a balance in seminal oxidative levels was achieved, and a marked decrease in SDF was observed [71]. However, critical questions about the ideal antioxidant, correct dosage, and treatment duration need resolution to ascertain therapeutic safety and effectiveness. Additionally, a profound understanding of environmental pollutants is of equal significance. Prospective investigations should endeavor to categorize the specific impacts of individual EDCs on SCC. This knowledge will be instrumental in devising targeted countermeasures and preventative methodologies, potentially curtailing the risks linked to aberrant SCC.

Role of Sperm Chromatin Condensation in Guiding ART Management

Assisted reproductive techniques require an optimal semen quality to achieve a desired success rate, and since a normal semen analysis cannot pertain a successful outcome, more complex testing is sought to undercover pathologic disease states including genetic abnormalities, which encompass various forms of aberrations including disorders of nuclear packaging and resultant sperm DNA aberrations [72]. Therefore, it is crucial to develop tools capable of assessing sperm chromatin integrity prior to use in ART. Duran et al., assessed the impact of DNA integrity on IUI cycles in a prospective study, and it was shown that patients with SDF>12% had no pregnancy occurring [73] which is also demonstrated in patients undergoing intracytoplasmic sperm injection (ICSI) cycles, where SDF was negatively correlated with ICSI fertilization ($r = -0.23$, $p = 0.017$) [74]. On the contrary it was shown in a different study that fertilization rate was not affected by SDF in IVF/ICSI patients, however, upon further analysis and among the same subjects, patients with SDF <10% had higher fertilization rate compared to those with SDF>10% (84.1 vs. 70.7%, $p < 0.05$) [75]. Though mild degrees of SDF are manageable through the oocyte repair mechanism, there is concern regarding the quality of the ICSI-related embryos when sperm with poor quality result in pregnancy [76]. Similarly, poor early embryo development and embryonic genetic aberrations may result from fertilization by sperm with poor chromatin condensation [43].

Sperm Selection in Patients with Abnormal Sperm Chromatin Condensation

Studies have demonstrated that centrifugation of sperm sample can be associated with increased rates of apoptosis and chromatin abnormalities [77]. Density gradient centrifugation (DGC) was shown to negatively affect sperm DNA integrity by increasing SDF rates in nearly half the cases of IVF/ICSI [78]. Another study has shown that in a multivariate analysis, performing DGC (600 × g for 15 min) resulted in higher rates of SDF when compared to swim up method (400 × g for 15 min) [79]. An alternative that is being sought when it comes to applying a non-destructive sperm selection tool in ART is intracytoplasmic morphologically selected sperm injection (IMSI), which could be considered as an alternative to ICSI in the context of elevated SDF and chromatin abnormalities. Intracytoplasmic morphologically selected sperm injection utilizes high magnification power to select the sperm with optimal nuclear morphology, head symmetry, and shape. When compared to ICSI, IMSI has been associated with higher implantation rate and better embryo quality and development [80]. In the latter study, the IMIS group had higher rate of implantation (57% vs. 27%; $P < 0.05$) [80]. On the contrary, a Cochrane review that included 13 randomized controlled trials involving 2775 couples divided between IMSI and ICSI cycles concluded that there is only very low-quality of evidence supporting the superiority of IMSI on pregnancy rates [81].

Take Home Message

- Sperm chromatin condensation plays an essential role in the fertilizing capacity of males.
- Defective SCC have been correlated with poor sperm quality and reproductive outcomes.
- The mechanisms of defective SCC and the etiological factors underlying these defects are not fully understood.
- Currently available tests for SCC evaluation relies on the assessment of sperm DNA strand breaks and/or abnormal nucleoprotein content. However, these tests are not standardized and their clinical utility is not clear.

- The latest 6th edition of the WHO manual of human semen analysis considers SCC evaluation as an advanced test of semen due to lack of robust data to suggest the routine use of SCC testing in the infertility practice.
- New research is warranted to determine reliable cutoff values that can differentiate between normal and abnormal sperm chromatin and to investigate the utility of this test in the clinical infertility practice.

References

1. Bonde JPE, Ernst E, Jensen TK, Hjollund NHI, Kolstad H, Scheike T, et al. Relation between semen quality and fertility: a population-based study of 430 first-pregnancy planners. Lancet. 1998;352(9135):1172–7.
2. Bichara C, Berby B, Rives A, Jumeau F, Letailleur M, Setif V, et al. Sperm chromatin condensation defects, but neither DNA fragmentation nor aneuploidy, are an independent predictor of clinical pregnancy after intracytoplasmic sperm injection. J Assist Reprod Genet. 2019;36:1387–99.
3. Colaco S, Sakkas D. Paternal factors contributing to embryo quality. J Assist Reprod Genet. 2018;35:1953–68.
4. World Health Organization. WHO laboratory manual for the examination and processing of human semen. Geneva: WHO; 2021.
5. Ward WS. Function of sperm chromatin structural elements in fertilization and development. MHR Basic Sci Reprod Med. 2009;16(1):30–6.
6. Oliva R, Castillo J. Proteomics and the genetics of sperm chromatin condensation. Asian J Androl. 2011;13(1):24.
7. Golan R, Cooper T, Oschry Y, Oberpenning F, Schulze H, Shochat L, et al. Andrology: changes in chromatin condensation of human spermatozoa during epididymal transit as determined by flow cytometry. Hum Reprod. 1996;11(7):1457–62.
8. Nagaki CAP, Hamilton TRS. What is known so far about bull sperm protamination: a review. Anim Reprod. 2022;19:e20210109.
9. Fujii J, Imai H. Redox reactions in mammalian spermatogenesis and the potential targets of reactive oxygen species under oxidative stress. Spermatogenesis. 2014;4(2):e979108.
10. Said S, Funahashi H, Niwa K. DNA stability and thiol-disulphide status of rat sperm nuclei during epididymal maturation and penetration of oocytes. Zygote. 1999;7(3):249–54.
11. Chapman JC, Michael SD. Proposed mechanism for sperm chromatin condensation/decondensation in the male rat. Reprod Biol Endocrinol. 2003;1(1):1–7.
12. Steven WW. Deoxyribonucleic acid loop domain tertiary structure in mammalian spermatozoa. Biol Reprod. 1993;48(6):1193–201.
13. Ward WS, Coffey DS. DNA packaging and organization in mammalian spermatozoa: comparison with somatic cells. Biol Reprod. 1991;44(4):569–74.
14. Ward WS. Regulating DNA supercoiling: sperm points the way. Biol Reprod. 2011;84(5):841–3.
15. Champroux A, Torres-Carreira J, Gharagozloo P, Drevet J, Kocer A. Mammalian sperm nuclear organization: resiliencies and vulnerabilities. Basic Clin Androl. 2016;26(1):1–22.
16. Lazaros LA, Vartholomatos GA, Hatzi EG, Kaponis AI, Makrydimas GV, Kalantaridou SN, et al. Assessment of sperm chromatin condensation and ploidy status using flow cytometry correlates to fertilization, embryo quality and pregnancy following in vitro fertilization. J Assist Reprod Genet. 2011;28:885–91.
17. Sifakis S, Androutsopoulos VP, Tsatsakis AM, Spandidos DA. Human exposure to endocrine disrupting chemicals: effects on the male and female reproductive systems. Environ Toxicol Pharmacol. 2017;51:56–70.

18. Tavalaee M, Razavi S, Nasr-Esfahani MH. Influence of sperm chromatin anomalies on assisted reproductive technology outcome. Fertil Steril. 2009;91(4):1119–26.
19. Spano M, Toft G, Hagmar L, Eleuteri P, Rescia M, Rignell-Hydbom A, et al. Exposure to PCB and p, p′-DDE in European and Inuit populations: impact on human sperm chromatin integrity. Hum Reprod. 2005;20(12):3488–99.
20. De Jager C, Aneck-Hahn NH, Bornman M, Farias P, Leter G, Eleuteri P, et al. Sperm chromatin integrity in DDT-exposed young men living in a malaria area in the Limpopo Province, South Africa. Hum Reprod. 2009;24(10):2429–38.
21. Agarwal A, Farkouh AA, Parekh N, Zini A, Arafa M, Kandil H, et al. Sperm DNA fragmentation: a critical assessment of clinical practice guidelines. World J Men's Health. 2022;40(1):30.
22. Gallegos G, Ramos B, Santiso R, Goyanes V, Gosálvez J, Fernández JL. Sperm DNA fragmentation in infertile men with genitourinary infection by chlamydia trachomatis and mycoplasma. Fertil Steril. 2008;90(2):328–34.
23. Dupont C, Faure C, Sermondade N, Boubaya M, Eustache F, Clément P, et al. Obesity leads to higher risk of sperm DNA damage in infertile patients. Asian J Androl. 2013;15(5):622.
24. Sepidarkish M, Maleki-Hajiagha A, Maroufizadeh S, Rezaeinejad M, Almasi-Hashiani A, Razavi M. The effect of body mass index on sperm DNA fragmentation: a systematic review and meta-analysis. Int J Obes. 2020;44(3):549–58.
25. Zhou L, Han L, Liu M, Lu J, Pan S. Impact of metabolic syndrome on sex hormones and reproductive function: a meta-analysis of 2923 cases and 14062 controls. Aging. 2021;13(2):1962.
26. Saleh RA, Agarwal A, Sharma RK, Said TM, Sikka SC, Thomas AJ Jr. Evaluation of nuclear DNA damage in spermatozoa from infertile men with varicocele. Fertil Steril. 2003;80(6):1431–6.
27. Ni K, Steger K, Yang H, Wang H, Hu K, Zhang T, et al. A comprehensive investigation of sperm DNA damage and oxidative stress injury in infertile patients with subclinical, normozoospermic, and astheno/oligozoospermic clinical varicocoele. Andrology. 2016;4(5):816–24.
28. Balhorn R. The protamine family of sperm nuclear proteins. Genome Biol. 2007;8(9):1–8.
29. Legube G, Trouche D. Regulating histone acetyltransferases and deacetylases. EMBO Rep. 2003;4(10):944–7.
30. Bao J, Bedford MT. Epigenetic regulation of the histone-to-protamine transition during spermiogenesis. Reproduction. 2016;151(5):R55.
31. Bisht S, Dada R. Oxidative stress: major executioner in disease pathology, role in sperm DNA damage and preventive strategies. Front Biosci. 2017;9(3):420–47.
32. Dutta S, Henkel R, Sengupta P, Agarwal A. Physiological role of ROS in sperm function. In: Parekattil SJ, Esteves SC, Agarwal A, editors. Male infertility: contemporary clinical approaches, andrology, ART and antioxidants. 2nd ed. Cham: Springer; 2020. p. 337–45.
33. Agarwal A, Sengupta P. Oxidative stress and its association with male infertility. In: Male infertility: contemporary clinical approaches, andrology, ART and antioxidants. Cham: Springer; 2020. p. 57–68.
34. Leisegang K, Dutta S. Do lifestyle practices impede male fertility? Andrologia. 2021;53(1):e13595.
35. Caliri AW, Tommasi S, Besaratinia A. Relationships among smoking, oxidative stress, inflammation, macromolecular damage, and cancer. Mutat Res. 2021;787:108365.
36. Jenkins T, James E, Alonso D, Hoidal J, Murphy P, Hotaling J, et al. Cigarette smoking significantly alters sperm DNA methylation patterns. Andrology. 2017;5(6):1089–99.
37. Das SK, Vasudevan D. Alcohol-induced oxidative stress. Life Sci. 2007;81(3):177–87.
38. Chaudhuri GR, Das A, Kesh SB, Bhattacharya K, Dutta S, Sengupta P, et al. Obesity and male infertility: multifaceted reproductive disruption. Middle East Fertil Soc J. 2022;27(1):8.
39. Boe-Hansen GB, Fedder J, Ersbøll AK, Christensen P. The sperm chromatin structure assay as a diagnostic tool in the human fertility clinic. Hum Reprod. 2006;21(6):1576–82.
40. Carrell DT, Emery BR, Hammoud S. Altered protamine expression and diminished spermatogenesis: what is the link? Hum Reprod Update. 2007;13(3):313–27.

41. Aoki VW, Emery BR, Liu L, Carrell DT. Protamine levels vary between individual sperm cells of infertile human males and correlate with viability and DNA integrity. J Androl. 2006;27(6):890–8.

42. Aoki VW, Moskovtsev SI, Willis J, Liu L, Mullen JBM, Carrell DT. DNA integrity is compromised in protamine-deficient human sperm. J Androl. 2005;26(6):741–8.

43. Jahmani M, Hammadeh M, Al Smadi M, Baller MK. Label-free evaluation of chromatin condensation in human normal morphology sperm using Raman spectroscopy. Reprod Sci. 2021;28:2527–39.

44. Sadek A, Almohamdy ASA, Zaki A, Aref M, Ibrahim SM, Mostafa T. Sperm chromatin condensation in infertile men with varicocele before and after surgical repair. Fertil Steril. 2011;95(5):1705–8.

45. Pratap H, Hottigoudar SY, Nichanahalli KS, Rajendran S, Bheemanathi HS. Sperm DNA integrity in leukocytospermia and its association with seminal adenosine deaminase. J Hum Reprod Sci. 2019;12(3):182.

46. Sánchez R, Villegas J, Peña P, Miska W, Schill W-B. Determination of peroxidase positive cells in semen: is it a secure parameter for the diagnosis of silent genital infections? Rev Med Chile. 2003;131(6):613–6.

47. Beaud H, Tremblay AR, Chan PT, Delbes G. Sperm DNA damage in cancer patients. In: Genetic damage in human spermatozoa. Cham: Springer; 2019. p. 189–203.

48. O'Hagan HM. Chromatin modifications during repair of environmental exposure-induced DNA damage: a potential mechanism for stable epigenetic alterations. Environ Mol Mutagen. 2014;55(3):278–91.

49. Di Santo M, Tarozzi N, Nadalini M, Borini A. Human sperm cryopreservation: update on techniques, effect on DNA integrity, and implications for ART. Adv Urol. 2012;2012:854837.

50. Petyim S, R C. Cryodamage on sperm chromatin according to different freezing methods, assessed by AO test. J Formos Med Assoc. 2006;89(3):306–13.

51. Duty S, Singh N. Ryan L, Chen Z, Lewis C, Huang T, et al. Reliability of the comet assay in cryopreserved human sperm. Hum Reprod. 2002;17(5):1274–80.

52. Erenpreiss J, Bars J, Lipatnikova V, Erenpreisa J, Zalkalns J. Comparative study of cytochemical tests for sperm chromatin integrity. J Androl. 2001;22(1):45–53.

53. Hodjat M, Akhondi M, Amirjanati N, Savadi Shirazi E, Sadeghi M. The comparison of four different sperm chromatin assays and their correlation with semen parameters. TUMJ. 2008;65(3):33–40.

54. Hekmatdoost A, Lakpour N, Sadeghi MR. Sperm chromatin integrity: etiologies and mechanisms of abnormality, assays, clinical importance, preventing and repairing damage. Avicenna J Med Biotechnol. 2009;1(3):147.

55. Dutta S, Henkel R, Agarwal A. Comparative analysis of tests used to assess sperm chromatin integrity and DNA fragmentation. Andrologia. 2021;53(2):e13718.

56. Evenson DP, Melamed MR. Rapid analysis of normal and abnormal cell types in human semen and testis biopsies by flow cytometry. J Histochem Cytochem. 1983;31(1):248–53.

57. Enciso M, Sarasa J, Agarwal A, Fernández JL, Gosálvez J. A two-tailed Comet assay for assessing DNA damage in spermatozoa. Reprod Biomed Online. 2009;18(5):609–16.

58. Foresta C, Zorzi M, Rossato M, Varotto A. Sperm nuclear instability and staining with aniline blue: abnormal persistance of histones in spermatozoa in infertile men. Int J Androl. 1992;15(4):330–7.

59. Hammadeh M, Zeginiadov T, Rosenbaum P, Georg T, Schmidt W, Strehler E. Predictive value of sperm chromatin condensation (aniline blue staining) in the assessment of male fertility. Arch Androl. 2001;46(2):99–104.

60. Beletti ME, Mello MLS. Comparison between the toluidine blue stain and the Feulgen reaction for evaluation of rabbit sperm chromatin condensation and their relationship with sperm morphology. Theriogenology. 2004;62(3-4):398–402.

61. Agarwal A, Damer M. Sperm chromatin assessment. In: Textbook of assisted reproduction techniques. London: Taylor & Francis Group; 2004.

62. Esterhuizen A, Franken D, Lourens J, Prinsloo E, Van Rooyen L. Sperm chromatin packaging as an indicator of in-vitro fertilization rates. Hum Reprod. 2000;15(3):657–61.
63. Jeng HA. Exposure to endocrine disrupting chemicals and male reproductive health. Front Public Health. 2014;2:55.
64. Pan D, Feng D, Ding H, Zheng X, Ma Z, Yang B, et al. Effects of bisphenol A exposure on DNA integrity and protamination of mouse spermatozoa. Andrology. 2020;8(2):486–96.
65. Giwercman A, Spanó M. Sperm chromatin and environmental factors. A clinician's guide to sperm DNA and chromatin damage. New York: Springer; 2018. p. 301–19.
66. Wright C, Milne S, Leeson H. Sperm DNA damage caused by oxidative stress: modifiable clinical, lifestyle and nutritional factors in male infertility. Reprod Biomed Online. 2014;28(6):684–703.
67. Majzoub A, Agarwal A, Esteves SC. Antioxidants for elevated sperm DNA fragmentation: a mini review. Transl Androl Urol. 2017;6(Suppl 4):S649.
68. Hamidian S, Talebi AR, Fesahat F, Bayat M, Mirjalili AM, Ashrafzadeh HR, et al. The effect of vitamin C on the gene expression profile of sperm protamines in the male partners of couples with recurrent pregnancy loss: a randomized clinical trial. Clin Exp Reprod Med. 2020;47(1):68.
69. Greco E, Iacobelli M, Rienzi L, Ubaldi F, Ferrero S, Tesarik J. Reduction of the incidence of sperm DNA fragmentation by oral antioxidant treatment. J Androl. 2005;26(3):349–53.
70. Mottola F, Iovine C, Carannante M, Santonastaso M, Rocco L. In vitro combination of ascorbic and ellagic acids in sperm oxidative damage inhibition. Int J Mol Sci. 2022;23(23):14751.
71. Caroppo E, Dattilo M. Sperm redox biology challenges the role of antioxidants as a treatment for male factor infertility. F&S Rev. 2022;3(1):90–104.
72. Emery BR, Carrell DT. The effect of epigenetic sperm abnormalities on early embryo-genesis. Asian J Androl. 2006;8(2):131–42.
73. Duran E, Morshedi M, Taylor S, Oehninger S. Sperm DNA quality predicts intrauterine insemination outcome: a prospective cohort study. Hum Reprod. 2002;17(12):3122–8.
74. Lopes S, Sun J-G, Jurisicova A, Meriano J, Casper RF. Sperm deoxyribonucleic acid fragmentation is increased in poor-quality semen samples and correlates with failed fertilization in intracytoplasmic sperm injection. Fertil Steril. 1998;69(3):528–32.
75. Benchaib M, Braun V, Lornage J, Hadj S, Salle B, Lejeune H, et al. Sperm DNA fragmentation decreases the pregnancy rate in an assisted reproductive technique. Hum Reprod. 2003;18(5):1023–8.
76. Mostafa Nayel D, El Din S, Mahrous H, El Din KE, Kholeif S, Mohamed EG. The effect of teratozoospermia on sex chromosomes in human embryos. The application of clinical genetics. New York: Springer; 2021. p. 125–44.
77. Saylan A, Erimsah S. High quality human sperm selection for IVF: a study on sperm chromatin condensation. Acta Histochem. 2019;121(7):798–803.
78. Muratori M, Tarozzi N, Cambi M, Boni L, Iorio AL, Passaro C, et al. Variation of DNA fragmentation levels during density gradient sperm selection for assisted reproduction techniques: a possible new male predictive parameter of pregnancy? Medicine. 2016;95:20.
79. Muratori M, Tarozzi N, Carpentiero F, Danti S, Perrone F, Cambi M, et al. Sperm selection with density gradient centrifugation and swim up: effect on DNA fragmentation in viable spermatozoa. Sci Rep. 2019;9(1):1–12.
80. Luna D, Hilario R, Dueñas-Chacón J, Romero R, Zavala P, Villegas L, et al. The IMSI procedure improves laboratory and clinical outcomes without compromising the aneuploidy rate when compared to the classical ICSI procedure. Clin Med Insights Reprod Health. 2015;9:S33032.
81. Teixeira DM, Miyague AH, Barbosa MA, Navarro PA, Raine-Fenning N, Nastri CO, et al. Regular (ICSI) versus ultra-high magnification (IMSI) sperm selection for assisted reproduction. Cochrane Database Syst Rev. 2020;2:CD010167.

Functional Analysis of Transmembrane Ion Flux and Transport in Sperm

L. Rocco and S. Darbandi

Abbreviations

AR	Acrosome reaction
BPA	Bisphenol A
CatSper	Sperm cation channel
Ccs	Cumulus cells
CFTR	Cystic fibrosis transmembrane conductance regulator
CNG	Cyclic nucleotide-gated
DDT	Dichlorodiphenyltrichloroethane
DGC	Density gradient centrifugation
DSD	Disorders of sexual development
DVF	Divalent-free
ED	Erectile dysfunction
Edcs	Endocrine disrupting chemicals
Ejd	Ejaculatory dysfunction
FDA	Food and Drug Administration
GH	Growth hormone
GPPPD	Genito-pelvic pain/penetration disorder
GΩ	Gigaohm
HCH	Hexachlorocyclohexane
ICSI	Intracytoplasmic sperm injection

L. Rocco (✉)
Department of Environmental, Biological and Pharmaceutical Sciences and Technologies, University of Campania "Luigi Vanvitelli", Caserta, Italy
e-mail: lucia.rocco@unicampania.it

S. Darbandi
Gene Therapy and Regenerative Medicine Research Center, Hope Generation Foundation, Tehran, Iran

A. Agarwal et al. (eds.), *Human Semen Analysis*, https://doi.org/10.1007/978-3-031-55337-0_15

293

MMP	Mitochondrial membrane potential
MSD	Male sexual dysfunction
mtDNA	Mitochondrial DNA
NO	Nitric oxide
NOS	Nitric oxide synthase
NOX5	NADPH oxidase
PCF	Patch-clamp fluorometry technique
PD	Peyronie's disease
Phgpx/Gpx4	Phospholipid hydroperoxide glutathione peroxidase
pHi	Intracellular pH
PMCA	PM Ca^{2+}-ATPase
pp'-DDE	P,P'-Dichlorodiphenyldichloroethylene
PPI	Proton-pump inhibitor
PRL	Pituitary hormone prolactin
RNS	Reactive nitrogen species
ROS	Reactive oxygen species
SB	Spina bifida
TDS	Testicular dysgenesis syndrome
TRP	Transient receptor potential
VCF	Voltage-clamp fluorometry
VGICs	Voltage-gated ion channels
XXY	Klinefelter syndrome

Introduction

Ion Channels, Transmembrane Ion Flux, and Transport That Regulate Sperm Functions

Ion channels are pore-forming transmembrane proteins that affect essential physiological functions such as rest and action potential, as well as ionic homeostasis through ion transport across the membrane. Their action is controlled by specific stimuli such as voltage, ligand binding, temperature, or mechanical stress. These stimuli create conformational rearrangements, leading to gate changes such as closure, opening, desensitization, and inactivation.

It is recommended that mitochondrial functional competence and mitochondrial membrane potential (MMP) of sperm can improve WHO semen analysis parameters such as sperm normal morphology, motility, quality, acrosome reaction (AR), and fertilizing potential. It has been suggested that sperm function characteristics affect the regulation of currents K^+, Na^+, Ca^{2+}, Zn^{2+}, Cu^{2+}, Fe^{2+}, Se^{2+}, H^+, Mg^{2+}, and Cl^- through ionic channels such as sperm cation channel (CatSper), voltage-gated ion channels (VGICs) like Ca^{2+}-activated Cl^- channels (CaCC), sodium channels (NaV1.1–1.9), potassium (Slo3/KCNU1), proton (HV1), cyclic nucleotide-gated (CNG), and the transient receptor potential (TRP) channel family (Fig. 15.1) [1]. Se^{2+} is one of the main trace elements that contribute to sperm function and fertility

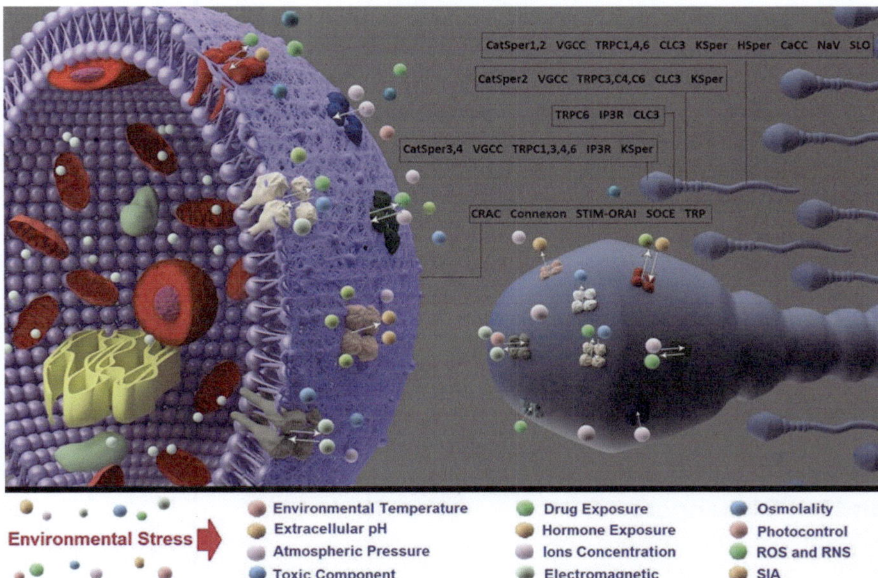

Fig. 15.1 Electrical events in capacitated sperm during fertilization. Modulation of ion channels, particularly Na^+, K^+, Cl^-, H^+, HCO^{3-}, and Ca^{2+} currents, directly/indirectly affect the fertilization process. Location of some ion channels such as Ca^{2+}-activated Cl^- channels (CaCC), Cl^- voltage-gated (CLC), H^+ channel of sperm (HSper), receptor-operated Ca^{2+} channel (ROCC-type IP3R), sperm cation channel (CatSper1-4), Sperm K^+ channel (Ksper), Sperm-specific K^+ channel (SLO), Transient Receptor Potential (TRP) channel, voltage-gated ion channel (VGIC) (voltage-gated Na^+ channel (NaV), and voltage-gated Ca^{2+} channel (VGCC)) **in sperm** and Ca^{2+} release-activated Ca^{2+} channels (CRAC), Large intracellular channels (connexon), store-operated ORAI calcium channels (STIM-ORAI channels), store-operated Ca^{2+} entry (SOCE), and TRP channel **in oocyte** is shown in the figure. Different spermatozoon–oocyte impact angles (SIA) and reactive oxygen and nitrogen species (ROS and RNS) cause different electrical changes in fertilization due to gamete localized contact stress and ZP deformations in the effect of sperm penetration. In addition, during fertilization cumulus cells that cover the oocyte produce and release progesterone, which increases sperm intracellular Ca^{2+} through progesterone-induced Ca^{2+} signaling to stimulate sperm motility and reorientation [1]

ability through two selenoproteins called selenoprotein P and phospholipid hydroperoxide glutathione peroxidase (PHGPx/GPx4) [1]. PHGPx/GPx4 is located in the mitochondria of testis germ cells and the midpiece of human sperm. So, a lower amount of mitochondrial PHGPx in sperm causes defects in sperm mitochondrial morphology, motility, and functions. Sperm motility is stimulated by ATP hydrolysis of dynein, which leads to axonemal bending that lowers intracellular pH (pHi) through H^+/Ca^{2+} exchange (CHX) and glycolysis. Similarly, many TRP channels, including TRPC1-C4, TRPV4, TRPM8, and TRPC6, are a superfamily of cation channels critical for human sperm motility. The HSper channel (H^+ channel of sperm) transmits H^+, is highly sensitive to Zn^{2+}, and mimics the HV1 channel in human sperm [1]. Although HV1 is not an ion channel, it provides a voltage-gated mechanism through the transporter and ion channel for H^+ to pass through a pore-less lipid bilayer [1]. In an ejaculation, SP contains about 2 mM of zinc, directly inhibiting the HV1 function. Sperm PMCA transporter, particularly PMCA4, can affect sperm motility, AR, and capacitation, possibly by interacting with nitric oxide synthase (NOS) at high cytosolic Ca^{2+} levels and preventing elevated nitric oxide (NO) levels and apoptosis. A Na^+-K^+-ATPase pump is also required for sperm motility and function. In mammals, adding Cu^{2+} to the IVF medium has been shown to increase sperm viability and motility. Many unexplained cases of sperm dysfunction, such as genetic abnormalities, may be due to the inadequate function of one or more of these proteins [2]. Therefore, functional analysis of transmembrane flux and ion transport in sperm may be a way to diagnose male infertility and genital diseases.

Physiology and Methodology of Testing

Strategies for Identifying Damaged Transporters and Ion Exchangers

X-ray crystallography and nuclear magnetic resonance spectroscopy study the apparent structural information of ion channels, and their role and regulation are studied using electrophysiological techniques. Voltage-clamp fluorometry (VCF) (cut-open or two-electrode techniques) is a combined technique of chemistry, molecular biology, electrophysiology, and fluorescence. It is used to analyze the voltage sensor data in the voltage gating process of channels [2]. It provides limited-resolution structural information, parallel recording of conformational changes and ion transport activity, and thus a direct link between structure and function. In addition, VCF can detect conformational changes associated with electrical off states (closed, inactive, and desensitizing states) and monitor the activity of transporters that are not electrogenic and cannot be detected by standard electrophysiological techniques. VCF is based on the sensitivity of specific fluorophores to hydrophobicity [2]. Conformational changes in the area around the fluorophore lead to changes in its environment and its diffusion spectra [2]. Compared to the standard voltage-clamps, VCF (cut-open or two-electrode techniques) increases the time resolution of electrophysiological measurements and the intracellular access of proteins [2]. The patch-clamp fluorometry technique (PCF) combines fluorescence and patch-clamp records in an in–out configuration. Compared to VCF, PCF provides direct and rapid intracellular access to ion channels (allowing the labeling of intracellular amino acids and the application of intracellular ligands and channel modulators to control the channel gate), better signal or noise of fluorescence (eliminating the intracellular environment that causes high autofluorescence), and high resolution of current recordings (Fig. 15.2). PCF can be used to study the biophysical properties of each ion channel expressed in the plasma membrane or in combination with other patch-clamp configurations (whole-cell and cell-attached) to investigate the relationship between gating rearrangements and activation in voltage-gated channels [2].

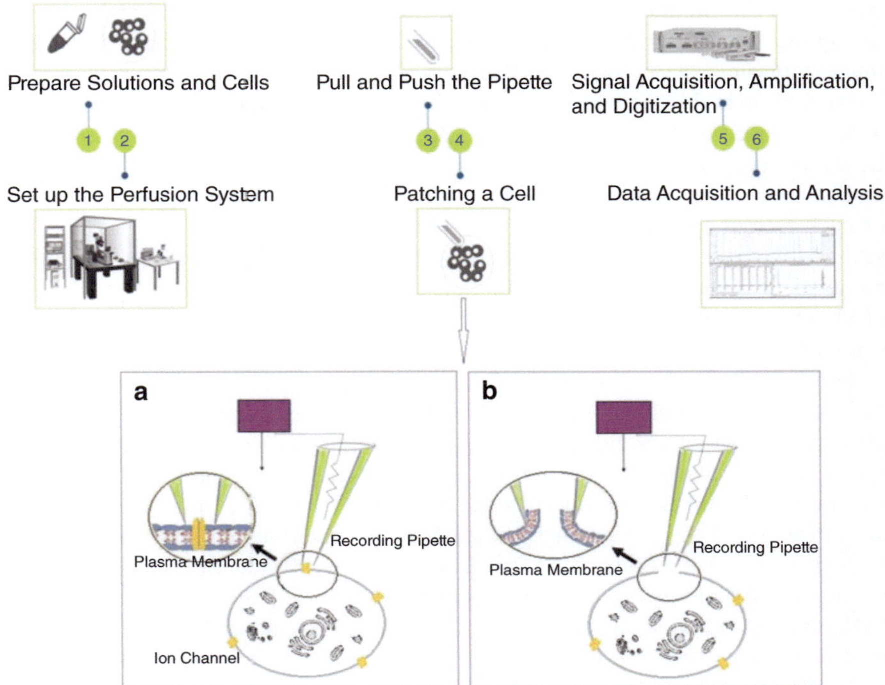

Fig. 15.2 Whole-cell and cell-attached patch-clamp techniques in electrophysiology: (**a**) To record the conductance of a single ion channel, cell-attached electrophysiology is performed by placing a recording pipette on the plasma membrane without rupture of the membrane. (**b**) To record the conductance of the entire cell, whole-cell electrophysiology is performed when a seal is established between the recording pipette and plasma membrane. After seal formation, negative pressure is used to rupture the plasma membrane using the recording pipette

Functional Tests of Transmembrane Ion Flux and Transport in Sperm for the Diagnosis of Fertility and Infertility

Although there is no standard diagnostic method for evaluating the function and the activity of ion channels and transporters in human sperm, clinical trial research has been developed to assess protocols. The two main methods of evaluating sperm ion channels are (a) electrophysiology and kinetic Ca^{2+} fluorometry methods to assess the performance of CatSper, and (b) electrophysiological and fluorometric methods for studying K^+ channel performance [3].

Electrophysiology and Kinetic Ca^{2+} Fluorometry Methods to Assess the Performance of CatSper

The function of the CatSper channel is to generate a current known as $I_{CatSper}$, which has been studied by electrophysiology and Ca^{2+} kinetic fluorometry in human sperm. The CatSper channel is activated by the progesterone released from CCs and affects the flow of Ca^{2+} in the flagellum, sperm swimming, and consequently male infertility. Studies show that sperm with defective CatSper can only be fertilized by using intracytoplasmic sperm injection (ICSI).

According to this method, human mobile sperm must first be purified by density gradient centrifugation (DGC) or swim-up methods. Then, in the whole-cell configuration, the CatSper current of purified sperm is electrophysiologically recorded in divalent ions-free solutions utilizing a glass electrode in the cytoplasmic droplets or neck area of sperm. Sperm are put on glass coverslips. When a gigaohm (GΩ) seal and the entire cell configuration are adjusted, the currents in the prototypical monovalent CatSper are induced using membrane voltage depolarization. The lack of significant reduction in these currents indicates the defective performance of CatSper [3].

For Ca^{2+} fluorometry, sperm are loaded onto the suspension with a fluorescent Ca^{2+} marker dye (such as Fura-2 or Fluo-4). To clear excess extracellular markers after loading, sperm should be centrifuged and suspended in a fresh buffer, and the sperm $[Ca^{2+}]_i$ evaluated by scanning the fluorescence emission markers. On microtiter plates or a cuvette, the fluorescence generated by the Ca^{2+} marker before and after injection of the CatSper agonist (such as progesterone, prostaglandin), buffer (negative control), and ionophore Ca^{2+} ionomycin (positive control) are respectively recorded by a fluorescence plate reader or spectrometer [4]. Studies have shown that CatSper dysfunction is due to a genetic disorder that affects CatSper. Recently, this method has identified two infertile men suffering from poor CatSper function. The result showed that less sensitivity to progesterone is common in infertile men and is associated with their fertilization rate [3, 4]. It is noteworthy that single sperm imaging $[Ca^{2+}]_i$ is also used to study CatSper in patients' sperm to obtain details about individual sperm.

Electrophysiological and Fluorometric Methods for Studying K⁺ Channel Performance

The function of K+ channels in human sperm can be scanned by documenting low and medium potency using whole-cell patch-clamp recording and membrane potential (Vm) fluorometry. Slo3 is the main K^+ channel of human sperm, which is activated by Ca^{2+} and controls the sperm membrane potential in a $[Ca^{2+}]_i$-dependent way. In whole-cell electrophysiological recordings, Slo_3 primary currents can be induced by depolarization of the sperm membrane using extracellular divalent ions solutions and a K^+-based pipette solution to stop CatSper currents. This led to the finding of disease with K^+ channel defects, the depolarization of the resting membrane potential, and low fertilization in IVF. A medium-potency screening for K^+ channel activity depends on voltage-sensitive fluorescent markers. These markers show changes in Vm as changes in their fluorescence emission. For screening, sperm (purified or diluted semen) are incubated with a marker for a few minutes. Then, the fluorescence is recorded in the population using a fluorescence plate reader or a spectrometer. As Valinomycin regulates sperm membrane potential to K^+ Nernst potential, the sperm are challenged with the K^+-ionophore valinomycin and solutions with different concentrations of K^+. Thus, you can convert fluorescence to

Vm conversion, which allows you to determine the membrane resting (V_{rest}) potential and indirect activity of the K^+ channel in human sperm and to show the relationship between V_{rest} and IVF rate [3].

Some Proposed Practical Protocols for Assessing Sperm Transmembrane Ion Flux and Transport

Protocol for the Sperm Flow Cytometry Analysis

1. Incubate the semen for 3 h in capacitating conditions
2. Centrifuge two aliquots containing 2×10^{-6} sperm at $0.3 \times g$ for 5 min.
3. Remove the supernatant.
4. Resuspend the pellets in a staining solution containing 10 µg/ml Alexa Fluor™ 647 conjugated peanut agglutinin (PNA-647, Life Technologies Ltd, Paisley, UK) and 0.8 µg/ml propidium iodide (Life Technologies Ltd) in supplemented Earls buffered salt solution (sEBSS).
5. Incubate control (1% DMSO) and trequinsin (10 µM) sperm at 37 °C and 5% CO_2 for 20 min before flow cytometry analysis.
6. To perform the AR and cell membrane damage, conduct paired positive controls in each experiment using control cells treated with the calcium ionophore A21387 (10 µM) and Triton X-100 (0.1%), respectively.
7. Assess the outcome of trequinsin on AR and membrane integrity using an Intellicyt iQue Screener equipped with a 488-nm laser.
8. Following Intellicyt guidelines, detect fluorescence emission using fluorescence detector 3 (670-nm LP filter) and 4 (675/25 nm) for propidium iodide and PNA-647, respectively.
9. Record forward scatter and side scatter fluorescence data from a minimum of 10,000 events per condition.
10. Select threshold levels to exclude cellular debris and set the gates to distinguish between live/dead and acrosome-reacted/non-reacted using positive control samples.
11. Analyze data using Intellicyt's proprietary Forecyt software [5].

Protocol for the $[Ca^{2-}]_i$ Fluorescence Measurements

1. Incubate the sample for 3 h in non-capacitating media (NCM), capacitating media (CM).
2. Incubate approximately 3×10^{-6} sperm per ml with 4.5 µM of FLUO-4 AM (Thermo Fisher Scientific, Oregon, USA) at 37 °C, 5% CO_2 for 20 min.
3. Centrifuge the sample at 500 g for 3 min.
4. Remove the supernatant and resuspend the pellet in sEBSS.
5. Measure the fluorescence on a FLUOstar Omega reader (BMG Labtech, Offenburg, Germany) at 37 °C; image 3×10^5 cells per well [6, 7].
6. To create the trequinsin dose-response curve, normalize the trequinsin data to the paired $[Ca^{2+}]_i$ response evoked by 3.4-µM progesterone (to prevent the extra sources of variation).

7. Perform desensitization tests using an established methodology [8–10].
8. Add the first mixture after recording the fluorescence for 1 min, then the second after 5 min.
9. Perform control tests to show that progesterone and PGE1 do not cross-desensitize.
10. Perform a control test to show desensitization by adding progesterone and then 17α hydroxyprogesterone or PGE1, followed by PGE2.
11. The protocol for evaluating the action mode of trequinsin is similar. Perform the first challenge cells with progesterone or PGE1, and after 5 min, with trequinsin.
12. Take readings from an additional time control well (baseline) as readings from a well exposed to a single agonist at the time point that matched the time point for adding the second agonist in desensitization tests.
13. Use all mixtures at a final concentration of 10 μM [5].

Protocol for the Measurement of pHi

1. Incubate the sample in CM for 3 h
2. Incubate the sperm (4×10^{-6} per ml) with 2-μM 20, 70 –bis (2-carboxyethyl)-5,6-carboxyfluorescein (ThermoFisher, Paisley, UK) for 30 min at 37 °C.
3. Centrifuge the sperm at 500 g for 3 min
4. Remove the supernatant and resuspend the sperm in sEBSS.
5. Use a FLUOstar Omega reader (BMG Labtech) to detect the emitted fluorescence (ratio of 440/490 nm excitation wavelength and 530 nm emission wavelength) [5].
6. Calibrate the cell after cell lysis by 1% Triton X-100
7. Read from each well
8. Create a calibration curve using 1-M HCl and 1-M NaOH.
9. Record fluorescence measurements for control (cells +1% DMSO), trequinsin (10 μM), and ammonium chloride (NH4Cl) as a positive control for a final concentration of 10-mM [5]

Protocol for Electrophysiology

1. Using the whole-cell patch-clamp electrophysiology, investigate the effect of trequinsin influence on the ion channels of a single sperm plasma membrane [5, 11]
2. Before placing sperm in the recording chamber perfused with a standard extracellular solution, allow them to settle on an untreated glass coverslip.
3. Perform gigaseals between cytoplasmic droplet/sperm midpiece and high resistance (3–12 MΩ) borosilicate glass pipettes filled with either quasi-physiological standard intracellular solution [11], Cs^+-based divalent-free (DVF) intracellular solution [11], or caesium methanesulphonate solution [12] for membrane slope conductance (Gm) analysis, which is mainly done by K^+ ions [11] and CatSper channels, respectively.
4. A seal is formed between the patch pipette and the cytoplasmic droplet/ sperm midpiece in a bath solution.
5. After the break-in, the bath solution can be changed.

(a) **For monovalent currents in DVF solution:** 150 mM sodium gluconate, 20 mM HEPES, and 5 mM Na_3HEDTA; pH7.4 with NaOH. In some studies, the DVF solution is modified by replacing 5 mM Na_3HEDTA with 2 mM Na_3HEDTA and 2 mM EGTA, or with 1 mM Na_3HEDTA and 1 mM EGTA.

    According to the WinMAXC v2.05 program (C. Patton, Stanford Univ.), CaCl2 can be added to the "2 mM Na_3HEDTA and 2 mM EGTA" DVF solution to achieve free $[Ca^{2+}]$ in the nM and low-μM ranges.

(b) **Bath solutions with different concentrations of Ca^{2+}, Ba^{2+}, and Mg^{2+} ions**: the mixture of nominal DVF bath solution (160 mM NMDG and 20 mM HEPES; pH7.4 with methanesulphonic acid) with 50 mM divalent solution (50 mM $Ca(OH)_2$, $Ba(OH)_2$ or $Mg(OH)_2$, 90 mM NMDG and 20 mM HEPES; pH 7.4 with methanesulphonic acid).

The solution's osmolarity is about 305 mmol/kg [12].

6. The access resistance in the whole-cell configuration is usually 25–80 MΩ [12].

7. On average, five successful daily attacks can be easily achieved. The cells are stimulated every 5 s.

8. Perform the transition to whole-cell configuration by using short suction.

9. To examine external membrane conductance, set a depolarizing ramp protocol (−92 to 68 mV) over 2500 ms and control membrane potential at −92 mV between test pulses [5].

10. Assess the effect of trequinsin on reversal potential and membrane slope conductance of external currents by regression analysis over the voltage range where membrane current crosses the x-axis ($I = 0$) and external current from 20 to 68 mV, respectively [5, 11].

11. After achieving the whole-cell configuration, record monovalent CatSper currents by superfusing sperm with Cs^+-based DVF bath solution.

12. Evoke currents by a ramp protocol (−80–80 mV over 1 s).

13. Control membrane potential at 0 mV between ramps.

14. Get a sample data at 2 kHz and filter at 1 kHz (PClamp 10 software, Axon Instruments, USA) [5] or a sample at 10 kHz and filter at 2 kHz (PClamp 9 software, Axon Instruments, USA) [12].

15. Perform the post-recording analysis to modify for liquid junction potential and normalize for cell size [5, 11, 13].

16. For perforated-patch recordings, pipettes solution is 130 mM caesium methanesulphonate, 8 mM NaCl, 10 mM HEPES, 10 mM Cs_4BAPTA, and 240 mg/ml of amphotericin B; pH7.2. Pipette resistance is 12–17 MΩ, and access resistance is 35–100 MΩ. Bath solutions are similar to conventional whole-cell configurations [12].

17. Some pipette solutions;

(a) To record monovalent ICatSper currents at pHi 7.2: 135 mM caesium methanesulphonate, 5 mM CsCl, 10 mM HEPES, 10 mM EGTA, 5 mM Na2ATP, and 0.5 mM Na2GTP (pH with CsOH). In some studies, Na2ATP and Na2GTP are removed from the pipette solution with no significant effect on ICatSper currents.

(b) To record monovalent ICatSper currents at pHi 6.0 and pHi 8.4: 140 mM caesium methanesulphonate, 5 mM CsCl, 20 MES (pH 6.0) or TrisBase (pH 8.4), and 10 mM EGTA (pH with CsOH).

(c) To record divalent ICatSper currents at pHi 7.0 and pHi 8.0: 150 mM NMDG, 5 mM CsCl, 10 mM HEPES, 10 mM EGTA, 5 mM Na2ATP, and 0.5 mM Na2GTP (pH with methanesulphonic acid). In some studies, Na2ATP and Na2GTP or CsCl are removed from the pipette solution with no significant effect on ICatSper currents.

(d) To record divalent ICatSper currents at pHi 6.0 and pHi 6.5: 165 mM NMDG, 10 mM MES, and 10 mM EGTA (pH with methanesulphonic acid).

(e) To record divalent ICatSper currents in symmetrical 50 mM Ba^{2+} conditions: 50 mM $Ba(OH)_2$, 90 mM NMDG, and 20 mM HEPES; pH 8.0 (with methanesulphonic acid).

In some studies, BAPTA solutions are used instead of EGTA solutions to remove divalent-dependent H^+ release by this chelator: 175 mM NMDG, 10 mM BAPTA, 10 mM HEPES, and 10 mM MES, pH 6.0 or pH 7.5 with methanesulphonic acid [12].

Interest in Evaluating Sperm Ion Channel Methods for the Diagnosis of Fertility and Infertility

Functional tests for evaluating sperm ion channel methods in the diagnosis of fertility and infertility are electrophysiology and kinetic Ca^{2+} fluorometry methods to assess the performance of CatSper and electrophysiological and fluorometric methods for studying K^+ channel performance, which has already been explained in detail.

Significant mutations in the cystic fibrosis transmembrane conductance regulator (CFTR) have been identified not only in men with cystic fibrosis but also in those with congenital bilateral absence of the vas deferens (CBAVD) and/or lower-quality sperm [14]. Although cystic fibrosis is a recessive disease, mutagenesis of one CFTR can lead to altered sperm parameters and be associated with CBAVD. There is a relationship between fertility and ciliopathies [14].

Mutations in the genes encoding PKD1 or PKD2, both located in primary cilia, can lead to autosomal dominant polycystic kidney disease (ADPKD), which is associated with infertility. Since the motility of cilia and flagella are both conferred by the same axoneme, it is tempting to speculate that similar axonemic defects could lead to similar phenotypes [14].

Because the Catsper complex is a sperm-specific ion channel, mutations in Catsper genes are less likely to cause broader health problems than changes in other ion channels such as CFTR. For example, deletion of 6 in-frame Catsper leads to normal sperm motility in humans, but fertilization fails due to defective hyperactivation and lack of Ca^{2+} response to progesterone [14].

Deafness-infertility syndrome is a sporadic syndrome characterized by deafness and male infertility associated with homozygous deletion of STRC (expressed in the inner ear) and Catsper2 on chromosome 15q15 [14].

These examples show the importance of diagnosing the mutations leading to channelopathies and the indications for checking them that can affect male fertility and other body systems.

The Na^+/K^+ ATPase generally maintains electrochemical gradients across the cell plasma membrane. The resting membrane potential is regulated mainly by K^+ channels and is typically around -70 mV in somatic cells without stimulation. However it is about -40 mV in mammalian sperm [1, 14]. During capacitation, the sperm membrane becomes hyperpolarized. K^+ current through the activated KSper is primarily responsible for this membrane potential change. Hyperpolarization regulates various membrane proteins, including the voltage-gated proton channel HV1, Ca^{2+} channels, and ion exchangers. Abnormal membrane potential depolarization, the molecular interactions and regulatory mechanisms of Na^+/K^+ exchange, Ksper, and mutations in genes encoding Na^+/K^+ ATPases and KSper are associated with male fertility defects and sperm physiology [1].

As already said, sperm capacitation involves a cascade of signaling pathways that directly or indirectly regulate CatSper [1]. During capacitation, an increase pHi activates CatSper and KSper. Activation of KSper hyperpolarizes the membrane to increase Ca^{2+} influx through CatSper in spermatozoa. It has been shown that HCO^{3-}, Ca^{2+}, and bovine serum albumin (BSA) are essential for sperm capacitation and fertilization in vitro and implicating signaling pathways that regulate CatSper-mediated Ca^{2+} influx [1].

Capacitation starts when spermatozoa are exposed to a high HCO^{3-} concentration in the female genital tract fluid, which also has a higher Ca^{2+} concentration than the epididymal fluid. HCO^{3-} enters sperm via HCO^{3-} transporters and increases cAMP levels. HCO^{3-} also stimulates the entry of Ca^{2+} into the sperm by increasing the pHi. However, the role of cAMP in regulating Ca^{2+} influx needs to be clarified. Membrane-permeable analogs of cyclic nucleotides stimulate Ca^{2+} entry in mouse and human sperm. Still, a series of studies have also shown that an increase in intracellular cAMP (stimulated by HCO^{3-}, 3-isobutyl-1-methylxanthine, cAMP release, or adenosine) cannot stimulate Ca^{2+} influx in rat and human spermatozoa. Thus, cAMP and PKA regulation of CatSper-mediated Ca^{2+} influx is likely species-specific and requires further elucidation [1, 14].

Serum albumin is also a key component in mammalian sperm capacitation in vivo and in vitro. Although BSA is known to induce Ca^{2+} influx in sperm in vitro, the molecular mechanism by which this occurs has not been fully elucidated. However, BSA-induced Ca^{2+} influx is obliterated in Catsper1-null spermatozoa. As cholesterol release from the sperm plasma membrane by BSA is associated with the activation of cAMP–PKA pathways during sperm capacitation in both mice and humans, lipid signaling by cholesterol efflux might participate in regulating CatSper-mediated Ca^{2+} signaling via the cAMP–PKA pathway [1, 14].

Mammalian sperms undergo intracellular alkalinization during their journey as they encounter the drastic change in extracellular pH in the female reproductive tract. During capacitation, the sperm membrane potential is hyperpolarized, mainly through KSper activation and K^+ efflux. An increase in intracellular Ca^{2+} is necessary to induce hypermotility and AR. CatSper is the major Ca^{2+} entry pathway in sperms and is organized into linear Ca^{2+} signaling nanodomains along flagella. CatSper-mediated Ca^{2+} signaling is integrated into other sperm capacitation signaling pathways, including phosphorylation cascades. An improved understanding of sperm ion channels and transporters will help elucidate the subtle and dynamic regulation of Ca^{2+} homeostasis in sperm motility and fertility [1].

Technical advances have significantly improved our understanding of the role of ion channels and membrane receptors in sperm function during fertilization. Current knowledge about ion channels and membrane transporters found in sperm has been shaped mainly by gene deletion studies in animals and human genetic evidence. In particular, our understanding of the molecular and spatial organization of the CatSper channel, the regulatory mechanism by which it is regulated, and the CatSper-based signaling pathways required to induce hypermotility are now well understood. However, this field is still subject to controversy, particularly regarding the way in vitro data can be applied in vivo and how data collected from one species can be extrapolated to other species. Many properties of ion channels are unique to sperm, as sperm-specific channel isoforms have unique properties not found in different cell types. Thus, understanding ion channel mechanisms in sperm cells will advance our knowledge of the treatments for male infertility and should inspire improvements in reproduction and the development of new contraceptives, and improved infertility diagnosis [14].

Sperm ion channels and membrane receptors are attractive targets for the development of contraceptives and infertility treatment drugs. Future studies should seek more evidence from in vivo studies and genetic studies to better understand the regulation and role of ion channels in sperm.

Furthermore, understanding the signaling processes implicated in defective sperm function, particularly those arising from genetic abnormalities is of the utmost importance. This should include identifying and analyzing of gene variants that underlie human infertility and researching fertility-related molecules and treatments.

The manipulation of ion channels to affect fertility could be leveraged for clinical applications such as producing male contraceptives or fertility treatments. About 15% of current drug targets are ion channels. G-protein-coupled receptors and ion channels are promising drug targets as they are implicated in various pathophysiologies and present druggable sites on cell surfaces [14]. Some compounds have been identified that inhibit CatSper. Still, they are non-specific and inhibit KSper with comparable potency, so they are probably not specific enough to be used as contraceptives. RU1968, a ligand of steroidal sigma receptors, has been shown to suppress progesterone-stimulated Ca^{2+} signaling and prostaglandin-stimulated Ca^{2+} signaling in human sperm. RU1968 has also been shown to inhibit human CatSper with about 15-fold higher potency than human KSper, and not to inhibit mouse KSper at all, demonstrating the specificity for CatSper inhibition. Hopefully, RU1968 and other CatSper inhibitors can be used as a template for the design of drugs that could be used in contraception. Many sperm ion channels have yet to be thoroughly explored as therapeutic targets, at least partially due to problems in establishing robustness [14].

Mouse genetic studies have led to an extensive list of genes encoding sperm ion channels and transporters involved in male infertility [14]. However, only a few of these genes, for example, and the genes encoding CFTR or CatSper, have been involved in human infertility but illustrate the practical difficulties of studying the inheritance of infertility. Humans' destructive mutations in the CatSper may have occurred and have been identified with increasing frequency due to the large number of genes required to form this channel complex. Targeted genomic analysis of large cohorts with a specific functional trait and analysis of large families showing Mendelian inheritance of these infertility traits can accelerate the finding of the tests that have the predictive value for the reproductive outcome.

Etiological Diagnosis of Male Reproductive Functions and Dysfunctions

Studies have shown that ions current flow through AQP, CaCC, CatSper1-4, CNG channels, GABA, HSper, IP3R, $K_{ATP,}$ KSper, membrane transporters CHX, Na^+-dependent Cl^-/HCO_3^- exchanger, Na^+-K^+-ATP_{ase}, NCX, NHX, NKCC, NKX, PMCA, ROCC, SLO, TRP channel, voltage-gated ion channels (VGICs) (HV, NaV, VGCC, CLC, and KV) in sperm (Fig. 15.1) [1, 6, 7]. Some SP factors such as pHi, Ca^{2+} concentration, Na^+ concentration, xenobiotics, reactive oxygen species (ROS), reactive nitrogen species (RNS), temperature, osmolality, negative and positive ion channel stimuli (elective, electromagnetic, and photocontrol), as well as the endocrine system, are the main factors can modulate ion channels, sperm Ca^{2+}, other ion concentrations, and protein phosphorylation levels, leading to changes in K^+ and Ca^{2+} input and affecting electrical changes during sperm motility, capacitation, and fertilization [1, 15, 16].

It has been suggested that sexual function between partners, patients' attachment styles, medical conditions, childhood experiences (including sexual abuse), psychological factors, interpersonal factors, sociocultural factors, relationship factors, initiation of sexual activity, personality, cognitive distraction and schemas, infertility concerns, sexual expectations, stress, substance use, post-traumatic stress disorders (and their medical treatments), the anxiety and/or depression, physical and mental illnesses commonly occurring at older age, low sexual desire, and eating disorders (EDs) have a long-term effect on the development and maintenance of male sexual problems [17–29]. Nervous and psychotic disorders, and sometimes prostatitis and hyperthyroidism in men, can cause infertility through erectile dysfunction (ED), ejaculatory dysfunction (EjD), and semen abnormalities [30, 31]. However, there are few studies on gender-incompatible children and adolescents to shed light on the specific developmental factors that shape the development of gender identity and sexual orientation [17, 18].

Congenital or genetic causes such as chromosomal abnormalities [Klinefelter syndrome (XXY), point mutations in the androgen receptor, and CFTR gene], monogenic disorders, multifactorial disorders, endocrine disorders of genetic origin, Y chromosome microdeletions in the AZF region, hypermethylation of the MTHFR (methylene tetrahydrofolate reductase) gene promoter, mitochondrial DNA (mtDNA) mutations, and mtDNA polymerase gene polymorphisms have been identified as a relatively common cause of male infertility. Numerous studies have shown the role of gross genomic rearrangements in male infertility, for example, constitutional aneuploidy, translocations, inversions, increased sperm disomy, and DNA damage [32, 33].

Non-genetic causes include lifestyle factors such as nutrition, balance diet, smoking, some medical causes such as weight, obesity, diabetes, cardiovascular disease, endocrine disorders [hypogonadism, pituitary hormone prolactin (PRL), growth hormone (GH), thyroid hormones, adrenal androgens, testosterone deficiency], hypogonadotrophic hypogonadism, testicular malformations, structural abnormalities of the male reproductive system (obstruction of spermatic ducts, sperm agglutination), infections and inflammation of the genital tract, impotence, varicoceles, chronic disease, gonadotoxic medication, immunological causes such as thyroid autoimmunity and mild hypothyroidism, ED, EjD, previous surgery of the scrotum or inguinal, pelvic and retroperitoneal surgery, pelvic floor muscles, Peyronie's disease (PD), testicular dysgenesis syndrome (TDS), disorders of sexual development (DSD), genito-pelvic pain/penetration disorder (GPPPD), congenital malformations of the spinal, spina bifida (SB), multiple sclerosis and spinal cord injury, anti-sperm antibodies, types of male infertility, male sexual dysfunction (MSD), low-level leukocytospermia, the environment to which the fetal testicle is exposed, and the precise transmission of epigenetic information also have a significant effect on male fertility and the fertility of their offspring [24, 30, 32, 34–42]. There is evidence that several reproductive problems in adult males, such as TDS, increase in the uterus due to the environment in which the fetal testicles are exposed. However, TDS may be caused by genetic mutations [42].

It has been shown that smoking can reduce fertilization capacity by impairing endocrine function, increasing serum LH and FSH levels, decreasing serum testosterone, reducing mitochondrial activity in sperm, increasing sperm ROS, damaging sperm DNA integrity, and resulting in cell apoptosis. Smoking also shows abnormalities in sperm motility count and morphology (astheno-, oligo—and teratozoospermia) [36, 43].

It has been suggested that environmental factors such as air pollution, electronic waste (e-waste), ecological pollution, environmental toxins such as cadmium, mercury, bisphenol A (BPA), and dioxin, endocrine disrupting chemicals (EDCs), and pesticides can also affect the adult endocrine system. These environmental factors may act directly through epigenetic mechanisms or indirectly disrupt the endocrine system, leading to male fertility complications [25, 36, 42, 44, 45]. Studies in the testis have shown the importance of ROS caused by environmental toxins in disrupting cell junctions, which are regulated by activating PI3K/c-Src/FAK and MAPK signaling pathways with the involvement of polarity proteins. This leads to reproductive dysfunction, such as decreased sperm count and semen quality [46]. Contaminants and drugs such as 4-aminopyridine, EDCs, endogenous steroids, endothelin-1, and plant triterpenoids can also significantly affect on fertilizing through selective channel inhibition [1, 47].

The timing and extent of exposure to different types of radiation can have lasting effects on humans. In particular, X-rays and gamma rays have lethal effects on the human body germ cells and Leydig cells [36]. These rays and the radiotherapy and chemotherapy treatments used for cancer, cause short-term or permanent dysfunction of the gonads and cytotoxic effects in male patients [36, 48]. The rate of loss of spermatogenesis is based on the fact that dividing sperm cells are susceptible to the lethal effect of cytotoxic chemotherapeutic and radiotherapeutic agents. Hence, the biological mechanism of sperm production remains unaffected after chemotherapy and radiotherapy. Decreased sperm count occurs due to the adverse effects of cytotoxic chemotherapy or radiotherapy treatment on the spermatogenic epithelium. However, if the sperm epithelium survives, there is a risk of reproduction because cancer treatment has mutagenic effects on the sperm [36, 48]. Low-frequency electromagnetic fields and cell phones show adverse effects on sperm count, viability, morphology, fertility, and increased ROS [36, 49]. It has been demonstrated that pulsed electric fields can create holes in VGICs voltage sensors and provide specific signals that regulate many intracellular processes [50]. Although many studies have shown that low-frequency electromagnetic fields have a positive effect on sperm fertility, it is not clear whether electromagnetic fields are beneficial or harmful [1, 49]. It has also been shown that photocontrol [51] and xenobiotics such as lead compound, phenylurea herbicide, zinc, and tin can affect VGICs in human sperm and reproductive processes [1, 52]. However, PM Ca^{2+}-ATPase (PMCA) has been reported to be involved in the removal of toxic heavy metal ions (such as Co^{2+} and Pb^{2+}) [1, 53].

Sperm membrane lipids and the migration of locally polarized surface essential antigens play an important role in regulating sperm interactions and stimulating sperm capacity in the sperm maturation process [1, 54]. Thus, peroxidation of sperm lipids by ROS and RNS can impair all sperm functions [1, 55]. During sperm activation, Ca^{2+}-dependent NADPH oxidase (NOX5), as a significant ROS generator, can pair with Ca^{2+} and disrupt AR and sperm fusion [1, 55].

It has been reported that the endocrine system can increase intracellular Ca^{2+} through the CatSper mechanism [1, 47, 56]. Cumulus cells (CCs) around the oocyte produce and release progesterone, which exposes human sperm to progesterone and increases its intracellular Ca^{2+} through progesterone-induced Ca^{2+} signaling. This causes sperm to undergo drastic changes necessary for sperm motility and reorientation [1, 6, 47, 57, 58].

Paternal aging can cause genetic and epigenetic changes in sperm through its adverse effects on sperm quality and count, as well as on the genitals and the hypothalamic-pituitary-gonadal axis, hormone production, spermatogenesis, and testes, which impair male reproductive functions. These small changes lead to a decrease in the quality and quantity of sperm. The children of older fathers show a high prevalence of genetic disorders, childhood cancers, and several neuropsychiatric disorders [59].

Planning of Further Investigations

As mentioned, mitochondrial functional competence, MMP and regulation of K^+, Na^+, Ca^{2+}, Zn^{2+}, Cu^{2+}, Fe^{2+}, Se^{2+}, H^+, Mg^{2+}, and Cl^- currents through ion channels such as CaCC, CLC, HSper, ROCC type IP3R, CatSper1-4, KSper, Slo, TRP, VGIC can improve WHO semen analysis parameters such as normal sperm morphology, motility, quality, AR, and fertilization potential.

The only solution currently proposed for diseases associated with sperm functional defects is ICSI, which involves invasive medical procedures for infertile male partners and in vitro culture of gametes. Therefore, the identification of potent strategies to stimulate sperm motility and fertilization potential, in vivo or in vitro, could lead to direct treatment of infertile men and become a more appropriate alternative to ICSI.

The study we performed here on sperm function endorses the existence of several ion-transmembrane channels that could be a good target for the development of such new therapeutic strategies soon. Importantly, targeting these proteins using specific inhibitory or enhancing compounds can also be a key point for male contraception.

It seems that choosing one of the tests to assess sperm transmembrane ion flux and transport, such as sperm flow cytometry analysis, $[Ca^{2+}]_i$ fluorescence measurements, pHi measurement, and electrophysiology, in addition to routine semen analysis tests, can provide more accurate information.

Since many male infertility diseases are related to defects in ion channels, several drugs that target ion channels and pumps can be developed and are known as proton-pump inhibitors (PPIs).

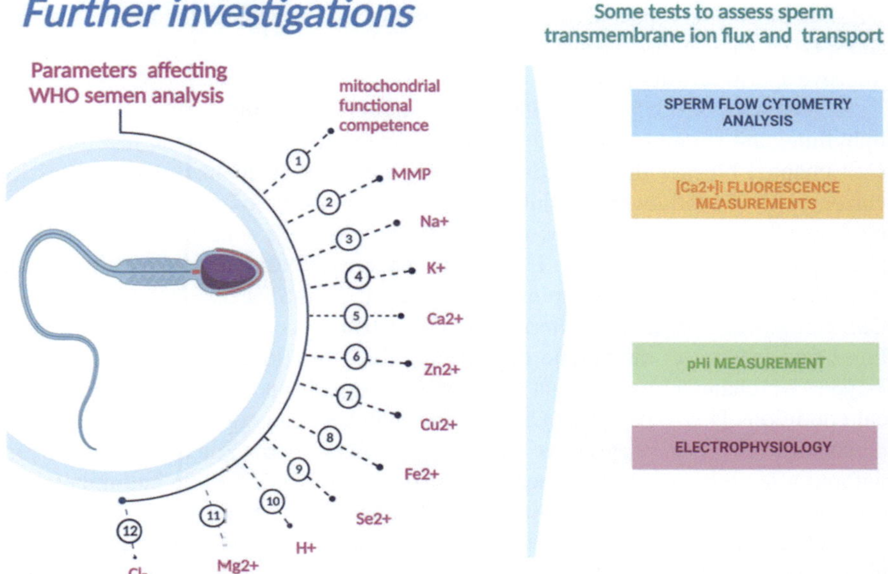

Fig. 15.3 Planning of further investigations

Further studies are needed to test drugs that act as agonists or inhibitors of CatSper to test the channel's potential role as a target for male infertility treatment and contraception. The US Food and Drug Administration (FDA) has approved several drugs for clinical treatment, most of which are in the laboratory testing phase, and a large part of them are natural extracts [60] (Fig. 15.3).

Non-ART Management: Treatment and Treatment Response Monitoring

One study suggested that PPI consumption may affect sperm physiology by inhibiting sperm ATP12A [61].

Studies reported that the concentration of organochlorine compounds such as dichlorodiphenyltrichloroethane (DDT) and its metabolites such as hexachlorocyclohexane (HCH), P,P'-dichlorodiphenyldichloroethylene (pp'-DDE) and pp'-DDD in the semen of infertile men is higher than that of fertile men. Anticholinesterases have been shown to affect male fertility by damaging the prostate [62–65]. However,

P,P′-DDE has been reported as a CatSper agonist that stimulates the opening of the CatSper channel and causes Ca^{2+} influx into sperm [66]. In So, P,P′-DDE may improve sperm fertility [60].

HC-056456, NNC55-0396, nifedipine, nimodipine, quinindium, clofilium, theophylline, and ketamine are Ca^{2+} channel blockers [60]. HC-056456 is a different Ca^{2+} channel blocker that selectively targets the CatSper channel and reduces its current. HC-056456 reversibly inhibits increased motility in capacitated sperm, so it is a capable compound that should be further studied as a male contraceptive [67]. Nifedipine and Nimodipine are L-type Ca^{2+} channel blockers that can induce male infertility [60, 68, 69]. Nifedipine also targets the CatSper channel and prevents Ca^{2+} influx into sperm, thus altering the cholestenone content of the sperm membrane and leading to membrane disruption. NNC55-0396 and mibefradil are two T-type Ca^{2+} channel blockers that suppress Ca^{2+} signals under standard physiological conditions [13]. These two Ca^{2+} channel blockers can significantly reduce the percentage of sperm progressive motility and other sperm kinematic parameters without affecting the rate of hyperactive sperm [60]. NNC55-0396 and mibefradil can increase pHi, and $[Ca^{2+}]_i$ and induce AR in human sperm [70].

Cyclamen and helional induce Ca^{2+} signals. These compounds are extracted from plants and bacteria and may act as potent molecules for treating CatSper-related male infertility [60]. Studies have shown that quinidine reversibly and *Clophyllum* irreversibly block Ca^{2+} currents in CatSper channels [13, 71, 72]. Ketamine has been shown to affect human sperm function and inhibit sperm progressive motility by reducing sperm Ca^{2+} influx [60, 73].

That being said, the mechanism of some drugs is not clearly understood. For example, emodin inhibits human sperm function by decreasing sperm $[Ca^{2+}]_i$ and tyrosine phosphorylation [60]. Some herbal compounds, such as Trigonellae Semen (TS) and Panax ginseng, induce sperm hyperactivity by regulating CatSper gene expression. Extraction of pure compounds from TS and Panax ginseng may treat oligoasthenospermia [60, 74]. In addition, matrine significantly inhibits progesterone-induced total sperm motility, linear velocity of capacitation, and AR by stimulating the CatSper channel [75]. Although further clinical trials and systematic evaluations of these molecules are necessary, it seems that matrine can be a potent drug for male contraceptive treatment [60].

So far, drugs targeting the CatSper channel are in preclinical research stages, and more intensive study of the CatSper channel as a target for therapy is needed (Fig. 15.4).

Non ART *and ART* *management with effect on sperm* *ATP12A* *and* *CatSper*

Effect on sperm ATP12A
Non-ART: Proton-pump inhibitor (PPI) consumption

Effect on sperm CatSper
Non-ART: Dichlorodiphenyltrichloroethane (DDT), Hexachlorocyclohexane (HCH), P,P'-Dichlorodiphenyldichloroethylene (pp '-DDE), p,p'-Dichlordiphenyldichlorethan (p,p'-DDD), HC-056456 , NNC55-0396, Nifedipine, Nimodipine, Quinindium, Clofilium, Theophylline, Ketamine, Cyclamen, Helional, Quinidine, Clophyllum, Emodin, Trigonellae Semen (TS), Panax ginseng, Matrine
ART: weakened responses to P4

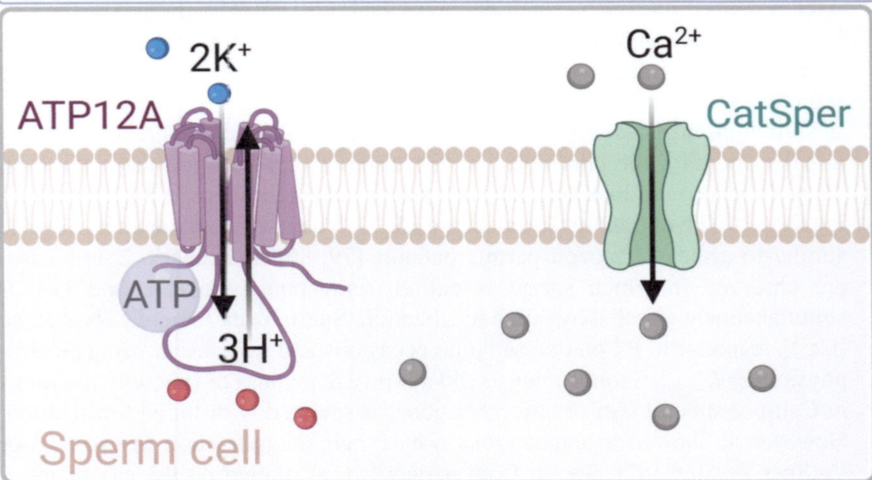

Fig. 15.4 Non-ART management and ART management

ART Management: Guide ART Choice

An unsuccessful or significantly weakened $[Ca^{2+}]_i$ response to P4 is common in sperm used for IVF and ICSI. However, the significance of this issue to CatSper performance has only recently been recognized [76–78].

Only the use of patch-clamp electrophysiology, in a limited number of cases, has definitely answered whether P4-insensitive sperm lack $I_{CatSper}$ (Fig. 15.4).

Clinical Scenarios

CatSper Null Sperm

1. These are three brothers with a complex medical history of congenital dyserythropoietic deafness, anemia type 1, and infertility [79]. Semen parameters are abnormal because the men suffer asthenoteratozoospermia [79]. There is a causative mutation for congenital dyserythropoietic anemia type 1. These males are also homozygous for a deletion of approximately 70 kb of the proximal copy of a 106 kb tandem repeat on chromosome 15q15 [79]. Chromosome 15q15 affects four genes, including CATSPER2, which is predicted to result in frameshifts and premature stop codons. An indirect method to identify patients with CatSper-null sperm is to use the $[Ca^{2+}]_i$ response induced by P4 to screen sperm from ART patients, followed by patch-clamp analysis [79, 80]. The absence of CatSper is subsequently confirmed in scenario 1 using sperm from one of the affected men [79]. Drug-induced Hyperactivation of Ca^{2+} was normal in these sperm cell samples [81].

2. In similar clinical cases of men with infertility and different degrees of hearing impairment [80], the chromosomal breakpoints vary between these families. They share a contiguous homozygous autosomal recessive gene deletion affecting the ~100 kb region on chromosome 15q15. Their semen parameters are also similar to asthenoteratozoospermic patients [79, 80]. In scenario 2, two cases are observed in which sperm is entirely unresponsive to P4, and IVF is simultaneously affected by failed fertilization. Sperm from Patient 1 showed no $[Ca^{2+}]_i$ response to P4 on two separate occasions and was absent using electrophysiology $I_{CatSper}$. Exome analysis did not reveal any loss of function mutations in CatSper subunit loci or any other genes associated with failed fertilization. However, it showed a homozygous 6-base pair microdeletion in exon 18 of CatSper Epsilon [82]. Sperm from patient 2 was studied on the day of treatment, and P4 had no $[Ca^{2+}]_i$ and fertilized zero out of nine eggs. However, when sperm from this patient was studied 7 months later (on the day of ICSI treatment) P4 induced a regular increase in $[Ca^{2+}]_i$, and fertilization resulted [82]. Drug-induced Hyperactivation of Ca^{2+} was normal in sperm cell samples from both patients [81, 82].

3. A case of a novel copy number variant at 15q15 (deafness–infertility locus), resulting in a ~55 kb heterozygous deletion causing total loss of CatSper2 [83]. Semen parameters are normal, but $I_{CatSper}$ is absent, and sperm function is affected, as previously reported for CatSper Epsilon deletion [84]. The reason for the profound effect of the heterozygous deletion is still unclear but may be related to mutations in additional gene regulatory elements [81, 83].

Take Home Message

- Conventional semen analysis is considered the initial step to investigate semen quality and male factor infertility; however, this method cannot always provide valid information regarding specific defects of sperm physiology.
- Some proposed practical protocols for assessing sperm transmembrane ion flux and transport are protocols for the sperm flow cytometry analysis, for the $[Ca^{2+}]_i$ fluorescence measurements, for the measurement of pHi, and protocol for electrophysiology, for monovalent currents in DVF solution, and bath solutions with different concentrations of Ca^{2+}, Ba^{2+}, and Mg^{2+} ions.
- Current techniques for evaluating the function of CatSper (or Slo3) are too challenging to implement in the clinical laboratory, and a routine semen analysis cannot detect the dysfunctions of these key signaling components.
- Only experimental research will allow us to implement our understanding of sperm transmembrane ion flux and transport.
- Furthermore, a set of new tests, easy to use and suitable for perfect integration in the framework of the current seminal fluid analysis, are necessary to obtain further helpful information.

References

1. Darbandi S, et al. Electrophysiology of human gametes: a systematic review. World J Men's Health. 2021;40(3):442–55.
2. Kusch J, Zifarelli G. Patch-clamp fluorometry: electrophysiology meets fluorescence. Biophys J. 2014;106(6):1250–7.
3. WHO. WHO laboratory manual for the examination and processing of human semen. Geneva: World Health Organization; 2021.
4. Kelly MC, et al. Single-cell analysis of $[Ca^{2+}]_i$ signalling in sub-fertile men: characteristics and relation to fertilization outcome. Hum Reprod. 2018;33(6):1023–33.
5. McBrinn RC, et al. Novel pharmacological actions of trequinsin hydrochloride improve human sperm cell motility and function. Br J Pharmacol. 2019;176(23):4521–36.
6. Mannowetz N, et al. Slo1 is the principal potassium channel of human spermatozoa. elife. 2013;2:e01009.
7. Lishko PV, et al. Acid extrusion from human spermatozoa is mediated by flagellar voltage-gated proton channel. Cell. 2010;140(3):327–37.
8. Brenker C, et al. Action of steroids and plant triterpenoids on CatSper Ca^{2+} channels in human sperm. Proc Natl Acad Sci. 2018;115(3):E344–6.
9. Schaefer M, et al. A new prostaglandin E receptor mediates calcium influx and acrosome reaction in human spermatozoa. Proc Natl Acad Sci. 1998;95(6):3008–13.
10. Strünker T, et al. The CatSper channel mediates progesterone-induced Ca^{2+} influx in human sperm. Nature. 2011;471(7338):382–6.
11. Brown SG, et al. Depolarization of sperm membrane potential is a common feature of men with subfertility and is associated with low fertilization rate at IVF. Hum Reprod. 2016;31(6):1147–57.
12. Kirichok Y, Navarro B, Clapham DE. Whole-cell patch-clamp measurements of spermatozoa reveal an alkaline-activated Ca^{2+} channel. Nature. 2006;439(7077):737–40.

13. Mansell S, et al. Patch clamp studies of human sperm under physiological ionic conditions reveal three functionally and pharmacologically distinct cation channels. Mol Hum Reprod. 2014;20(5):392–408.
14. Wang H, McGoldrick LL, Chung J-J. Sperm ion channels and transporters in male fertility and infertility. Nat Rev Urol. 2021;18(1):46–66.
15. Brown SG, et al. Complex CatSper-dependent and independent $[Ca^{2+}]_i$ signalling in human spermatozoa induced by follicular fluid. Hum Reprod. 2017;32(10):1995–2006.
16. Mundt N, Spehr M, Lishko PV. TRPV4 is the temperature-sensitive ion channel of human sperm. elife. 2018;7:e35853.
17. Gomes ALQ, Nobre P. Personality traits and psychopathology on male sexual dysfunction: an empirical study. J Sex Med. 2011;8(2):461–9.
18. McCabe M, et al. Psychological and interpersonal dimensions of sexual function and dysfunction. J Sex Med. 2010;7(1):327–36.
19. Fanni E, et al. The role of somatic symptoms in sexual medicine: somatization as important contextual factor in male sexual dysfunction. J Sex Med. 2016;13(9):1395–407.
20. Brotto L, et al. Psychological and interpersonal dimensions of sexual function and dysfunction. J Sex Med. 2016;13(4):538–71.
21. Castellini G, et al. Sexuality in eating disorders patients: etiological factors, sexual dysfunction and identity issues. A systematic review. Horm Mol Biol Clin Invest. 2016;25(2):71–90.
22. Nobre P. Male sexual dysfunctions. In: Hofmann SG, Dozois DJA, Rief W, Smits JAJ, editors. The Wiley handbook of cognitive behavioral therapy. Hoboken: Wiley; 2014. p. 645–71.
23. Rubio-Aurioles E, Bivalacqua TJ. Standard operational procedures for low sexual desire in men. J Sex Med. 2013;10(1):94–107.
24. Bilgutay AN, Pastuszak AW. Peyronie's disease: a review of etiology, diagnosis, and management. Curr Sex Health Rep. 2015;7(2):117–31.
25. Nordkap L, et al. Regional differences and temporal trends in male reproductive health disorders: semen quality may be a sensitive marker of environmental exposures. Mol Cell Endocrinol. 2012;355(2):221–30.
26. Hamada A, et al. Unexplained male infertility: diagnosis and management. Int Braz J Urol. 2012;38(5):576–94.
27. Lee NG, et al. The effect of spinal cord level on sexual function in the spina bifida population. J Pediatr Urol. 2015;11(3):142.e1–6.
28. Berger MH, et al. Association between infertility and sexual dysfunction in men and women. Sex Med Rev. 2016;4(4):353–65.
29. Cohen D, Gonzalez J, Goldstein I. The role of pelvic floor muscles in male sexual dysfunction and pelvic pain. Sex Med Rev. 2016;4(1):53–62.
30. Fode M, et al. Male sexual dysfunction and infertility associated with neurological disorders. Asian J Androl. 2012;14(1):61.
31. McMahon CG, et al. The pathophysiology of acquired premature ejaculation. Transl Androl Urol. 2016;5(4):434.
32. Poongothai J. Etiology, investigation and treatment of human men's infertility. J Infertil Reprod Biol. 2013;1(2):31–6.
33. García-Acero M, et al. Disorders of sexual development: current status and progress in the diagnostic approach. Curr Urol. 2019;13(4):169–78.
34. Rusz A, et al. Influence of urogenital infections and inflammation on semen quality and male fertility. World J Urol. 2012;30(1):23–30.
35. Schuppe H-C, et al. Urogenital infection as a risk factor for male infertility. Dtsch Arztebl Int. 2017;114(19):339.
36. Muhammad H, et al. Male infertility: etiological factors. Am Eurasian J Toxicol Sci. 2015;7:95–103.
37. Lewis RW, et al. Definitions/epidemiology/risk factors for sexual dysfunction. J Sex Med. 2010;7(4):1598–607.
38. Maggi M, et al. Hormonal causes of male sexual dysfunctions and their management (hyperprolactinemia, thyroid disorders, GH disorders, and DHEA). J Sex Med. 2013;10(3):661–77.

39. Buvat J, et al. Endocrine aspects of male sexual dysfunctions. J Sex Med. 2010;7(4):1627–56.
40. Krysiak R, Szkróbka W, Okopień B. The effect of l-thyroxine treatment on sexual function and depressive symptoms in men with autoimmune hypothyroidism. Pharmacol Rep. 2017;69(3):432–7.
41. Celik O, et al. To evaluate the etiology of erectile dysfunction: what should we know currently? Arch Ital Urol Androl. 2014;86(3):197–201.
42. Skakkebaek NE, et al. Male reproductive disorders and fertility trends: influences of environment and genetic susceptibility. Physiol Rev. 2016;96(1):55–97.
43. Dai J-B, Wang Z-X, Qiao Z-D. The hazardous effects of tobacco smoking on male fertility. Asian J Androl. 2015;17(6):954.
44. Sidorkiewicz I, et al. Endocrine-disrupting chemicals—mechanisms of action on male reproductive system. Toxicol Ind Health. 2017;33(7):601–9.
45. Xu X, et al. Increase male genital diseases morbidity linked to informal electronic waste recycling in Guiyu, China. Environ Sci Pollut Res. 2014;21(5):3540–5.
46. Wong EW, Cheng CY. Impacts of environmental toxicants on male reproductive dysfunction. Trends Pharmacol Sci. 2011;32(5):290–9.
47. Mannowetz N, Miller MR, Lishko PV. Regulation of the sperm calcium channel CatSper by endogenous steroids and plant triterpenoids. Proc Natl Acad Sci. 2017;114(22):5743–8.
48. Kenney LB, et al. Male reproductive health after childhood, adolescent, and young adult cancers: a report from the Children's Oncology Group. J Clin Oncol. 2012;30(27):3408.
49. Darbandi M, et al. The effects of exposure to low frequency electromagnetic fields on male fertility. Altern Ther Health Med. 2017;23:24–9.
50. Rems L, et al. Pulsed electric fields can create pores in the voltage sensors of voltage-gated ion channels. Biophys J. 2020;119(1):190–205.
51. Rennhack A, et al. Photocontrol of the Hv1 proton channel. ACS Chem Biol. 2017;12(12):2952–7.
52. Gallo A. Toxicity of marine pollutants on the ascidian oocyte physiology: an electrophysiological approach. Zygote. 2018;26(1):14–23.
53. Andrews RE, Galileo DS, Martin-DeLeon PA. Plasma membrane Ca^{2+}-ATPase 4: interaction with constitutive nitric oxide synthases in human sperm and prostasomes which carry Ca^{2+}/CaM-dependent serine kinase. Mol Hum Reprod. 2015;21(11):832–43.
54. Kawano N, et al. Lipid rafts: keys to sperm maturation, fertilization, and early embryogenesis. J Lipids. 2011;2011:264706.
55. Darbandi M, et al. Reactive oxygen species and male reproductive hormones. Reprod Biol Endocrinol. 2018;16(1):87.
56. Lishko PV, Botchkina IL, Kirichok Y. Progesterone activates the principal Ca^{2+} channel of human sperm. Nature. 2011;471(7338):387–91.
57. Smith JF, et al. Disruption of the principal, progesterone-activated sperm Ca^{2+} channel in a CatSper2-deficient infertile patient. Proc Natl Acad Sci. 2013;110(17):6823–8.
58. Brenker C, et al. The Ca^{2+}-activated K^+ current of human sperm is mediated by Slo3. elife. 2014;3:e01438.
59. Gunes S, et al. Effects of aging on the male reproductive system. J Assist Reprod Genet. 2016;33(4):441–54.
60. Sun X-H, et al. The Catsper channel and its roles in male fertility: a systematic review. Reprod Biol Endocrinol. 2017;15(1):1–12.
61. Cavarocchi E, et al. Sperm ion transporters and channels in human asthenozoospermia: genetic etiology, lessons from animal models, and clinical perspectives. Int J Mol Sci. 2022;23(7):3926.
62. Dallinga JW, et al. Decreased human semen quality and organochlorine compounds in blood. Hum Reprod. 2002;17(8):1973–9.
63. Pant N, et al. Correlation of chlorinated pesticides concentration in semen with seminal vesicle and prostatic markers. Reprod Toxicol. 2004;19(2):209–14.
64. Younglai E, et al. Levels of environmental contaminants in human follicular fluid, serum, and seminal plasma of couples undergoing in vitro fertilization. Arch Environ Contam Toxicol. 2002;43(1):121–6.

65. Kumar R, Pant N, Srivastava S. Chlorinated pesticides and heavy metals in human semen. Int J Androl. 2000;23(3):145–9.
66. Tavares RS, et al. p,p′-DDE activates CatSper and compromises human sperm function at environmentally relevant concentrations. Hum Reprod. 2013;28(12):3167–77.
67. Carlson AE, et al. Pharmacological targeting of native CatSper channels reveals a required role in maintenance of sperm hyperactivation. PLoS One. 2009;4(8):e6844.
68. Li L, et al. Pharmacological investigation of voltage-dependent Ca^{2+} channels in human ejaculatory sperm in vitro. J Huazhong Univ Sci Technol. 2006;26(5):607–9.
69. Saha L, et al. Effect of nimodipine on male reproductive functions in rats. Indian J Physiol Pharmacol. 2000;44(4):449–55.
70. Chávez JC, et al. Acrosomal alkalization triggers Ca^{2+} release and acrosome reaction in mammalian spermatozoa. J Cell Physiol. 2018;233(6):4735–47.
71. Navarro B, Kirichok Y, Clapham DE. KSper, a pH-sensitive K^+ current that controls sperm membrane potential. Proc Natl Acad Sci. 2007;104(18):7688–92.
72. Zeng X-H, et al. Deletion of the Slo3 gene abolishes alkalization-activated K^+ current in mouse spermatozoa. Proc Natl Acad Sci. 2011;108(14):5879–84.
73. He Y, et al. Ketamine inhibits human sperm function by Ca^{2+}-related mechanism. Biochem Biophys Res Commun. 2016;478(1):501–6.
74. Park EH, et al. Panax ginseng induces the expression of CatSper genes and sperm hyperactivation. Asian J Androl. 2014;16(6):845.
75. Luo T, et al. Matrine compromises mouse sperm functions by a $[Ca^{2+}]_i$-related mechanism. Reprod Toxicol. 2016;60:69–75.
76. Falsetti C, et al. Decreased responsiveness to progesterone of spermatozoa in oligozoospermic patients. J Androl. 1993;14(1):17–22.
77. Krausz C, et al. Intracellular calcium increase and acrosome reaction in response to progesterone in human spermatozoa are correlated with in-vitro fertilization. Hum Reprod. 1995;10(1):120–4.
78. Krausz C, et al. Andrology: two functional assays of sperm responsiveness to progesterone and their predictive values in in-vitro fertilization. Hum Reprod. 1996;11(8):1661–7.
79. Avidan N, et al. CATSPER2, a human autosomal nonsyndromic male infertility gene. Eur J Hum Genet. 2003;11(7):497–502.
80. Zhang Y, et al. Sensorineural deafness and male infertility: a contiguous gene deletion syndrome. J Med Genet. 2007;44(4):233–40.
81. Brown SG, et al. Human sperm ion channel (dys) function: implications for fertilization. Hum Reprod Update. 2019;25(6):758–76.
82. Williams HL, et al. Specific loss of CatSper function is sufficient to compromise fertilizing capacity of human spermatozoa. Hum Reprod. 2015;30(12):2737–46.
83. Luo T, et al. A novel copy number variation in CATSPER2 causes idiopathic male infertility with normal semen parameters. Hum Reprod. 2019;34(3):414–23.
84. Brown SG, et al. Homozygous in-frame deletion in CATSPERE in a man producing spermatozoa with loss of CatSper function and compromised fertilizing capacity. Hum Reprod. 2018;33(10):1812–6.

Computer-Assisted Semen Analysis (CASA)

16

Marion Bendayan and Florence Boitrelle

Introduction

Semen analysis (SA) is part of the first line of investigations for an infertile couple [1]. SA assesses various parameters such as sperm volume, pH, sperm concentration and sperm count, sperm motility, sperm vitality, and sperm morphology. SA provides valuable information in the male infertility work-up such as: (1) assessment of male reproductive health and function, (2) diagnosis of male infertility and guidance of its management, (3) the choice of assisted reproductive technique (ART), (4) monitoring the response to male infertility treatment, and (5) assessment of the efficacy of different male contraceptive tools [2, 3]. When these semen analyses are performed on a semen fraction prepared for ART (e.g., by density gradient or swim-up), they could provide information on the choice of the ART technique to use.

The technical procedures are described by the WHO laboratory manual for the examination and processing of human semen in the chapter "Basic Semen Examination" and are updated regularly [2, 4]. The technical procedures described in the current version of the WHO manual are all manual procedures. Automated techniques are currently considered as "non-routine" techniques and are described in the chapter "Advanced Examinations." However, more and more computer-assisted sperm analysis (CASA) systems are on the market and are being used by laboratories to increase the speed of analysis and reduce inter-operator variability.

M. Bendayan
Reproductive Biology, Fertility Preservation, Andrology, CECOS, Poissy Hospital, Poissy, France

Paris Saclay University, UVSQ, INRAE, BREED, Jouy-en-Josas, France

F. Boitrelle (✉)
ART and Andrology Center, Centre Hospitalier Intercommunal de Pois, Poissy, France

In this chapter, we will detail the different CASA systems and their potential clinical applications.

Physiology: Methodology of Testing

There are two types of CASA systems: systems using phase contrast microscopy and systems using an electro-optical technique.

The first CASA system dates back to the 1980s and consisted in the acquisition of successive images of a semen sample with a camera connected to a phase contrast microscope. The integrated software allowed the measurement of sperm concentration and sperm motility. The sperm trajectory was also evaluated, bringing an added value compared to the manual technique where this parameter is not measurable with the naked eye. CASA systems using this technique have subsequently improved and can now differentiate sperm from cell debris. An operator usually has to adjust the optical settings, choose the fields, and validate the consistency of the final result. Among the models using this technique, the best known are those from Hamilton Thorne Research (IVOS and CEROS models) and Microptic Automatic Systems (SCA model). The current versions also allow for additional analyses such as the study of sperm morphology and sperm DNA fragmentation.

Another method consists of the analysis of a light signal passing through the semen sample with a spectrophotometer. The sperm concentration is measured in this way. Sperm motility is also measured through light disturbances induced by the movement of spermatozoa. Sperm morphology is estimated from the concentration and motility results using specific algorithms. The best-known model using this methodology is the SQA from medical electronic systems.

Utility of CASA for the Diagnosis of Male Fertility and Infertility

CASA systems allow the analysis of different sperm parameters, and thus help to establish a diagnosis of infertility linked to a male cause. The main parameters analyzed are sperm concentration, quantitative sperm motility, and sperm morphology. These machines can also assess the qualitative sperm motility, measuring velocity parameters, which cannot be measured by the manual method.

Sperm Concentration

Many studies have focused on comparing the efficacy of sperm concentration measurement by CASA versus the standard manual method (Table 16.1). In 2014, Lammers' Team compared the analyses performed with SQA-V and CASA CEROS versus the manual method on 250 semen samples and showed no significant difference between these three methods, apart from samples with severe oligozoospermia

Table 16.1 Studies comparing sperm concentration analysis between CASA systems and the manual method

Study	Number of samples analyzed	CASA system	Results automated method (M/ml)	Results manual method (M/ml)	Conclusion
Lammers et al. [5]	250	SQA-V Gold CASA-CEROS	32.6 (NS) 2.0 (OS) 32.0 (NS) 7.4 (OS)	28.1 (NS) 1.6 (OS)	No significant difference for patient NS Significant difference for CASA-CEROS for patients OS
Dearing et al. [6]	352	SCA (4.0)	No data	No data	No significant difference
Talarczyk-Desole et al. [7]	184	SCA (5.4)	39	34	Significant difference ($p < 0.0001$)
Schubert et al. [8]	150	SCA (5.4)	No data	No data	No difference
Engel et al. [9]	100	SQA-vision	58.6	59.0	No significant difference except for cryptozoospermia

NS normozoospermic patients, *OS* oligozoospermic patients

Table 16.2 Studies comparing sperm motility analysis between CASA systems and the manual method

Study	Number of samples analyzed	CASA system	Result automated method Total motility	Result manual method Total motility	Result automated method Progressive motility	Result manual method Progressive motility	Conclusion
Lammers et al. [5]	250	SQA-V Gold CASA-CEROS	54.7% NS 38.9% OS 57.0% NS 22% OS	58.3% NS 48% OS	40.1% NS 40.8% NS	40.6% NS	No significant difference for patients NS Significant difference fort patients OS
Talarczyk-Desole et al. [7]	184	SCA (5.4)			34%	30%	Significant difference for progressive motility ($p <$ 0.0001)
Schubert et al. [8]	150	SCA (5.4)	No data	No data	No data	No data	No significant difference
Engel et al. [9]	100	SQA-vision	47.0%	49.6%	33.1%	40.2%	No difference for total motility but significant difference for progressive motility
Dearing et al. [6]	255	SCA (4.1)	No data	No data	No data	No data	Significant difference

NS normozoospermic patients, *OS* oligozoospermic patients

[5]. Dearing's Team found the same result with the SCA (version 4.0) [6]. Similarly, in 2019, the Schubert and Engels teams did not find a significant difference on this parameter using SCA (version 5.4) and SQA-V, respectively [8, 9]. However, Engel's team noted a difference for samples with cryptozoospermia. In contrast, the Talarczyk-Desole study shows a significant difference in sperm concentration analysis of 184 samples with SCA (version 5.4) compared to the manual method [7]. In their study, CASA overestimated sperm concentration compared to the manual method (mean on 184 samples: 39M/ml vs 34M/ml, $p < 0.0001$). To summarize, according to the literature, there is a good correlation of the automatons in the measurement of the sperm concentration compared to the manual method. In the most severe cases of male infertility (severe oligozoospermia, cryptozoospermia), differences between CASA systems are important to take into account. To diagnose cryptozoospermia, for example, the laboratory needs to equip itself with high-performance equipment and/or check their results manually.

Sperm Motility

In the same way, the studies described above have also investigated the analysis of sperm mobility by automate (Table 16.2). Concerning total motility, most studies agree in finding no significant difference whatever the automate used [5, 8, 9]. However, when we are interested in the analysis of progressive mobility, differences are found.

Engel et al. found a significant difference in the analysis of progressive motility with the SQA-V automate [9]. Similarly, the Talarczyk-Desole study shows a significant difference for progressive motility [7]. Dearing et al. in 2019 also finds a significant difference for this parameter [6]. The analysis of total sperm motility by automaton seems to be well correlated with the manual method. Concerning progressive motility, the results are conflicting.

Sperm Morphology

Depending on the CASA system used, the method of analysis of sperm morphology is not the same. Most CASA systems measure sperm morphology by analyzing sperm images and performing morphometric measurements via software. In contrast, the SQA system estimates morphology using algorithms that take into account sperm motility and sperm concentration to deduce the percentage of typically shaped spermatozoa. In the literature, sperm morphology analysis by CASA systems is controversial (Table 16.3).

In 2014, Lammers' team showed a significant difference between the manual method and the automated method using the SQA-V Gold and CASA-CEROS for morphology evaluation [5]. Talarczyk-Desole's 2017 and Engel's 2018 studies also found significant differences between the manual and automated methods [7, 9].

Table 16.3 Studies comparing sperm morphology analysis between CASA systems and the manual method.

Study	Number of samples analyzed	CASA system	Result automated method	Result manual method	Conclusion
Singh et al. [11]	201	SQA-V			Good correlation for the detection of teratozoospermia
Lammers et al. [5]	250	SQA-V Gold CASA-CEROS	10.6% NS 2.8% OS 5.0% NS 3% OS	7% NS 3% OS	Significant difference ($P < 0.05$) for patients NS No significant difference for patients OS
Talarczyk-Desole et al. [7]	184	SCA (5.4)	4%	3%	Significant difference ($p < 0.0001$)
Schubert et al. [8]	150	SCA (5.4)	No data	No data	No significant difference
Engel et al. [9]	100	SQA-vision	7.3%	2.5%	Significant difference

Only the study by Schubert in 2019 showed an acceptable agreement between the manual and automated methods (SCA 5.4) [8].

In 2011, Singh's Team compared morphology analysis on 201 semen samples between the manual method and the SQA-V [10]. The SQA-V analysis showed a sensitivity and specificity of more than 85% for the detection of teratozoospermia (typical form less than 30% with WHO criteria). While the authors confirm that this automate is reliable as a screening test, they note that the gold standard for the analysis of sperm morphology remains the manual method.

Thus, at present, the automated method does not appear to be sufficiently efficient to perform a fine analysis of sperm morphology.

Standardization and Quality Control

For sperm concentration and sperm motility, CASA systems correlate well with the manual method. This seems to be less the case for the analysis of sperm morphology. CASA systems also, in theory, improves the accuracy of the results obtained, as they analyze a large number of cells [11, 12]. Furthermore, once CASA system is well-mastered, it results in saving of time and reduction in operator failure and certainly a better analysis yield.

Since the 5th edition of WHO laboratory manual for the examination and processing of human semen [4], great importance has been given to quality control and standardization of semen analysis so that it is reproducible from one laboratory to another. It is surprising to note that the CASA systems, which perfectly meet these criteria, have not been included in routine analysis systems. If the literature continues to show the value of automated systems, it is likely that the 7th edition of the WHO manual will include them in routine use.

Etiological Diagnosis of Male Reproductive Functions and Dysfunctions

One of the great advantages of automated systems such as CASA is the ability to analyze the quality of sperm movement. The velocity parameters are additional information provided by the automated method that cannot be measured by the manual method. They are mainly the following parameters, as described in the WHO manual [2]:

- VCL, velocity along the curvilinear path (μm/s)
- VSL, velocity along the straight-line path (μm/s)
- VAP, velocity along the average path (μm/s)
- ALH, the amplitude of the lateral displacement of the head (μm)
- MAD, mean angular displacement (degrees)

These measurements provide additional information to the analysis of sperm motility and in particular to assess sperm hyperactivation and thus diagnose abnormalities of hyperactivation of spermatozoa and thus to determine their capacity to cross the cervical mucus and fertilize the oocyte.

Flagellar dyskinesias are indeed difficult to diagnose, are not necessarily coupled with a decrease in spermatic motility and the analysis of spermatic morphology is not always sufficient for the diagnosis, especially when the detail of the abnormalities is not rendered. These parameters can allow diagnosis, as shown in the 1985 study by Feneux, where the authors present the case of patients with a form of flagellar dyskinesia called slippery spermatozoa, which is not detectable by the manual method [13].

ART Management: Guide ART Choice

During an ART attempt, the automated analysis of sperm parameters will allow to easily and quickly orient the choice of the technique. The analyses are performed on the migrated fraction of the semen, which limits the biases linked to the sample, such as cellular debris or viscosity, which can distort the results.

In intrauterine insemination (IUI), the automated measurement of sperm parameters allows for a rapid determination of the number of inseminated motile spermatozoa. In addition, Shibahara's study carried out on 662 IUI cycles showed that motility and velocity parameters performed with the CASA system (Hamilton) are correlated with clinical pregnancy rates [14].

Similarly, during in invitro fertilization (IVF), the sperm parameters will condition the choice of the technique. Indeed, sperm concentration and sperm motility are the parameters mainly used for the choice between conventional IVF and intracytoplasmic sperm injection (ICSI) and are reliable parameters when they are measured with an automatic machine. In addition, a study showed a correlation between mobility and velocity parameters of the CASA system (Hamilton) and fertilization rates in conventional IVF [15].

In the case of ICSI, the usefulness of automated systems seems more questionable. Most reading systems fail at low sperm concentrations. It is important to be familiar with the characteristics and performance of the system used, and it is often necessary to check results manually.

Thus, further studies seem necessary to determine the role of automated systems in the choice of the technique in ART.

Emerging Technologies

More and more companies are developing artificial intelligence (AI) systems that will be linked to CASA. Using algorithms and increasingly powerful image analysis, sperm can be classified according to their motility and DNA integrity [16–18]. Studies by Agarwal et al. [19, 20] using a new AI system based on optical microscopy technology (LensHooke® X1 PRO device) have shown a high correlation with

IVOS® CASA and manual methods with respect to sperm concentration, total and progressive motility. Other studies focus on the use of AI to obtain better determination of sperm morphology [17, 21–25] but large-scale studies are needed to validate these tools before routine use.

There are also many commercially available kits for the general public. They allow semen analysis at home, generally using the camera of smartphones. Depending on the system, they determine an estimate of sperm concentration and motility and allow a quick and less expensive diagnosis than sperm analysis performed in the laboratory. There is also an immunochromatographic test (SpermCheck Fertility®, Princeton BioMeditech Corp., Monmouth Junction, NJ) which allows the detection of spermatozoa in human semen, via a strip which is colored in case of a concentration higher than 2.1M/ml.

However, these technologies have not yet proven their effectiveness and cannot be used in a medical setting at the present time. These remain innovative technologies that deserve to be further developed to allow screening in certain regions where access to care is complicated. Moreover, it could allow patients who cannot afford a complete sperm analysis to have a first idea of their fertility.

Conclusion

CASA systems are equipment that use different methodologies and some systems are very good at assessing sperm motility and count. In the context of ART, these systems optimize technical time and can provide a standardized assessment of sperm parameters (before IUI and IVF). These tools still need to be improved but currently allow reliable routine use subject to validation of results by an accredited and qualified person.

Take Home Messages
- CASA systems allow a quick and standardized analysis of sperm parameters.
- There are different CASA systems, each with its own advantages and disadvantages.
- CASA systems are a diagnostic tool for semen abnormalities but need to be used by trained and qualified personnel
- CASA analysis of sperm morphology is not yet perfectly reliable for routine use.
- CASA systems have the advantage of providing standardized results and eliminating inter-operator variability.

References

1. Schlegel PN, Sigman M, Collura B, De Jonge CJ, Eisenberg ML, Lamb DJ, et al. Diagnosis and treatment of infertility in men: AUA/ASRM guideline part II. Fertil Steril. 2021;115(1):62–9.
2. World Health Organization. WHO laboratory manual for the examination and processing of human semen. 6th ed. Geneva: World Health Organization; 2021. https://apps.who.int/iris/handle/10665/343208.

3. Boitrelle F, Shah R, Saleh R, Henkel R, Kandil H, Chung E, et al. The sixth edition of the WHO manual for human semen analysis: a critical review and SWOT analysis. Life. 2021;11(12):1368.

4. World Health Organization. WHO laboratory manual for the examination and processing of human semen. 5th ed. Geneva: World Health Organization; 2010. p. 271.

5. Lammers J, Splingart C, Barrière P, Jean M, Fréour T. Double-blind prospective study comparing two automated sperm analyzers versus manual semen assessment. J Assist Reprod Genet. 2014;31(1):35–43.

6. Dearing CG, Kilburn S, Lindsay KS. Validation of the sperm class analyser CASA system for sperm counting in a busy diagnostic semen analysis laboratory. Hum Fertil. 2014;17(1):37–44.

7. Talarczyk-Desole J, Berger A, Taszarek-Hauke G, Hauke J, Pawelczyk L, Jedrzejczak P. Manual vs. computer-assisted sperm analysis: can CASA replace manual assessment of human semen in clinical practice? Ginekol Pol. 2017;88(2):56–60.

8. Schubert B, Badiou M, Force A. Computer-aided sperm analysis, the new key player in routine sperm assessment. Andrologia. 2019;51(10):e13417. https://doi.org/10.1111/and.13417. Epub 2019 Sep 2. PMID: 31475742.

9. Engel KM, Grunewald S, Schiller J, Paasch U. Automated semen analysis by SQA Vision® versus the manual approach-a prospective double-blind study. Andrologia. 2019;51(1):e13149.

10. Singh S, Sharma S, Jain M, Chauhan R. Importance of papanicolaou staining for sperm morphologic analysis: comparison with an automated sperm quality analyzer. Am J Clin Pathol. 2011;136(2):247–51.

11. Garrett C, Baker HW. A new fully automated system for the morphometric analysis of human sperm heads. Fertil Steril. 1995;63(6):1306–17.

12. Menkveld R, Stander FSH, Kotze TJ, Kruger TF, van Zyl JA. The evaluation of morphological characteristics of human spermatozoa according to stricter criteria. Hum Reprod. 1990;5(5):586–92.

13. Feneux D, Serres C, Jouannet P. Sliding spermatozoa: a dyskinesia responsible for human infertility? Fertil Steril. 1985;44(4):508–11.

14. Shibahara H, Obara H, Ayustawati N, Hirano Y, Suzuki T, Ohno A, et al. Prediction of pregnancy by intrauterine insemination using CASA estimates and strict criteria in patients with male factor infertility. Int J Androl. 2004;27(2):63–8.

15. Hirano Y, Shibahara H, Obara H, Suzuki T, Takamizawa S, Yamaguchi C, et al. Relationships between sperm motility characteristics assessed by the computer-aided sperm analysis (CASA) and fertilization rates in vitro. J Assist Reprod Genet. 2001;18(4):213–8.

16. Hicks SA, Andersen JM, Witczak O, Thambawita V, Halvorsen P, Hammer HL, et al. Machine learning-based analysis of sperm videos and participant data for male fertility prediction. Sci Rep. 2019;9(1):16770.

17. Ilhan HO, Sigirci IO, Serbes G, Aydin N. A fully automated hybrid human sperm detection and classification system based on mobile-net and the performance comparison with conventional methods. Med Biol Eng Comput. 2020;58(5):1047–68.

18. McCallum C, Riordon J, Wang Y, Kong T, You JB, Sanner S, et al. Deep learning-based selection of human sperm with high DNA integrity. Commun Biol. 2019;2:250.

19. Agarwal A, Panner Selvam MK, Ambar RF. Validation of LensHooke® X1 PRO and computer-assisted semen analyzer compared with laboratory-based manual semen analysis. World J Mens Health. 2021;39(3):496–505.

20. Agarwal A, Henkel R, Huang CC, Lee MS. Automation of human semen analysis using a novel artificial intelligence optical microscopic technology. Andrologia. 2019;51(11):e13440.

21. Wei SY, Chao HH, Huang HP, Hsu CF, Li SH, Hsu L. A collective tracking method for preliminary sperm analysis. Biomed Eng Online. 2019;18(1):112.

22. Movahed RA, Mohammadi E, Orooji M. Automatic segmentation of sperm's parts in micro-scopic images of human semen smears using concatenated learning approaches. Comput Biol Med. 2019;109:242–53.
23. Ilhan HO, Serbes G. Sperm morphology analysis by using the fusion of two-stage fine-tuned deep networks. Biomed Signal Process Control. 2022;71:103246.
24. Chandra S, Gourisaria MK, Gm H, Konar D, Gao X, Wang T, et al. Prolificacy assessment of spermatozoan via state-of-the-art deep learning frameworks. IEEE Access. 2022;10:13715–27.
25. Chang V, Garcia A, Hitschfeld N, Härtel S. Gold-standard for computer-assisted morphologi-cal sperm analysis. Comput Biol Med. 2017;83:143–50.

Part V

Sperm Preparation for ART

Sperm Preparation and Sperm Selection Techniques

17

Roberto Bagaskara Indy Christanto, Missy Savira, and Ponco Birowo ⓘ

Key Points
- Sperm preparation and sperm selection techniques should be done to effectively retrieve the functional sperm, prevent DNA impairment, and eliminate debris.
- Sperm preparation and selection is critical for further diagnostic and research purposes and for optimizing the success of assisted reproductive techniques.
- A number of sperm preparation and selection techniques are available at the moment. Understanding their advantages and disadvantages are crucial in selecting the best techniques for each patient.

Introduction

Intracytoplasmic sperm injection (ICSI) is a type of assisted reproductive technique (ART) first developed by Palermo et al. [1]. It was in 1992 that the first human birth using this method [1, 2]. At the beginning, patients were stimulated using a combination of gonadotropin-releasing hormone analog (GnRHa) and human menopausal gonadotropin (HMG) to promote superovulation. On the other hand, spermatozoa were collected from semen samples and prepared to retrieve acrosome-reacted spermatozoa [3]. These spermatozoa would then be injected into the prepared oocyte using a microinjection needle and pipette [2, 3]. Fertilization was achieved on 66% of oocytes, where more than half of those were able to develop into embryos, and four pregnancies were achieved [2]. A clinical study was conducted on 227 couples, resulting in a 37% pregnancy rate per retrieval [4]. A more recent review indicated that the fertilization rate of ICSI ranged between 70 and 80% [5]. Meanwhile, the

R. B. I. Christanto · M. Savira · P. Birowo (✉)
Department of Urology, Faculty of Medicine, Universitas Indonesia, Dr. Cipto Mangunkusumo Hospital, Jakarta, Indonesia

© The Author(s), under exclusive license to Springer Nature Switzerland AG 2024
A. Agarwal et al. (eds.), *Human Semen Analysis*,
https://doi.org/10.1007/978-3-031-55337-0_17

pregnancy rate of ICSI reached up to 45%. Maternal age has been found highly influential to pregnancy rate.

Following the implementation of ICSI, sperm collection of testicular and epididymal spermatozoa was also done in combination to achieve a higher rate of in vitro fertilization [6, 7]. Cryopreserved spermatozoa and oocytes were also usable for ICSI [8–10]. Due to cryopreservation, the zona surrounding oocytes becomes hardened, impeding sperm entry through natural methods. This is not a problem for ICSI patients, as sperm entry is done manually using microinjection [10]. In vitro fertilization using ICSI has also been shown to reduce the likelihood of contamination of sperm DNA, making ICSI preferable to be done to generate embryos particularly when pre-implantation genetic diagnosis (PGD) and pre-implantation genetic screening (PGS) are needed [11]. Studies on ICSI have also been shown to reduce the risk of transmission of sexually transmitted diseases [12, 13].

Over the years, ICSI had become the most frequently used ART in around 60 countries by 2010. However, a disparity of ICSI usage exists within different regions, where 55% of ART in Asia involves ICSI, compared to 60% in Europe and nearly 100% in the Middle East. Meanwhile, the efficacy of ICSI remained consistent from 2008 to 2010. This can be seen through the pregnancy rate (25.4–26.1%) and the delivery rate (18.9–19.1%) per aspiration. Within the same period, efficacy using frozen embryo transfer had a slightly higher pregnancy rate (27.3–29.1%) and delivery rate (18.8–20.7%). On the other hand, a rising pattern in the global proportion of single embryo transfer (SET) was also found, from 25.7% in 2008 to 28.3% in 2009 and 30.0% in 2010. Among these, the rate of SET is higher in patients with frozen embryo transfer compared to fresh embryo transfer [14].

The aim of this chapter is to provide detailed explanation on sperm preparation and selection technique including its pros and cons, complimenting the principle aspects that have been provided in the WHO 6th ed manual of semen analysis. Through a more comprehensive discussion, we aim to give a clearer interpretation on the WHO manual to be applied in daily practice both for laboratory and clinical personnel.

Indications of ICSI

As with other ARTs, the primary indication for ICSI is to treat subfertility, particularly male factor subfertility, as ICSI enables surgically retrieved spermatozoa to be used [1, 15]. In addition, ICSI is recommended in some cases of female factor subfertility, such as having dysmorphic oocytes, low oocyte yield, poor oocyte maturity, and in patients with low fertilization rates despite undergoing other IVF methods [1]. Other indications include reducing the risk of disease transmission [12, 13, 16]. ICSI indications can be classified into two major groups: male and nonmale. Male factors could be further classified according to the examined sample: ejaculated, testicular, and epididymal spermatozoa. Meanwhile, non-male factors include oocyte abnormalities, transmissible diseases among the couple [human immune deficiency virus (HIV), hepatitis B, or hepatitis C], intention to conduct PGD/PGS, and restrictive legislation toward other ART methods [1].

During the early development of ICSI, oligozoospermia was one of the primary indications of ICSI. Multiple studies indicated that both fertilization and pregnancy rates are unaffected by sperm count within the semen [2, 17]. However, a more recent study showed a significant reduction in fertilization and pregnancy rates, accompanied by an increased rate of abortion, among patients with cryptozoospermic cases [18]. This was presumed to be affected by the different severities of oligospermia between study samples. A very low sperm count may increase the difficulty in finding viable sperm for microinjection [19, 20]. To counteract this, testicular sperm is used instead of an ejaculated sperm sample, which has proven to show significant improvement in the outcome of ICSI [21]. This finding might be related to the reduced DNA fragmentation among testicular spermatozoa samples [22].

In the event of asthenoteratozoospermia, ICSI was shown to be superior to intrauterine insemination (IUI) and IVF in terms of pregnancy rate [23]. As asthenozoospermia and teratozoospermia would hinder sperm binding and penetration of the zona pellucida, ICSI would not be affected as the procedure bypasses this process. Additionally, ICSI also allows the manual selection of the most favorable sperm [24]. During the early development of ICSI, this technique was developed for patients with unfavorable semen parameters, including asthenozoospermia patients. This makes sense as ICSI directly injects spermatozoa into the oocyte [2]. In teratozoospermia cases, ICSI has been proven to have no significant difference in fertility and pregnancy outcomes compared to control groups by multiple studies [24–26]. These results also apply to those with severe teratozoospermia, with 0% of sperm with normal morphology [25]. Additionally, there was no difference in embryo quality and risk of birth defects [24, 26]. Results of ICSI may be unaffected by sperm morphology as fertilization rate as normal fertilization dependent on the oocyte activating factor, which is located inside the sperm head and is unaffected by abnormal sperm morphology [27, 28].

Male-factor infertility caused by anti-sperm antibodies (ASA) is also indicated to perform ICSI, as both fertilization and pregnancy outcomes of ICSI are similar to male patients without ASA [29]. Results remained consistent in multiple studies, showing no statistically significant difference in the outcome of ICSI in correlation to ASA status. As such, it can be concluded that ICSI nullified any negative impact caused by ASA [30].

Fertility preservation using cryopreservation is an integral part of ART as it allows preventive measures for individuals whose fertility may be compromised in the future. This includes aging, surgical interventions involving the reproductive system, PGD/PGS, autoimmune disorders, and patients about to undergo cancer therapy [31]. As previously discussed, cryopreserved oocytes and spermatozoa have been used since the early development stages [8–10]. A more recent study observed a significant increase in successful fertilization when frozen sperm was used with ICSI compared to conventional IVF. Meanwhile, the difference in the fertility rate from fresh sperm between the two procedures was non-significant. In addition, lower embryo fragmentation was observed among ICSI procedures [32]. Similar study regarding cryopreserved oocytes is unavailable, however, multiple arguments suggest that ICSI would be the preferred ART method as the zona pellucida hardens after cryopreservation [10, 33]. Cryopreservation of oocytes has also been shown to hinder in vitro aging, preserving the integrity of the meiotic spindles and maturation-promoting factor. If ICSI preparation is completed in under an hour, the loss of maturation-promoting factor and the meiotic spindle is minimal, thus maintaining oocyte viability [33]. In the event of prior failed IVF, ICSI was shown to be efficient in rescuing both total and partial fertilization failure when combined with frozen embryo transfer compared to fresh embryo transfer [34].

Ejaculatory disorder or dysfunction comprises a broad spectrum of diseases, ranging from premature ejaculation—to anorgasmia—to retrograde ejaculation and anejaculation. Among these disorders, ART, such as ICSI, may be indicated for patients with retrograde ejaculation and anejaculation [35]. Successful fertilization through ICSI can be done for anejaculation as long as a single motile sperm can be obtained [36]. Spermatozoa can be collected using electroejaculation or testicular sperm extraction [35, 36].

Human immunodeficiency virus, hepatitis B virus, and hepatitis C virus are diseases that have been known to be transmissible through sexual intercourse and can be vertically transmitted [12, 13, 37]. However, studies have shown that these infections are not transmitted to the offspring despite having male or female carriers [12, 13]. Nevertheless, it was found that among males with active hepatitis B virus infection, ICSI outcomes were not affected when ejaculated sperm was used. On the other hand, if testicular or epididymal spermatozoa were used, reduced fertilization and live birth rate and increased miscarriage rate can be found [38].

The above-mentioned indications of ICSI underline the variation of ICSI use worldwide, for managing both male factor and non-male factor issues. With the importance of ICSI, a proper technique of sperm preparation and selection is imperative before ICSI and ART to maximize the success rate.

Sperm Preparation Techniques

The WHO Manual of Human Semen Processing had a dedicated chapter on sperm preparation techniques [39]. The Editors of the manual emphasized the importance of preparation to recover a highly functional sperm while preserving the quality and not inducing any dysfunction that may be detrimental for fertilization. A number of techniques are viable for sperm preparation and should be chosen based on the objectives and condition of semen sample. One of general principles of sperm preparation is to provide a culture medium with supporting environmental conditions using a sterile techniques and materials. Specific for testicular and epididymal sperm, a special handling will be needed to prepare the sperm. The present section will give a better description in the indication, advantages and limitations of sperm preparation techniques [40].

Advantages and Disadvantages of Sperm Preparation Techniques

Upon ejaculation, the spermatozoa suspended in the epididymis are mixed with the secretions of the accessory glands to form semen. The prostate and seminal vesicles comprise most of these glands, with the bulbourethral glands and the epididymis making up a minor portion of the ejaculate [39]. Human ejaculation is not homogenous and consists of two primary parts. The first part is the prostatic fraction containing a high concentration of spermatozoa and the second part is the vesicular fraction, which consists of fewer spermatozoa. Thus, the collection of the whole ejaculate is imperative before sperm preparation [41].

The term sperm preparation is defined as procedures to isolate functional, motile spermatozoa, which are deemed viable candidates for assisted reproduction, from non-motile spermatozoa and other debris [39, 41]. This separation within an in vivo setting also occurs through the migration of motile spermatozoa across cervical mucus [42]. During this phase, progressively motile sperm are selected, and they undergo capacitation, a crucial physiological change required to initiate the acrosome reaction. This reaction enables the sperm to penetrate the zona pellucida and fuse with the oocyte membrane [43].

There are currently numerous sperm preparation procedures that are available. Nevertheless, these methods could be divided into three main categories: simple washing, swim-up, and density gradients technique [39].

Simple Washing

Simple washing is an approach where centrifugal force is applied to the semen sample while allowing the spermatozoa to settle after diluting the semen with two or more times the amount of culture medium required (Fig. 17.1). Afterward, the pellet is extracted and diluted with a small quantity of the medium. This sample is incubated until the designated time of insemination using ART [39].

Swim-Up Technique

The swim-up technique is the most conventional sperm preparation technique, first developed by Mahadevan and Baker in 1984 [44]. Nevertheless, it is still widely used as it is a cost-effective and uncomplicated procedure [42]. In principle, this technique utilizes functional spermatozoa's inept ability to swim. The standard swim-up process is based on the active movement of spermatozoa from the pre-washed cell pellet into an overlying medium. The incubation period usually lasts 60 min, where motile spermatozoa are expected "swim" to the richer overlaying medium. This method stands out for its highly high motile sperm content (>90%), preferential enrichment of morphologically intact spermatozoa, and absence of other cells and detritus. The yield of motile spermatozoa is constrained since the

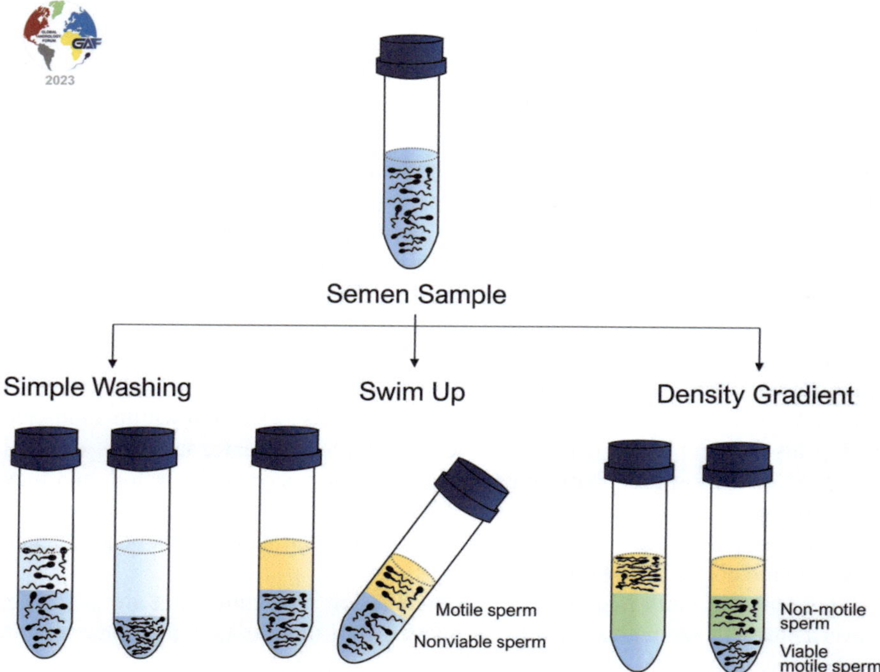

Fig. 17.1 Overview of sperm preparation techniques: simple washing, swim-up, and density gradients method. Source: Nordhoff V, Kliesch S. Sperm Preparation for Therapeutic IVF. In: Morbeck DE, Montag MHM, editors. Principles of IVF Laboratory Practice: Optimizing Performance and Outcomes. Cambridge: Cambridge University Press; 2017. p. 97–105

approach's effectiveness depends on the cell pellet's surface and the initial sperm motility in the ejaculate [42, 45]. However, several potentially motile spermatozoa with normal chromatin layers may not have reached the culture medium, thus wasting viable male germ cells [45]. Additionally, close contact between spermatozoa and other cells or debris within the pellet would increase the production of reactive oxygen species (ROS), leading to a decline in sperm motility [46]. As a solution, liquified semen could be used directly instead of cell pellets placed in multiple small tubes to maximize interface area. This modification has been shown to increase the number of spermatozoa recovered [47].

Density Gradient Technique

Density gradients are the second option for spermatozoa selection. The density column is placed on top of the pipetted semen sample and is subsequently centrifuged. Spermatozoa would be separated by density gradient centrifugation based on the difference in density. After sperm cells are isolated, the motile spermatozoa with normal morphology can be chosen and aspirated for further usage from the solution with the highest concentration of gradient [48]. There are two types of density gradient centrifugation: continuous and discontinuous gradient [49, 50]. Continuous gradients would result in a diffused sample with a progressive increase in density from top to bottom [49]. Using centrifugation, particles with higher density would sediment faster. Depending on the time and the centrifugal force, the isolation of certain cells is possible by extracting the suspension. A series of differential centrifugation is generally performed to reduce contamination of other biological particles within the extracted sample [51]. Whereas samples of discontinuous gradients would comprised of layers filled with different components, each with distinct boundaries between them [50]. Similar to continuous gradient, centrifugation is done to segregate particles, pushing those with higher density to the bottom of the tube. However, particles with different densities and/or sizes will be partitioned into different layers using density mediums [51]. A number of materials can be used for density gradient material used to prepare spermatozoa, one of the most widely available materials are silane-coated silica particles [42]. Apart from the type of density gradient centrifugation, the density media would be put above the semen sample and centrifuged for approximately 15–30 min. As a result, sperm cells would be collected within the sampled sediment. Within the sedimentation, motile sperm could penetrate the boundary produced by density gradient media at a faster rate than less motile or immotile spermatozoa. As a result, spermatozoa with high motility are gathered and extractable from the bottom of the sediment [48].

Comparison of the Three Methods of Sperm Preparation

Swim-Up Vs. Simple Washing Technique

No significant difference between swim-up and simple washing techniques was found in clinical and multiple pregnancy rates. Unfortunately, the lack of high-quality evidence with adequate sample size causes uncertainty to take any [39].

Density Gradient Vs. Simple Washing Technique

No significant difference was found in two randomized controlled trials comparing clinical pregnancy rates between density gradient and simple washing technique. The difference between both miscarriage rates and multiple pregnancy rates also remains unclear [39].

Swim-Up Vs. Density Gradient Technique

Neither the swim-up nor density gradient technique was found to have a significantly higher clinical pregnancy rate. However, this might be caused by the need for more high-quality evidence in current studies. Similarly, non-significant differences were found in terms of multiple pregnancy rates and miscarriage rates. On the other hand, the ongoing pregnancy rate is significantly higher among couples using the swim-up technique. Despite that, with a pooled OR of 0.39 originating from only one randomized controlled trial with poor quality evidence, a clinically significant difference between the two techniques remain inconclusive [39].

Advantages and Disadvantages of Sperm Preparation Techniques

Each of these sperm preparation methods has its advantages and disadvantages, which play a crucial role in selecting the best for each patient (Table 17.1). Nevertheless, both sperm washing and swim-up procedure are preferred for sperm samples that have a normal count, good motility, and normal morphology. Meanwhile, in cases with poor quality of sperm samples, density gradient centrifugation is preferred instead, as it allows segregation between functional and non-functional spermatozoa [52].

Different contamination levels in the sample are produced during the final preparation of both density gradient centrifugation and the swim-up procedure. Compared to density gradient centrifugation, the swim-up approach yields a more significant

Table 17.1 Advantages and disadvantages of sperm collection procedures

Procedures	Advantages	Disadvantages
Simple washing	– Simple procedure – Most affordable sperm preparation method	– Highly motile, poorly motile, and immotile spermatozoa are clumped together within the pellet
Swim-up method	– Easily executed – Cost-effective – Sperm fragment usually consist of spermatozoa with high motility	– Low quantity of sperm extracted – Can be only done in ejaculated sperm samples with high sperm count and motility
Density gradients	– Spermatozoa are set apart according to DNA integrity, maturity, and morphology – Removal of unwanted particles: debris, virus, bacteria, leukocytes – Results in good sperm yield for patients who have low sperm count, abnormal morphology, or poor sperm motility – Shorter duration of procedure compared to swim-up	– Lower yield in general compared to swim-up – Higher risk of iatrogenic damage due to higher force for centrifugation – Most expensive compared to the other procedures

Source: Boomsma CM, Cohlen BJ, Farquhar C. Semen preparation techniques for intrauterine insemination. Cochrane Database Syst Rev. 2019;10(10):Cd004507; Nordhoff V, Kliesch S. Sperm Preparation for Therapeutic IVF. In: Morbeck DE, Montag MHM, editors. Principles of IVF Laboratory Practice: Optimizing Performance and Outcomes. Cambridge: Cambridge University Press; 2017. p. 97–105; Henkel RR, Schill WB. Sperm preparation for ART. Reprod Biol Endocrinol. 2003;1:108

amount of non-sperm components (such as detritus and bacteria) and the diffusion of other compounds (such as prostatic zinc) from the semen into the overlaying media [53].

Sperm Selection Techniques

Selection of Viable Sperm

Sperm samples retrieved by testicular aspiration (TESA) or other retrieval procedures usually have immotile spermatozoa. This happens due to incomplete sperm maturation in the epididymis. Swim-up and continuous or discontinuous density gradient techniques are unsuitable for immotile sperm because these techniques exploit dynamic characteristics for sperm separation. Thus, several sperm selection techniques were developed to sort out viable sperm [42, 54]. The WHO manual for the human semen examination and processing mentioned that the typical indicators to evaluate the efficacy of sperm selection technique are based on the recovery of morphologically normal motile spermatozoa, the total number of motile spermatozoa, or the absolute sperm number. A number of techniques are described on the manual including their efficacy. The current sections will provide detailed description of indication for each technique (Fig. 17.2).

Mechanical Touch Technique (MTT)

Mechanical touch is a technique proposed by Marques De Oliveira and colleagues for the selection of viable immotile sperm before ICSI [55]. Sperm tail touched by ICSI injection needle, and if it is still flexible and can return to its original position, the sperm is viable. Non-viable sperm tails are rigid and not capable of retaining their position. However, this technique heavily relies on biologist proficiency and expertise [55, 56].

Hypo-osmotic Swelling Test (HOST)

Hypo-osmotic swelling test (HOST) principle is to introduce sperm into a hypo-osmotic environment. The activity of the osmo-sensitive calcium membrane channels causes the viable sperm tails to swell and bend [57, 58]. Furthermore, the chromatin integrity of viable sperm can be assessed by HOST through seven distinct patterns of swelling. Thus, sperm cells with better nuclear material for ICSI can be observed through a microscope [59, 60]. World Health Organization laboratory manual for examining and processing human semen recommended HOST for asthenozoospermia patients before ICSI [61].

Existing studies about HOST are still controversial. A study suggested that HOST should be used in a future ICSI cycle following the complete failure of

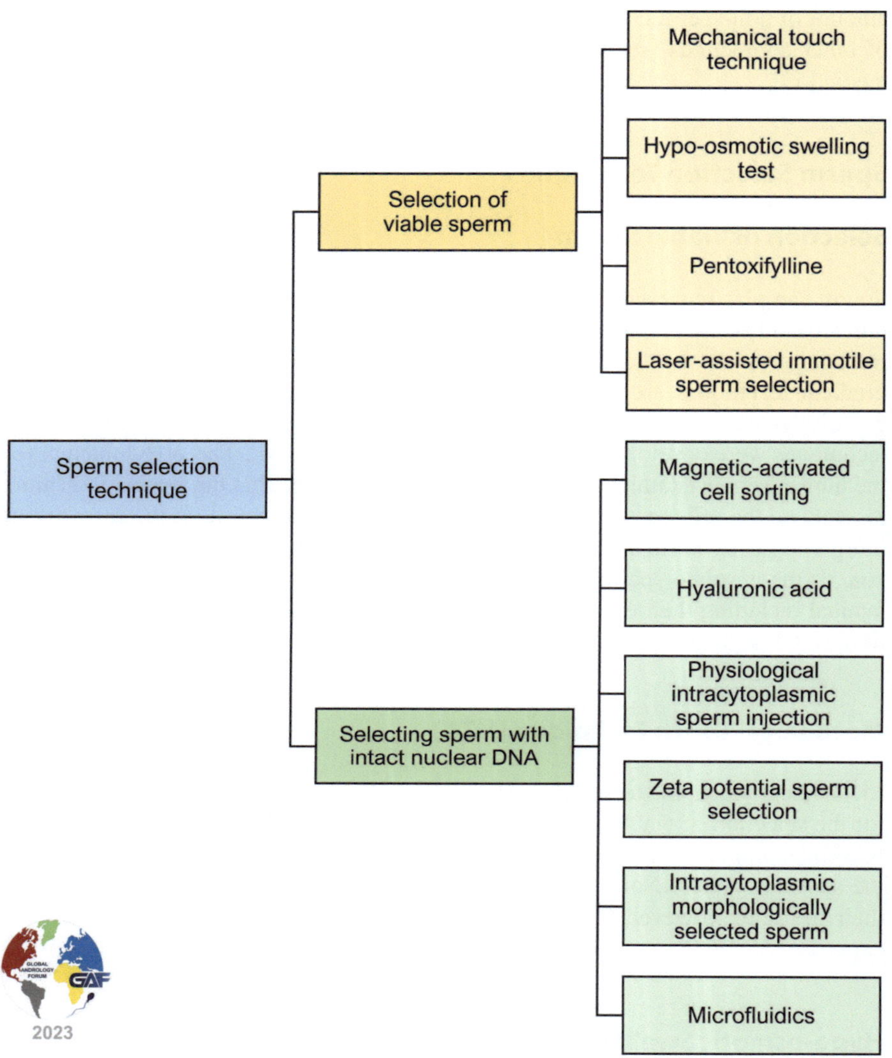

fertilization. However, some conflicting research argues that using the HOST is linked to a poor rate of fertilization and sperm survivability after 30 minutes of incubation in a hypo-osmotic solution [62]. Moreover, the HOST test requires diluting the material, and researchers often have to work with minimal volumes of testicular sperm.

Consequently, based on the specific ART laboratory condition and the number of sperm samples available, this procedure should be considered [63].

Fig. 17.2 Sperm selection techniques. Source: Henkel RR, Schill WB. Sperm preparation for ART. Reprod Biol Endocrinol. 2003;1:108; Baldini D, Ferri D, Baldini GM, Lot D, Catino A, Vizziello D, et al. Sperm Selection for ICSI: Do We Have a Winner? Cells. 2021;10(12); de Oliveira NM, Vaca Sanchez R, Rodriguez Fiesta S, Lopez Salgado T, Rodriguez R, Bethencourt JC, et al. Pregnancy with frozen-thawed and fresh testicular biopsy after motile and immotile sperm microinjection, using the mechanical touch technique to assess viability. Hum Reprod. 2004;19(2):262–5; Nassar A, Morshedi M, Mahony M, Srisombut C, Lin MH, Oehninger S. Pentoxifylline stimulates various sperm motion parameters and cervical mucus penetrability in patients with asthenozoospermia. Andrologia. 1999;31(1):9–15; Aktan TM, Montag M, Duman S, Gorkemli H, Rink K, Yurdakul T. Use of a laser to detect viable but immotile spermatozoa. Andrologia. 2004;36(6):366–9; Dirican EK, Ozgun OD, Akarsu S, Akin KO, Ercan O, Ugurlu M, et al. Clinical outcome of magnetic activated cell sorting of non-apoptotic spermatozoa before density gradient centrifugation for assisted reproduction. J Assist Reprod Genet. 2008;25(8):375–81; Miller D, Pavitt S, Sharma V, Forbes G, Hooper R, Bhattacharya S, et al. Physiological, hyaluronan-selected intracytoplasmic sperm injection for infertility treatment (HABSelect): a parallel, two-group, randomised trial. Lancet. 2019;393(10170):416–22; Nasr Esfahani MH, Deemeh MR, Tavalaee M, Sekhavati MH, Gourabi H. Zeta Sperm Selection Improves Pregnancy Rate and Alters Sex Ratio in Male Factor Infertility Patients: A Double-Blind, Randomized Clinical Trial. Int J Fertil Steril. 2016;10(2):253–60; Smith GD, Takayama S. Application of microfluidic technologies to human assisted reproduction. Mol Hum Reprod. 2017;23(4):257–68

Pentoxifylline

A methylxanthine derivative known as pentoxifylline is a nonspecific inhibitor of phosphodiesterase. Pentoxifylline has been approved for human administration by the Food and Drug Administration. The medication is used to treat individuals with cardiovascular disorders on a systemic level.

Pentoxifylline has been shown to improve sperm motility and motion traits such as sperm velocity or hyperactivity in both fresh and cryopreserved spermatozoa, according to several studies [64–69]. Conflicting findings exist on its effect on stimulating sperm motility. Yovich et al., Rees et al., and Lewis et al. found no impact in patients who had normozoospermia. However, other researchers discovered that asthenozoospermic individuals had higher motility and quantity of motile spermatozoa [65, 69, 70]. In a condition of necrozoospermia, pentoxifylline or theophylline also have a role for vitality test in immobile spermatozoa. As mentioned earlier, these substances can have an impact to sperm motility, one of which is to induce flagellar movement in immotile yet alive spermatozoa [71].

There is also some concern regarding the method revolves mainly around compounds' inherent toxicity to genetic material. However, research shows that in vitro treatment of immotile sperm may increase motility effectively while preventing acrosome reaction, DNA damage, and viability loss [72, 73]. Furthermore, researchers found that this method had a greater rate of fertilization and pregnancy (32% vs. 16%) compared to HOST [74]. Therefore, when using pentoxifylline or theophylline for sperm selection, rinsing the spermatozoa prior to injecting it to the oocyte is a must.

Laser Assisted Immotile Sperm Selection (LAISS)

The immotile sperm cell tail can be hit using a laser built into the magnification system further to reactivate motility (LAISS laser-assisted immotile sperm selection) [75]. Laser irradiation results in the release of second messengers like Ca^{2+} or ROS in the cytosol and an increase in ATP synthesis, which may result in a subtle movement of the tail [76]. When the sperm cell's tail coils up following the laser blast, it is deemed viable [77]. However, other scientists contend that excessive amounts of possibly harmful ROS are produced when laser doses are excessive [78]. Additionally, increased Ca^{2+} inflow causes Ca^{2+}-ATPase calcium channels to become hyperactive and depletes the cell's ATP stores.

Due to a decrease in cell channel activity and a rise in internal osmotic pressure, this process may cause the sperm cell to enlarge and eventually burst its plasma membrane [79]. On the other hand, other scientists believe this procedure has no adverse effects on the spermatic membrane or the degree of genetic material fragmentation [80]. The chemical motility activators, which can be hazardous, can alternatively be substituted with LAISS [81]. Additionally, compared to control groups, it dramatically raises the embryonic segmentation and post-ICSI birth rate utilizing testicular or ejaculated spermatozoa [82]. When a patient has Kartagener's syndrome or primary ciliary dyskinesia, LAISS is the technique that is recommended [83, 84].

Despite the method's considerable promise, its complexity and expensive cost are the primary barriers to its adoption in ART laboratories for everyday use.

Selection Based on Sperm Nuclear Quality

Magnetic-Activated Cell Sorting (MACS)

Since it is initially used in many fertilization elements, such as oocyte binding, and acrosome response, the outer sperm membrane is essential for their function. Methods that consider its membrane's properties have been researched to select high-quality sperm cells.

Magnetic-activated cell sorting is another approach that uses the membrane's properties (MACS). With the help of this technology, it is possible to choose the non-apoptotic portion of a sample [85]. It uses magnetic microspheres attached to Annexin V and has a strong affinity for phosphatidyl-serine (AV-MACS) [86]. When the sperm cells are in an apoptotic condition, phosphatidyl-serine is often visible on the membrane's outer side [87]. The viable spermatozoa are extracted while the non-viable spermatozoa are retained inside the column, enhancing the vitality properties of the initial sample.

Numerous studies have proven the efficacy of the MACS technique in individuals with varicocele, high nuclear fragmentation, and idiopathic infertility [88, 89]. The recovered spermatozoa showed an even lower proportion of fragmentation when this approach was used in conjunction with traditional techniques like swim-up or density gradient centrifugation [90, 91]. When compared to conventional centrifugation on a density gradient, research on a group of oligoasthenozoospermia patients found that seminal samples exposed to MACS increased embryonic segmentation and conception rates [92]. However, the amount of live births research still needs to be improved in this scenario. MACS procedure does not allow for differentiation between the types of motile spermatozoa chosen (progressive or non-progressive).

Hyaluronic Acid

The primary element of the extracellular matrix surrounding the cumulus-oocyte complex is hyaluronic acid [93]. The hyaluronic-binding receptors on sperm cells' outer membranes can only be seen in mature sperm cells that have completed spermatogenesis and maturation [94, 95]. Additionally, they often have a normal shape and a low level of nuclear material fragmentation [96]. Utilizing these traits, spermatozoa are cultured in conditions containing hyaluronic acid or on plates as part of a methodology for sperm cell selection. A swim-up straight from semen into a hyaluronic acid solution produced a much more significant proportion of motile spermatozoa than the conventional swim-up from a washed pellet, which eventually led to a higher pregnancy rate in a clinical IVF procedure [97]. While it has been demonstrated that highly pure hyaluronic acid increases the calcium influx into spermatozoa and subsequently causes an acrosome response, it is also costly. It has been shown that the acrosome response is impacted by elevated local concentrations of hyaluronic acid in the cumulus oophorus [98]. Therefore, it needs to be clarified whether this chemical benefits IVF.

Furthermore, it is unclear if hyaluronate or a different technique that did not involve the initial pelleting of unselected spermatozoa was responsible for the enhanced sperm motility outcomes. However, hyaluronic acid has been suggested as a successful substitute to evaluate sperm penetration into human cervical mucus [99, 100].

Physiological Intracytoplasmic Sperm Injection (PICSI)

A physiological intracytoplasmic sperm injection (PICSI) dish and a commercially available hyaluronic acid containing media are the two techniques most frequently used to include hyaluronic acid in ART [101]. In PICSI, mature sperm can adhere to immobilized hyaluronic acid patches in the petri dish, and the adhering sperm are chosen for ICSI usage. The selection should lead to a higher incidence of fertilization; however, the clinical evidence could be more evident in this situation. While several studies did not necessarily support the benefits of this technique, others suggest that the procedure increases both the fertilization rate and the proportion of high-quality embryos [102, 103].

According to research comprising 16 assisted reproductive centers in the UK, there was no discernible difference between the live birth rate of PICSI and normal ICSI ($P = 0.18$). Because of this, PICSI and hyaluronic acid-containing media are rarely used and still need to be studied more [102].

Zeta Potential Sperm Selection

According to studies, the sperm cell membrane has a negative charge. This characteristic is used by the Zeta technique to distinguish between sperm cells carrying the Y chromosome and those carrying the X chromosome. Two different methodologies, one utilizing a positively charged centrifuge tube and the other utilizing migration in an electrophoretic field, have been developed by two research groups. Both allow the collection of live spermatozoa with normal morphology and a high percentage of the genetic material's integrity. Spermatozoa chosen using the Zeta technique with ICSI have only been reported in one randomized trial [104].

Intracytoplasmic Morphologically Selected Sperm (IMSI)

The morphological assessment of spermatozoa has long been linked to the measurement of semen quality. Because of the development of digital microscopy, it is now possible to examine the ultrastructural traits of motile spermatozoa, Motile Sperm Organelle Morphology Examination (MSOME) [105]. A high-magnification microinjection is potential because of MSOME's inclusion into the ICSI procedure (IMSI) [106]. A 6000-magnification system linked with the micromanipulation system makes it possible to choose motile spermatozoa with few vacuoles and proper nuclear morphology [107]. However, contradicting scientific evidence is presented. Using this technique, several studies have found a correlation between a high amount of nuclear fragmentation and large vacuoles in the sperm nucleus [108]. The IMSI approach has been recommended as preferred if the ICSI method repeatedly fails to achieve fertilization. However, several publications could not discover any noteworthy distinctions between ICSI and IMSI in terms of fragmentation or pregnancy rates [109]. Recently, no association between the existence of vacuoles in the nucleus and DNA fragmentation was discovered in research on a sizable sample of semen evaluated using MSOME [110]. According to the authors, vacuoles are biologically present in the sperm head and have no bearing on how it performs its activities. Unfortunately, the IMSI approach has yet to be fully included in the standard operating procedures of ART clinics due to a lack of literature, the timing of the test, and the expense of the instrument.

Microfluidics

Microfluidics-related technologies are expanding quickly in ART facilities. Smith and Takayama released a series of publications proving the procedure's effectiveness in selecting high-quality spermatozoa as one of the initial trials using this technology [111]. In millimeter-diameter capillaries, fluid dynamics may be controlled to simulate the natural pH and temperature of the female genital tract [112]. So, we can choose spermatozoa with greater motility using flows, chemical gradients, or electrophoretic fields. The Smith and Takayama technique makes use of two parallel laminar flow channels. While the immotile cells and detritus are passively conveyed from the capillary canal's entry to its exit, the motile spermatozoa can travel through the flows and be eluted individually. The chosen spermatozoa had considerably improved morphology and motility (98% and 22%) compared to a conventional density gradient centrifugation [111]. According to research by Parrella et al. on a small sample of couples having ICSI, spermatozoa chosen using these technologies may be associated with a higher pregnancy rate (71%).

Another technique is a microfluidic chip technology, known as Fertile Chip® (Koek Biotechnology, Izmir, Turkey). It is a revolutionary technique for extracting spermatozoa from the ejaculate that have DNA double-stranded fragmentation. The success rate of the various assisted reproduction procedures is increased in this way. The original goal of the fertile chip was to choose spermatozoa with a reduced level of DNA fragmentation. It has been demonstrated, however, that sperm chosen using this technology also has superior motility and less reactive oxygen species (ROS). It is a slide with an inlet, an exit, and a microfluidic channel connecting the two chambers. The device's input chamber receives the sample of sperm, and after some time, the spermatozoa that have made it to the collecting chamber are selected.

Conclusion

For more than 30 years, ARTs—specifically, ICSI have been utilized globally to treat infertility resulting from a variety of problems. The preparation and selection of sperm is a significant step in increasing the success rate of ICSI. In sperm preparation, the process includes separating viable candidates for assisted reproduction; that is, motile, functioning spermatozoa, from non-motile spermatozoa and other waste. Additionally, sperm samples may need to be retrieved by sperm retrieval techniques in certain situations of infertility, which increases the incidence of immotile spermatozoa. Numerous techniques for selecting sperm were developed as a result. Weighing the pros and cons of each process helps choose the best sperm selection method for each patient.

References

1. O'Neill CL, Chow S, Rosenwaks Z, Palermo GD. Development of ICSI. Reproduction. 2018;156(1):51–8.
2. Palermo G, Joris H, Devroey P, Van Steirteghem AC. Pregnancies after intracytoplasmic injection of single spermatozoon into an oocyte. Lancet. 1992;340(8810):17–8.
3. Palermo G, Joris H, Devroey P, Van Steirteghem AC. Induction of acrosome reaction in human spermatozoa used for subzonal insemination. Hum Reprod. 1992;7(2):248–54.
4. Palermo GD, Cohen J, Alikani M, Adler A, Rosenwaks Z. Intracytoplasmic sperm injection: a novel treatment for all forms of male factor infertility. Fertil Steril. 1995;63(6):1231–40.
5. Palermo GD, Neri QV, Takeuchi T, Rosenwaks Z. ICSI: where we have been and where we are going. Semin Reprod Med. 2009;27(2):191–201.
6. Schoysman R, Vanderzwalmen P, Nijs M, Segal L, Segal-Bertin G, Geerts L, et al. Pregnancy after fertilisation with human testicular spermatozoa. Lancet. 1993;342(8881):1237.
7. Tournaye H, Devroey P, Liu J, Nagy Z, Lissens W, Van Steirteghem A. Microsurgical epididymal sperm aspiration and intracytoplasmic sperm injection: a new effective approach to infertility as a result of congenital bilateral absence of the vas deferens. Fertil Steril. 1994;61(6):1045–51.
8. Podsiadly B, Woolcott R, Stanger J, Stevenson K. Pregnancy resulting from intracytoplasmic injection of cryopreserved spermatozoa recovered from testicular biopsy. Hum Reprod. 1996;11:1306–8.
9. Porcu E, Fabbri R, Seracchioli R, Ciotti P, Magrini O, Flamigni C. Birth of a healthy female after intracytoplasmic sperm injection of cryopreserved human oocytes. Fertil Steril. 1997;68:724–6.
10. Beckers NG, Pieters MH, Ramos L, Zeilmaker GH, Fauser BC, Braat DD. Retrieval, maturation, and fertilization of immature oocytes obtained from unstimulated patients with polycystic ovary syndrome. J Assist Reprod Genet. 1999;16(2):81–6.
11. Harton G, Magli M, Lundin K, Montag M, Lemmen J, Harper J. ESHRE PGD Consortium/ Embryology Special Interest Group – best practice guidelines for polar body and embryo biopsy for pre-implantation genetic diagnosis/screening (PGD/PGS). Hum Reprod. 2011;26:41–6.
12. Garrido N, Meseguer M, Bellver J, Remohí J, Simón C, Pellicer A. Report of the results of a 2 year programme of sperm wash and ICSI treatment for human immunodeficiency virus and hepatitis C virus serodiscordant couples. Hum Reprod. 2004;19:2581–6.
13. Wu M, Ho H. Cost and safety of assisted reproductive technologies for human immunodeficiency virus-1 discordant couples. World J Virol. 2015;4:142–6.
14. Dyer S, Chambers GM, de Mouzon J, Nygren KG, Zegers-Hochschild F, Mansour R, et al. International Committee for monitoring assisted reproductive technologies world report: assisted reproductive technology 2008, 2009 and 2010. Hum Reprod. 2016;31(7):1588–609.
15. Practice Committees of the American Society for Reproductive Medicine and the Society for Assisted Reproductive Technology. Intracytoplasmic sperm injection (ICSI) for non-male factor indications: a committee opinion. Fertil Steril. 2020;114(2):239–45.
16. Palermo G, Neri Q, Rosenwaks Z. To ICSI or not to ICSI. Semin Reprod Med. 2015;33:92–102.
17. Nagy ZP, Liu J, Joris H, Verheyen G, Tournaye H, Camus M, et al. The result of intracytoplasmic sperm injection is not related to any of the three basic sperm parameters. Hum Reprod. 1995;10(5):1123–9.
18. Strassburger D, Friedler S, Raziel A, Schachter M, Kasterstein E, Ronel R. Very low sperm count affects the result of intracytoplasmic sperm injection. J Assist Reprod Genet. 2000;17(8):431–6.
19. Zini A, Bach PV, Al-Malki AH, Schlegel PN. Use of testicular sperm for ICSI in oligozoospermic couples: how far should we go? Hum Reprod. 2016;32(1):7–13.
20. De Braekeleer M, Dao TN. Cytogenetic studies in male infertility: a review. Hum Reprod. 1991;6(2):245–50.

21. Esteves SC, Sánchez-Martín F, Sánchez-Martín P, Schneider DT, Gosálvez J. Comparison of reproductive outcome in oligozoospermic men with high sperm DNA fragmentation undergoing intracytoplasmic sperm injection with ejaculated and testicular sperm. Fertil Steril. 2015;104(6):1398–405.
22. Mehta A, Bolyakov A, Schlegel PN, Paduch DA. Higher pregnancy rates using testicular sperm in men with severe oligospermia. Fertil Steril. 2015;104(6):1382–7.
23. Mangoli V, Dandekar S, Desai S, Mangoli R. The outcome of ART in males with impaired spermatogenesis. J Hum Reprod Sci. 2008;1(2):73–6.
24. Zhou W-J, Huang C, Jiang S-H, Ji X-R, Gong F, Fan L-Q, et al. Influence of sperm morphology on pregnancy outcome and offspring in in vitro fertilization and intracytoplasmic sperm injection: a matched case-control study. Asian J Androl. 2021;23(4):421–8.
25. Pereira N, Neri QV, Lekovich JP, Spandorfer SD, Palermo GD, Rosenwaks Z. Outcomes of intracytoplasmic sperm injection cycles for complete teratozoospermia: a case-control study using paired sibling oocytes. Biomed Res Int. 2015;2015:470819.
26. Demir B, Arikan II, Bozdag G, Esinler I, Karakoc Sokmensuer L, Gunalp S. Effect of sperm morphology on clinical outcome parameters in ICSI cycles. Clin Exp Obstet Gynecol. 2012;39(2):144–6.
27. Palermo GD, Avrech OM, Colombero LT, Wu H, Wolny YM, Fissore RA, et al. Human sperm cytosolic factor triggers Ca^{2+} oscillations and overcomes activation failure of mammalian oocytes. Mol Hum Reprod. 1997;3(4):367–74.
28. Neri QV, Lee B, Rosenwaks Z, Machaca K, Palermo GD. Understanding fertilization through intracytoplasmic sperm injection (ICSI). Cell Calcium. 2014;55(1):24–37.
29. Check ML, Check JH, Katsoff D, Summers-Chase D. ICSI as an effective therapy for male factor with antisperm antibodies. Arch Androl. 2000;45(3):125–30.
30. Zini A, Fahmy N, Belzile E, Ciampi A, Al-Hathal N, Kotb A. Antisperm antibodies are not associated with pregnancy rates after IVF and ICSI: systematic review and meta-analysis. Hum Reprod. 2011;26(6):1288–95.
31. Hussein RS, Khan Z, Zhao Y. Fertility preservation in women: indications and options for therapy. Mayo Clin Proc. 2020;95(4):770–83.
32. Luna JJ, Garrido N, Muñoz M, Rocha F, Cuapio P, Meseguer M. Fertilization rate and embryo quality is affected by sperm cryopreservation depending on fertilization procedure (IVF or ICSI). Fertil Steril. 2009;92(3):S74.
33. Iussig B, Maggiulli R, Fabozzi G, Bertelle S, Vaiarelli A, Cimadomo D, et al. A brief history of oocyte cryopreservation: arguments and facts. Acta Obstet Gynecol Scand. 2019;98(5):550–8.
34. Paffoni A, Reschini M, Pisaturo V, Guarneri C, Palini S, Viganò P. Should rescue ICSI be re-evaluated considering the deferred transfer of cryopreserved embryos in in-vitro fertilization cycles? A systematic review and meta-analysis. Reprod Biol Endocrinol. 2021;19(1):121.
35. Otani T. Clinical review of ejaculatory dysfunction. Reprod Med Biol. 2019;18(4):331–43.
36. Komiya A, Sato K, Ishidoh T, Tanaka K, Tomoda T. Clinical results of infertility treatment to male patients with spinal cord injury. Hinyokika Kiyo. 2004;50(1):21–3.
37. Lutgens SPM, Nelissen ECM, van Loo IHM, Koek GH, Derhaag JG, Dunselman GAJ. To do or not to do: IVF and ICSI in chronic hepatitis B virus carriers. Hum Reprod. 2009;24(11):2676–8.
38. Zheng Z, Zhao X, Hong Y, Xu B, Tong J, Xia L. The safety of intracytoplasmic sperm injection in men with hepatitis B. Arch Med Sci. 2016;12(3):587–91.
39. World Health Organization. WHO laboratory manual for the examination and processing of human semen. 6th ed. Geneva: WHO Press; 2021.
40. Boomsma CM, Cohlen BJ, Farquhar C. Semen preparation techniques for intrauterine insemination. Cochrane Database Syst Rev. 2019;10(10):Cd004507.
41. Björndahl L, Kvist U. Sequence of ejaculation affects the spermatozoon as a carrier and its message. Reprod Biomed Online. 2003;7(4):440–8.
42. Henkel RR, Schill WB. Sperm preparation for ART. Reprod Biol Endocrinol. 2003;1:108.

43. Bedford JM. Significance of the need for sperm capacitation before fertilization in eutherian mammals. Biol Reprod. 1983;28(1):108–20.

44. Mahadevan M, Baker G. Clinical in vitro fertilization. Cham: Springer; 1984.

45. Henkel RR, Franken DR, Lombard CJ, Schill WB. Selective capacity of glass-wool filtration for the separation of human spermatozoa with condensed chromatin: a possible therapeutic modality for male-factor cases? J Assist Reprod Genet. 1994;11(8):395–400.

46. Mortimer D. Sperm preparation techniques and iatrogenic failures of in-vitro fertilization. Hum Reprod. 1991;6(2):173–6.

47. Al Hasani S, Küpker W, Baschat AA, Sturm R, Bauer O, Diedrich C, et al. Mini-swim-up: a new technique of sperm preparation for intracytoplasmic sperm injection. J Assist Reprod Genet. 1995;12(7):428–33.

48. WHO. WHO laboratory manual for the examination of human semen and sperm-cervical mucus interaction. Cambridge: Cambridge University Press; 1999.

49. Bolton VN, Braude PR. Preparation of human spermatozoa for in vitro fertilization by isopycnic centrifugation on self-generating density gradients. Arch Androl. 1984;13(2-3):167–76.

50. Pousette A, Akerlöf E, Rosenborg L, Fredricsson B. Increase in progressive motility and improved morphology of human spermatozoa following their migration through Percoll gradients. Int J Androl. 1986;9(1):1–13.

51. Carmignac DF. Biological centrifugation. Cell Biochem Funct. 2002;20(4):357.

52. Canale D, Giorgi PM, Gasperini M, Pucci E, Barletta D, Gasperi M, et al. Inter and intra-individual variability of sperm morphology after selection with three different techniques: layering, swimup from pellet and percoll. J Endocrinol Investig. 1994;17(9):729–32.

53. Björndahl L, Mohammadieh M, Pourian M, Söderlund I, Kvist U. Contamination by seminal plasma factors during sperm selection. J Androl. 2005;26(2):170–3.

54. Baldini D, Ferri D, Baldini GM, Lot D, Catino A, Vizziello D, et al. Sperm selection for ICSI: do we have a winner? Cell. 2021;10(12):3566.

55. de Oliveira NM, Vaca Sanchez R, Rodriguez Fiesta S, Lopez Salgado T, Rodriguez R, Bethencourt JC, et al. Pregnancy with frozen-thawed and fresh testicular biopsy after motile and immotile sperm microinjection, using the mechanical touch technique to assess viability. Hum Reprod. 2004;19(2):262–5.

56. Soares JB, Glina S, Galuppo AG. Pregnancy with frozen-thawed and fresh testicular biopsy after motile and immotile sperm microinjection, using the mechanical touch technique to assess viability. Hum Reprod. 2005;20(2):569; author reply.

57. Jeyendran RS, Van der Ven HH, Perez-Pelaez M, Crabo BG, Zaneveld LJ. Development of an assay to assess the functional integrity of the human sperm membrane and its relationship to other semen characteristics. J Reprod Fertil. 1984;70(1):219–28.

58. Rossato M, Di Virgilio F, Foresta C. Involvement of osmo-sensitive calcium influx in human sperm activation. Mol Hum Reprod. 1996;2(12):903–9.

59. Bloch A, Rogers EJ, Nicolas C, Martin-Denavit T, Monteiro M, Thomas D, et al. Detailed cell-level analysis of sperm nuclear quality among the different hypo-osmotic swelling test (HOST) classes. J Assist Reprod Genet. 2021;38(9):2491–9.

60. Bassiri F, Tavalaee M, Shiravi AH, Mansouri S, Nasr-Esfahani MH. Is there an association between HOST grades and sperm quality? Hum Reprod. 2012;27(8):2277–84.

61. World Health Organization. WHO laboratory manual for the examination and processing of human semen. 5th ed. Geneva: World Health Organization; 2010. p. 271.

62. Casper RF, Meriano JS, Jarvi KA, Cowan L, Lucato ML. The hypo-osmotic swelling test for selection of viable sperm for intracytoplasmic sperm injection in men with complete asthenozoospermia. Fertil Steril. 1996;65(5):972–6.

63. Tsai YL, Liu J, Garcia JE, Katz E, Compton G, Baramki TA. Establishment of an optimal hypo-osmotic swelling test by examining single spermatozoa in four different hypo-osmotic solutions. Hum Reprod. 1997;12(5):1111–3.

64. Nassar A, Morshedi M, Mahony M, Srisombut C, Lin MH, Oehninger S. Pentoxifylline stimulates various sperm motion parameters and cervical mucus penetrability in patients with asthenozoospermia. Andrologia. 1999;31(1):9–15.

65. Rees JM, Ford WC, Hull MG. Effect of caffeine and of pentoxifylline on the motility and metabolism of human spermatozoa. J Reprod Fertil. 1990;90(1):147–56.
66. Sharma RK, Agarwal A. Influence of artificial stimulation on unprocessed and Percoll-washed cryopreserved sperm. Arch Androl. 1997;38(3):173–9.
67. Stanic P, Sonicki Z, Suchanek E. Effect of pentoxifylline on motility and membrane integrity of cryopreserved human spermatozoa. Int J Androl. 2002;25(3):186–90.
68. Yovich JM, Edirisinghe WR, Cummins JM, Yovich JL. Preliminary results using pentoxifylline in a pronuclear stage tubal transfer (PROST) program for severe male factor infertility. Fertil Steril. 1988;50(1):179–81.
69. Yovich JM, Edirisinghe WR, Cummins JM, Yovich JL. Influence of pentoxifylline in severe male factor infertility. Fertil Steril. 1990;53(4):715–22.
70. Lewis SE, Moohan JM, Thompson W. Effects of pentoxifylline on human sperm motility in normospermic individuals using computer-assisted analysis. Fertil Steril. 1993;59(2):418–23.
71. Agarwal A, Sharma RK, Gupta S, Boitrelle F, Finelli R, Parekh N, et al. Sperm vitality and necrozoospermia: diagnosis, management, and results of a global survey of clinical practice. World J Mens Health. 2022;40(2):228–42.
72. Ibis E, Hayme S, Baysal E, Gul N, Ozkavukcu S. Efficacy and safety of papaverine as an in vitro motility enhancer on human spermatozoa. J Assist Reprod Genet. 2021;38(6):1523–37.
73. Sandi-Monroy NL, Musanovic S, Zhu D, Szabo Z, Vogl A, Reeka N, et al. Use of dimethyl-xanthine theophylline (SpermMobil) does not affect clinical, obstetric or perinatal outcomes. Arch Gynecol Obstet. 2019;300(5):1435–43.
74. Mangoli V, Mangoli R, Dandekar S, Suri K, Desai S. Selection of viable spermatozoa from testicular biopsies: a comparative study between pentoxifylline and hypoosmotic swelling test. Fertil Steril. 2011;95(2):631–4.
75. Aktan TM, Montag M, Duman S, Gorkemli H, Rink K, Yurdakul T. Use of a laser to detect viable but immotile spermatozoa. Andrologia. 2004;36(6):366–9.
76. Park YJ, Pang MG. Mitochondrial functionality in male fertility: from spermatogenesis to fertilization. Antioxidants. 2021;10(1):98.
77. Birowo P, Tendi W, Rasyid N, Turek PJ, Sini IR, Rizal M. Successful targeted testicular sperm extraction using microsurgical technique (microTESE) following fine needle aspiration (FNA) mapping in a non-obstructive azoospermia (NOA) patient: a case report. J Reprod Infertil. 2021;22(1):65–9.
78. Salman Yazdi R, Bakhshi S, Jannat Alipoor F, Akhoond MR, Borhani S, Farrahi F, et al. Effect of 830-nm diode laser irradiation on human sperm motility. Lasers Med Sci. 2014;29(1):97–104.
79. Montag M, Rink K, Delacretaz G, van der Ven H. Laser-induced immobilization and plasma membrane permeabilization in human spermatozoa. Hum Reprod. 2000;15(4):846–52.
80. Ebner T, Moser M, Tews G. Possible applications of a non-contact 1.48 micron wavelength diode laser in assisted reproduction technologies. Hum Reprod Update. 2005;11(4):425–35.
81. Tarlatzis BC, Kolibianakis EM, Bontis J, Tousiou M, Lagos S, Mantalenakis S. Effect of pentoxifylline on human sperm motility and fertilizing capacity. Arch Androl. 1995;34(1):33–42.
82. Nordhoff V, Schuring AN, Krallmann C, Zitzmann M, Schlatt S, Kiesel L, et al. Optimizing TESE-ICSI by laser-assisted selection of immotile spermatozoa and polarization microscopy for selection of oocytes. Andrology. 2013;1(1):67–74.
83. Gerber PA, Kruse R, Hirchenhain J, Krussel JS, Neumann NJ. Pregnancy after laser-assisted selection of viable spermatozoa before intracytoplasmatic sperm injection in a couple with male primary cilia dyskinesia. Fertil Steril. 2008;89(6):1826.
84. Ozkavukcu S, Celik-Ozenci C, Konuk E, Atabekoglu C. Live birth after laser assisted viability assessment (LAVA) to detect pentoxifylline resistant ejaculated immotile spermatozoa during ICSI in a couple with male Kartagener's syndrome. Reprod Biol Endocrinol. 2018;16(1):10.
85. Plouffe BD, Murthy SK, Lewis LH. Fundamentals and application of magnetic particles in cell isolation and enrichment: a review. Rep Prog Phys. 2015;78(1):016601.

86. Vermes I, Haanen C, Steffens-Nakken H, Reutelingsperger C. A novel assay for apoptosis. Flow cytometric detection of phosphatidylserine expression on early apoptotic cells using fluorescein labelled Annexin V. J Immunol Methods. 1995;184(1):39–51.

87. Arends MJ, Wyllie AH. Apoptosis: mechanisms and roles in pathology. Int Rev Exp Pathol. 1991;32:223–54.

88. Degheidy T, Abdelfattah H, Seif A, Albuz FK, Gazi S, Abbas S. Magnetic activated cell sorting: an effective method for reduction of sperm DNA fragmentation in varicocele men prior to assisted reproductive techniques. Andrologia. 2015;47(8):892–6.

89. Lee TH, Liu CH, Shih YT, Tsao HM, Huang CC, Chen HH, et al. Magnetic-activated cell sorting for sperm preparation reduces spermatozoa with apoptotic markers and improves the acrosome reaction in couples with unexplained infertility. Hum Reprod. 2010;25(4):839–46.

90. Nadalini M, Tarozzi N, Di Santo M, Borini A. Annexin V magnetic-activated cell sorting versus swim-up for the selection of human sperm in ART: is the new approach better then the traditional one? J Assist Reprod Genet. 2014;31(8):1045–51.

91. Tavalaee M, Deemeh MR, Arbabian M, Nasr-Esfahani MH. Density gradient centrifugation before or after magnetic-activated cell sorting: which technique is more useful for clinical sperm selection? J Assist Reprod Genet. 2012;29(1):31–8.

92. Dirican EK, Ozgun OD, Akarsu S, Akin KO, Ercan O, Ugurlu M, et al. Clinical outcome of magnetic activated cell sorting of non-apoptotic spermatozoa before density gradient centrifugation for assisted reproduction. J Assist Reprod Genet. 2008;25(8):375–81.

93. Dandekar P, Aggeler J, Talbot P. Structure, distribution and composition of the extracellular matrix of human oocytes and cumulus masses. Hum Reprod. 1992;7(3):391–8.

94. Cayli S, Jakab A, Ovari L, Delpiano E, Celik-Ozenci C, Sakkas D, et al. Biochemical markers of sperm function: male fertility and sperm selection for ICSI. Reprod Biomed Online. 2003;7(4):462–8.

95. Huszar G, Ozkavukcu S, Jakab A, Celik-Ozenci C, Sati GL, Cayli S. Hyaluronic acid binding ability of human sperm reflects cellular maturity and fertilizing potential: selection of sperm for intracytoplasmic sperm injection. Curr Opin Obstet Gynecol. 2006;18(3):260–7.

96. Jakab A, Sakkas D, Delpiano E, Cayli S, Kovanci E, Ward D, et al. Intracytoplasmic sperm injection: a novel selection method for sperm with normal frequency of chromosomal aneuploidies. Fertil Steril. 2005;84(6):1665–73.

97. Wikland M, Wik O, Steen Y, Qvist K, Soderlund B, Janson PO. A self-migration method for preparation of sperm for in-vitro fertilization. Hum Reprod. 1987;2(3):191–5.

98. Slotte H, Akerlof E, Pousette A. Separation of human spermatozoa with hyaluronic acid induces, and Percoll inhibits, the acrosome reaction. Int J Androl. 1993;16(6):349–54.

99. Aitken RJ, Bowie H, Buckingham D, Harkiss D, Richardson DW, West KM. Sperm penetration into a hyaluronic acid polymer as a means of monitoring functional competence. J Androl. 1992;13(1):44–54.

100. Mortimer D, Mortimer ST, Shu MA, Swart R. A simplified approach to sperm-cervical mucus interaction testing using a hyaluronate migration test. Hum Reprod. 1990;5(7):835–41.

101. Miller D, Pavitt S, Sharma V, Forbes G, Hooper R, Bhattacharya S, et al. Physiological, hyaluronan-selected intracytoplasmic sperm injection for infertility treatment (HABSelect): a parallel, two-group, randomized trial. Lancet. 2019;393(10170):416–22.

102. Parmegiani L, Cognigni GE, Bernardi S, Troilo E, Ciampaglia W, Filicori M. "Physiologic ICSI": hyaluronic acid (HA) favors selection of spermatozoa without DNA fragmentation and with normal nucleus, resulting in improvement of embryo quality. Fertil Steril. 2010;93(2):598–604.

103. Van Den Bergh MJ, Fahy-Deshe M, Hohl MK. Pronuclear zygote score following intracytoplasmic injection of hyaluronan-bound spermatozoa: a prospective randomized study. Reprod Biomed Online. 2009;19(6):796–801.

104. Nasr Esfahani MH, Deemeh MR, Tavalaee M, Sekhavati MH, Gourabi H. Zeta sperm selection improves pregnancy rate and alters sex ratio in male factor infertility patients: a double-blind, randomized clinical trial. Int J Fertil Steril. 2016;10(2):253–60.

105. Bartoov B, Berkovitz A, Eltes F. Selection of spermatozoa with normal nuclei to improve the pregnancy rate with intracytoplasmic sperm injection. N Engl J Med. 2001;345(14):1067–8.
106. Lo Monte G, Murisier F, Piva I, Germond M, Marci R. Focus on intracytoplasmic morphologically selected sperm injection (IMSI): a mini-review. Asian J Androl. 2013;15(5):608–15.
107. Franco JG Jr, Baruffi RL, Mauri AL, Petersen CG, Oliveira JB, Vagnini L. Significance of large nuclear vacuoles in human spermatozoa: implications for ICSI. Reprod Biomed Online. 2008;17(1):42–5.
108. Shalom-Paz E, Anabusi S, Michaeli M, Karchovsky-Shoshan E, Rothfarb N, Shavit T, et al. Can intra cytoplasmatic morphologically selected sperm injection (IMSI) technique improve outcome in patients with repeated IVF-ICSI failure? A comparative study. Gynecol Endocrinol. 2015;31(3):247–51.
109. Teixeira DM, Hadyme Miyague A, Barbosa MA, Navarro PA, Raine-Fenning N, Nastri CO, et al. Regular (ICSI) versus ultra-high magnification (IMSI) sperm selection for assisted reproduction. Cochrane Database Syst Rev. 2020;2:CD010167.
110. Fortunato A, Boni R, Leo R, Nacchia G, Liguori F, Casale S, et al. Vacuoles in sperm head are not associated with head morphology, DNA damage and reproductive success. Reprod Biomed Online. 2016;32(2):154–61.
111. Smith GD, Takayama S. Application of microfluidic technologies to human assisted reproduction. Mol Hum Reprod. 2017;23(4):257–68.
112. Sackmann EK, Fulton AL, Beebe DJ. The present and future role of microfluidics in biomedical research. Nature. 2014;507(7491):181–9.

Sperm Banking

18

Parviz K. Kavoussi and Murat Gül

Introduction

Cryopreservation and storage of sperm has been standard practice for preserving a man's reproductive potential for the future. Patients are offered the option of storing one or more samples before undergoing potentially fertility adverse therapies such chemotherapy, radiation therapy (RT), or certain surgeries, and while the specifics may vary from center to center and country to country, the premise is consistent. In addition, men frequently store surplus cryopreserved spermatozoa for use in assisted reproductive techniques (ARTs) as a "back-up" sample in case the primary sample is not usable at the time of collection. In this chapter, we outline the indications of sperm banking along with its utilization in ART.

Indications for Sperm Banking

Sperm Banking in Cancer Patients

Every year, cancer is diagnosed in more than 70,000 teenagers and young adults between the ages of 15 and 39 in the USA alone. About 10,000 children under the age of 15 are diagnosed with cancer each year [1, 2]. Physicians involved in the care of young patients with cancer today are concerned not only with achieving cure or remission, but also with preserving an optimal quality of life after cancer therapy, thanks to advances in treatment regimens and supportive care measures. It is

P. K. Kavoussi (✉)
Department of Reproductive Urology, Austin Fertility and Reproductive Medicine/Westlake IVF, Austin, TX, USA

M. Gül
Department of Urology, School of Medicine, Selcuk University, Konya, Turkey

A. Agarwal et al. (eds.), *Human Semen Analysis*,
https://doi.org/10.1007/978-3-031-55337-0_18

estimated that there are currently between 300,000 and 500,000 childhood cancer survivors in Europe [3]. This has resulted in a greater awareness of the significance of cancer treatment's long-term side effects. For example, it is known that high-dose alkylating chemicals used in chemotherapy and radiotherapy treatment may cause infertility. Risk factors for gonadal dysfunction and reduced fertility in men due to the exposure to alkylating agents in chemotherapy, high-dose cranial radiotherapy are the disruption of the hypothalamic pituitary gonadal axis function, and targeted RT to the testes [4–8]. Therefore, adolescent and young adult males who have survived cancer and would like the opportunity to build a family with the use of their own gametes, may permanently have lost this ability due to the side effects of cancer treatment [9, 10].

The age of the patient at the time of diagnosis and therapy, as well as the agent, duration of therapy, and severity of the treatment; all may affect the patient's fertility [11]. Cytotoxic destruction to differentiating spermatogonia is a typical side effect of many chemotherapeutic drugs used to treat cancer and can result in temporary or permanent infertility in male patients. A person's sperm count is at its lowest 6 months after therapy is completed, and the temporary impairment may last for up to 2 years post treatment [12]. Both quantitative and qualitative damage to spermatogenic stem cells may lead to permanent infertility in some men [13, 14].

The level of destruction to the spermatogenic system varies depending on the age of the patient, the agent, dose, and schedule of chemotherapy [11, 15]. Higher doses of alkylating drugs such cisplatin, busulfan, chlorambucil, procarbazine, and cyclophosphamide are the most frequently linked agents to the onset of long term or irreversible infertility [16]. On the other hand, doxorubicin, vinblastine, dacarbazine, and bleomycin (without a high-dose alkylating drug) treatment which are used to treat Hodgkin's disease typically results in a stable spermiogram and gonadotrophin levels in most individuals beyond the time of chemotherapy. Vinca alkaloids (vincristine, vinblastine), anti-metabolites (methotrexate, mercaptopurine), and low-dose alkylating drugs pose a similarly low risk of irreversible infertility in patients with standard-risk non-Hodgkin lymphoma or acute lymphoblastic leukemia [17–20].

Radiation therapy is also extremely harmful to the testicular germinal epithelium, leading to loss of germ cells at doses as low as 0.1–0.2 Gy [21]. Exposure of the testes to radiation at a dose of 1.2 Gy or more may result in infertility [22]. High-dose conditioning with total body irradiation (TBI) before a hematopoietic stem cell transplant can cause damage to the testes, resulting in permanent infertility in most young adult men [23]. Hypothalamic pituitary axis dysfunction caused by cranial radiation of 35–40 Gy or greater may adversely impact male fertility, just as it does in women [24]. It is also known that azoospermia may precede the start of therapy in some diseases, such as Hodgkin's lymphoma and testicular cancer due to the pathology itself [25, 26].

Cryopreservation of spermatozoa before the start of cytotoxic treatment is the most consistent and well-established method of preserving fertility in adolescent and young males, as the quantity and health of sperm cryopreserved after the start of therapy may be hampered [27, 28]. Pregnancies conceived from sperm that had been frozen and preserved for 10–28 years have been shown to be successful in long-term follow-up investigations [14, 29–31]. Abstinence for at least 48 h before to ejaculation and the collection of several samples are recommended in order to increase the number of viable spermatozoa for cryopreservation [32]. Age, stress response, or having any disease that prevent people from masturbating or ejaculating are the limitations of this intervention's applicability [33]. Some young males, especially those who have been diagnosed with testicular cancer and Hodgkin's lymphoma, are at risk for azoospermia due to their pathology, even before they start potentially gonadotoxic treatments [25, 26, 34].

If masturbation is not possible for collection of a sample, sperm counts are poor, or the individual has obstructive azoospermia, there are a number of alternative interventions for obtaining sperm [35]. Options include microsurgical epididymal sperm aspiration (MESA), in which sperm is extracted from the epididymal tubule, testicular sperm extraction (TESE), which is conducted via direct extraction from the testis, and electroejaculation, which is performed under anesthesia due to the placement of an electric probe into the rectum. With advancements such as intracytoplasmic sperm injection (ICSI), which requires only a few number of viable sperm, these techniques may provide the potential of fatherhood with their own sperm to men with low sperm counts or obstructive azoospermia[35].

Cryopreservation of Spermatogonial Stem Cells in Prepubertal Children

The standard fertility preservation technique for adult men is cryopreservation of ejaculated semen. This approach is impossible in prepubertal boys and can be difficult for some pubertal boys, making prepubertal and pubertal fertility preservation challenging. In this group of patients, cryopreservation and subsequent transplantation of spermatogonial stem cells and testicular tissue, although still experimental, may provide alternatives for fertility preservation and restoration in the future [20, 36–38]. Initial animal research involving the use of stem cells and testicular tissue to regenerate spermatogenesis have shown promising results [39–41]. It seems that patients and/or guardians are willing to pursue an experimental fertility preservation procedure when no alternatives are available [42]. Therefore, several clinics across the globe are conserving testicular samples for patients who cannot maintain sperm in the hope that cell-based or tissue-based therapies will 1 day be used to create sperm and offspring [42].

Prior to undergoing orchiectomy or gonadotoxic treatment, the American Society of Clinical Oncology strongly recommends informing patients about the possibility of cryopreservation techniques [43]. Unfortunately, this recommendation is not implemented by all health care providers caring for patients with malignancies, leaving many patients unadvised on the subject [44].

Sperm Banking in Patients with Other Medical Conditions

Gonadotoxic therapies may be administered to patients with non-malignant diseases. Sickle cell disease (SCD) is a hereditary red blood cell abnormality and represents a substantial population of patients worldwide for whom low-dose TBI is required for allogeneic hematopoietic stem cell transplantation [45–47]. Patients with SCD suffer from vaso-occlusion, which leads to organ damage and hypoxia in the tissues. The anticancer medication hydroxyurea, an antimetabolite that inhibits ribonucleotide reductase and DNA replication, and can lessen the occurrence of vasoocclusion [48]. Boys getting this treatment are eligible for fertility preservation; however, the majority of boys will have already had treatment before a testicular tissue sample is provided [19]. Other blood disorders, including thalassemia, chronic granulomatous diseases, and idiopathic medulla aplasia, may necessitate irradiation treatment before hydroxyurea regimens and hemopoietic stem cell transplantation [49].

Allogeneic hematopoietic stem cell transplantation is linked with a substantial risk of germ cell loss, including resulting in complete azoospermia in 72–85% of males and oligozoospermia in the remainder [15, 50, 51]. Some rare syndromes such as Wiskott–Aldrich syndrome, high IgM syndrome, Farber disease, severe combined immune deficiency syndrome, IPEX syndrome, and DOCK8 immunodeficiency syndrome have also been identified as potential indications for spermatogonial stem cell/ testicular tissue cryopreservation [42].

Sperm Banking for ART Indications

In some circumstances when a difficult sperm retrieval is anticipated, it is preferable to begin testicular sperm retrieval at least 8 h prior to ovum retrieval to prevent post-mature oocyte damage [52]. Nonetheless, this can result in scheduling conflicts (operating room availability and the urologist may change his time schedule). Also, men who travel for work may not be physically available on the day of oocyte retrieval for in vitro fertilization (IVF) or the day of ovulation for intrauterine insemination (IUI) to provide a semen sample. Some men who are physically available but psychologically distressed by the process may find it difficult to provide a sample at the time of IUI/IVF. Another alternative is to undertake the surgical sperm retrieval on a separate day from the ovum retrieval and to freeze the testicular sperm. A benefit of this is that the pair will know in advance that testicular sperm is accessible, eliminating the risk of ovarian stimulation failure and financial loss. Before oocyte retrieval, the embryologist can also determine whether healthy sperm are available for ART using cryopreserved sperm. Fertilization and clinical pregnancy rates achieved using frozen sperm from men are comparable to those obtained using fresh sperm [53].

Sperm Cryopreservation Technique: Strengths and Weaknesses

Assisted reproductive technology commonly involves cryopreserved spermatozoa for various situations including fertility preservation, anxiety induced challenges with semen collection at the time of need, the presence of very low numbers of spermatozoa in the ejaculate or poor semen parameters, and surgically retrieved spermatozoa [54–56]. Assisted reproductive technology using donor sperm also requires cryopreserved spermatozoa during the quarantine period [57]. Different techniques have been evaluated for cryopreserving spermatozoa with the intent for use with ART. As the spermatozoa being cryopreserved are intended to ultimately be used to create embryos, all cryopreservation procedures, when possible, should be performed under a class A hood in a classified room or laboratory. Regardless of the cryopreservation technique, after the semen has been mixed with the cryoprotectant of choice for the laboratory, it is aspirated in plastic straws. A heat sealer is used to seal both ends of the straws and straws are correctly labeled. For fast vapor freezing, the straws are placed in liquid nitrogen 10 cm above the level of liquid nitrogen at –80 °C for 8–10 min for slow-freezing. The straws are then plunged into liquid nitrogen immediately after that timeframe [58].

Slow-freezing is the conventional technique for sperm cryopreservation [59, 60]. The recovery rate of cryopreserved spermatozoa is typically around 50%, but there is a great deal of interindividual variability [54, 61]. Slow-freezing of sperm has been shown to result in dramatic structural and functional qualitative changes in sperm [62–64]. Slow-freezing can result in the formation of ice crystals which may also damage the sperm cytoskeleton, membrane, and DNA [63, 65, 66]. The damaging effect of slow-freezing is more pronounced in the semen sample with severe oligoasthenoteratozoospermia than normospermic samples [67, 68]. However, sperm vitrification protocols have not been widely used in sperm banks or IVF laboratories and slow-freezing has remained the standard for sperm cryopreservation for ART use.

The technique of vitrification for sperm cryopreservation refers to ultrafast freezing of a small volume of semen with direct contact with contaminant-free liquid nitrogen which reduces osmotic damage by preventing ice formation. Per the WHO 6th edition laboratory manual for examination and processing of human spermatozoa, sperm vitrification should be considered an experimental procedure as improved post thaw semen parameters after vitrification in comparison to conventional cryopreservation techniques has limited data to support it [58, 69]. However, there are studies suggesting that vitrification offers advantages over slow-freezing including higher recovery rates and better motility [70]. Zhou et al. reported that vitrification resulted in higher sperm recovery rates, motility, morphology, and velocity than slow-freezing. In the latter study, the rate of recovery of motile sperm was 65.8% in the vitrification samples in comparison to 59.3% in the slow-freeze samples. The vitrification group in this study revealed a lower sperm DNA fragmentation (SDF) index than the slow-freeze group, 13.1% versus 16.5%, respectively [71]. Vitrification has specifically been advocated to cryopreserve small numbers of spermatozoa with reported higher recovery rates and motility [72, 73]. Other studies have also reported a lower SDF index with vitrified sperm in comparison to slow-freeze [74]. Conflicting studies have reported no advantage in SDF with vitrification [75]. Some studies reveal inconsistent results with sperm vitrification showing non-superiority and some reporting worsened motility with vitrification compared to slow-freeze [76–78]. A systematic review and meta-analysis of studies comparing slow-freeze versus vitrification of spermatozoa including 13 randomized controlled trials revealed significantly higher total motility and progressive motility of thawed sperm after vitrification compared to conventional cryopreservation. SDF and morphology were similar between the two groups. Vitrification had a better ability to preserve high quality spermatozoa than vitrification with low quality spermatozoa [69].

As far as actual ART outcomes with sperm cryopreserved by vitrification in comparison to slow-freeze, there is not reliable data to direct clinicians. It has been established that higher SDF indices contribute to worsened ART outcomes, particularly miscarriage rates, but it would be considered extrapolation of data to correlate the potential for lower SDF with vitrification to improve ART outcomes. In addition, there is some conflict in the medical literature on whether vitrification actually results in lower SDF than slow-freeze.

Cryopreservation of Testicular Sperm

In the era of ART, cryopreserved spermatozoa are frequently used for multiple clinical scenarios as described in this chapter. Arguably the most challenging scenario in reproductive care is managing couples with a male partner with non-obstructive azoospermia (NOA). Approximately 1% of men in the general population and 15% of men presenting for infertility evaluations are azoospermic [79, 80]. Microdissection testicular sperm extraction (microTESE) allows for retrieval of the largest number of spermatozoa for use for IVF/ICSI in men with NOA [81–84]. In the past, micro-TESE was performed with the intent to retrieve fresh sperm to use just prior to oocyte retrieval after controlled ovarian stimulation for the IVF/ICSI cycle. This posed a number of real-world challenges. One was scheduling for the microTESE with minimal lead-time notice and coordinating the timing for the reproductive urologist, the patient, the laboratory team, anesthesia, and the surgical facility. Fresh microTESE cycles also necessitated that the couple would have to take care of each other in a short period of time following microTESE and oocyte retrieval and would typically require more support at home. Another challenge includes the emotional, physical, and financial burdens of an IVF cycle with uncertainly of having spermatozoa from the male partner available for ICSI. This means that prior to microTESE the couple had to decide an alternative plan if spermatozoa were not isolated at the time of microTESE including cancelation of the IVF cycle, retrieving and cryopreserving oocytes without a sperm source and if so for what reason, or having a donor sperm source available as a back-up plan. In the latter case, many of these couples would not have needed IVF/ICSI but rather a much less costly and much less involved therapeutic donor insemination if they knew they needed a donor sperm source prior to the initiation of the IVF cycle. Fresh microTESE was historically the preference as there was concern for survivability of cryopreserved spermatozoa from microTESE specimens and loss of cells with freeze-thaw. However, over the years multiple studies evaluating large numbers of such microTESE/IVF/ICSI cycles have demonstrated equivalent outcomes of fertilization, pregnancy rates, and live birth rates with fresh versus frozen microTESE retrieved spermatozoa for IVF/ICSI [85, 86]. The American Urological Association/American Society for Reproductive Medicine guidelines for the diagnosis and treatment of male infertility states, "In men undergoing surgical sperm retrieval, either fresh or cryopreserved sperm may be used for ICSI" [87]. The question arises that if it is known that not all spermatozoa survive freeze-thaw, and at times very few sperm cells are isolated in men with NOA that undergo microTESE, how can the clinical outcomes be equivalent with fresh versus frozen sperm? The hypothesis is that the spermatozoa that do not survive freeze-thaw may be less robust cells and the ones that would perform poorly and not provide good outcomes even if used fresh. The use of previously retrieved cryopreserved spermatozoa from microTESE in men with NOA allows for the couple to make decisions with knowledge of the presence of absence of spermatozoa prior to initiating an IVF cycle.

Take Home Message

- Sperm banking is indicated in men prior to undergoing cancer treatment, including cryopreservation of testicular tissue for spermatogonial stem cells in prepubertal males, other medical conditions that require gonadotoxic treatment, and when the male partner is not physically present to provide a sample or has severe psychological distress inhibiting sample collection for a timed fertility treatment.
- Sperm banking is also indicated in men with disease processes that may diminish spermatogenesis.
- There is conflicting data regarding the benefit of vitrification of spermatozoa versus standard slow-freeze technique. Currently, the WHO 6th edition of human semen analysis manual considers vitrification of spermatozoa as experimental.
- In men undergoing surgical sperm retrieval either fresh or cryopreserved sperm may be used for ICSI.

References

1. Coccia PF, Pappo AS, Altman J, et al. Adolescent and young adult oncology, version 2.2014. J Natl Compr Cancer Netw. 2014;12(1):21–32. quiz 32
2. Coccia PF, Pappo AS, Beaupin L, et al. Adolescent and young adult oncology, version 2.2018, NCCN clinical practice guidelines in oncology. J Natl Compr Cancer Netw. 2018;16(1):66–97.
3. Hjorth L, Haupt R, Skinner R, et al. Survivorship after childhood cancer: PanCare: a European Network to promote optimal long-term care. Eur J Cancer. 2015;51(10):1203–11.

4. Wallace W, Anderson R, Irvine D. Fertility preservation for young patients with cancer: who is at risk and what can be offered? Lancet Oncol. 2005;6:209–18.
5. Darzy K. Radiation-induced hypopituitarism after cancer therapy: who, how and when to test. Nat Clin Pract Endocrinol Metab. 2009;5:88–99.
6. Chemaitilly W, Mertens A, Mitby P. Acute ovarian failure in the childhood cancer survivor study. J Clin Endocrinol Metab. 2006;91:1723–8.
7. Green D, Sklar C, Boice J. Ovarian failure and reproductive outcomes after childhood cancer treatment: results from the Childhood Cancer Survivor Study. J Clin Oncol. 2009;27:2374–81.
8. Green D, Kawashima T, Stovall M. Fertility of male survivors of childhood cancer: a report from the Childhood Cancer Survivor Study. J Clin Oncol. 2010;28:332–9.
9. Metzger M, Meacham L, Patterson B. Female reproductive health after childhood, adolescent, and young adult cancers: guidelines for the assessment and management of female reproductive complications. J Clin Oncol. 2013;31:1239–47.
10. Kenney L, Cohen L, Shnorhavorian M. Male reproductive health after childhood, adolescent, and young adult cancers: a report from the Children's Oncology Group. J Clin Oncol. 2012;30:3408–16.
11. Fallat ME, Hutter J. Preservation of fertility in pediatric and adolescent patients with cancer. Pediatrics. 2008;121(5):1461–9.
12. Hart R. Preservation of fertility in adults and children diagnosed with cancer. BMJ. 2008;337:2045.
13. Shetty G, Meistrich ML. Hormonal approaches to preservation and restoration of male fertility after cancer treatment. J Natl Cancer Inst Monogr. 2005;34:36–9.
14. Feldschuh J, Brassel J, Durso N, Levine A. Successful sperm storage for 28 years. Fertil Steril. 2005;84(4):1017.
15. Rovó A, Tichelli A, Passweg JR, et al. Spermatogenesis in long-term survivors after allogeneic hematopoietic stem cell transplantation is associated with age, time interval since transplantation, and apparently absence of chronic GvHD. Blood. 2006;108(3):1100–5.
16. Levine J, Canada A, Stern CJ. Fertility preservation in adolescents and young adults with cancer. J Clin Oncol. 2010;28(32):4831–41.
17. Anderson RA, Mitchell RT, Kelsey TW, Spears N, Telfer EE, Wallace WH. Cancer treatment and gonadal function: experimental and established strategies for fertility preservation in children and young adults. Lancet Diab Endocrinol. 2015;3(7):556–67.
18. Colpi GM, Contalbi GF, Nerva F, Sagone P, Piediferro G. Testicular function following chemoradiotherapy. Eur J Obstet Gynecol Reprod Biol. 2004;113(1):2–6.
19. Jahnukainen K, Mitchell RT, Stukenborg JB. Testicular function and fertility preservation after treatment for haematological cancer. Curr Opin Endocrinol Diabetes Obes. 2015;22(3):217–23.
20. Gul M, Hildorf S, Dong L, et al. Review of injection techniques for spermatogonial stem cell transplantation. Hum Reprod Update. 2020;26(3):368–91.
21. Howell SJ, Shalet SM. Spermatogenesis after cancer treatment: damage and recovery. J Natl Cancer Inst Monogr. 2005;34:12–7.
22. Howell S, Shalet S. Gonadal damage from chemotherapy and radiotherapy. Endocrinol Metab Clin N Am. 1998;27(4):927–43.
23. Socié G, Salooja N, Cohen A, et al. Nonmalignant late effects after allogeneic stem cell transplantation. Blood. 2003;101(9):3373–85.
24. Littley MD, Shalet SM, Beardwell CG, Ahmed SR, Applegate G, Sutton ML. Hypopituitarism following external radiotherapy for pituitary tumours in adults. Q J Med. 1989;70(262):145–60.
25. Vigersky RA, Chapman RM, Berenberg J, Glass AR. Testicular dysfunction in untreated Hodgkin's disease. Am J Med. 1982;73(4):482–6.
26. Petersen PM, Skakkebaek NE, Vistisen K, Rørth M, Giwercman A. Semen quality and reproductive hormones before orchiectomy in men with testicular cancer. J Clin Oncol. 1999;17(3):941–7.
27. Chung K, Irani J, Knee G, Efymow B, Blasco L, Patrizio P. Sperm cryopreservation for male patients with cancer: an epidemiological analysis at the University of Pennsylvania. Eur J Obstet Gynecol Reprod Biol. 2004;113(1):7–11.

28. Lass A, Akagbosu F, Abusheikha N, et al. A programme of semen cryopreservation for patients with malignant disease in a tertiary infertility centre: lessons from 8 years' experience. Hum Reprod. 1998;13(11):3256–61.
29. Horne G, Atkinson AD, Pease EH, Logue JP, Brison DR, Lieberman BA. Live birth with sperm cryopreserved for 21 years prior to cancer treatment: case report. Hum Reprod. 2004;19(6):1448–9.
30. Sanger WG, Olson JH, Sherman JK. Semen cryobanking for men with cancer–criteria change. Fertil Steril. 1992;58(5):1024–7.
31. Scammell GE, White N, Stedronska J, Hendry WF, Edmonds DK, Jeffcoate SL. Cryopreservation of semen in men with testicular tumour or Hodgkin's disease: results of artificial insemination of their partners. Lancet. 1985;2(8445):31–2.
32. Shin D, Lo KC, Lipshultz LI. Treatment options for the infertile male with cancer. J Natl Cancer Inst Monogr. 2005;34:48–50.
33. Pacey AA. Fertility issues in survivors from adolescent cancers. Cancer Treat Rev. 2007;33(7):646–55.
34. Rueffer U, Breuer K, Josting A, et al. Male gonadal dysfunction in patients with Hodgkin's disease prior to treatment. Ann Oncol. 2001;12(9):1307–11.
35. Park YS, Lee SH, Song SJ, Jun JH, Koong MK, Seo JT. Influence of motility on the outcome of in vitro fertilization/intracytoplasmic sperm injection with fresh vs. frozen testicular sperm from men with obstructive azoospermia. Fertil Steril. 2003;80(3):526–30.
36. Jensen CFS, Dong L, Gul M, et al. Fertility preservation in boys facing gonadotoxic cancer therapy. Nat Rev Urol. 2022;19(2):71–83.
37. Dong L, Gul M, Hildorf S, et al. Xeno-free propagation of spermatogonial stem cells from infant boys. Int J Mol Sci. 2019;20(21):5390.
38. Dong L, Kristensen SG, Hildorf S, et al. Propagation of spermatogonial stem cell-like cells from infant boys. Front Physiol. 2019;10:1155.
39. Brinster RL, Avarbock MR. Germline transmission of donor haplotype following spermatogonial transplantation. Proc Natl Acad Sci USA. 1994;91(24):11303–7.
40. Zhang X, Ebata KT, Nagano MC. Genetic analysis of the clonal origin of regenerating mouse spermatogenesis following transplantation. Biol Reprod. 2003;69(6):1872–8.
41. Fayomi AP, Peters K, Sukhwani M, et al. Autologous grafting of cryopreserved prepubertal rhesus testis produces sperm and offspring. Science. 2019;363(6433):1314–9.
42. Valli-Pulaski H, Peters KA, Gassei K, et al. Testicular tissue cryopreservation: 8 years of experience from a coordinated network of academic centers. Hum Reprod. 2019;34(6):966–77.
43. Oktay K, Harvey BE, Partridge AH, et al. Fertility preservation in patients with cancer: ASCO clinical practice guideline update. J Clin Oncol. 2018;36(19):1994–2001.
44. Del-Pozo-Lérida S, Salvador C, Martínez-Soler F, Tortosa A, Perucho M, Giménez-Bonafé P. Preservation of fertility in patients with cancer. Oncol Rep. 2019;41(5):2607–14.
45. Horan JT, Liesveld JL, Fenton P, Blumberg N, Walters MC. Hematopoietic stem cell transplantation for multiply transfused patients with sickle cell disease and thalassemia after low-dose total body irradiation, fludarabine, and rabbit anti-thymocyte globulin. Bone Marrow Transplant. 2005;35(2):171–7.
46. Strouse J. Sickle cell disease. Handb Clin Neurol. 2016;138:311–24.
47. Gül M, Luca B, Dimitropoulos K, et al. What is the effectiveness of surgical and non-surgical therapies in the treatment of ischemic priapism in patients with sickle cell disease? A systematic review by the EAU Sexual and Reproductive Health Guidelines Panel. Int J Impot Res. 2022;36(1):20–35.
48. DeBaun MR. Hydroxyurea therapy contributes to infertility in adult men with sickle cell disease: a review. Expert Rev Hematol. 2014;7(6):767–73.
49. Picton HM, Wyns C, Anderson RA, et al. A European perspective on testicular tissue cryopreservation for fertility preservation in prepubertal and adolescent boys. Hum Reprod. 2015;30(11):2463–75.

50. Anserini P, Chiodi S, Spinelli S, et al. Semen analysis following allogeneic bone marrow transplantation. Additional data for evidence-based counselling. Bone Marrow Transplant. 2002;30(7):447–51.
51. Kassim AA, Sharma D. Hematopoietic stem cell transplantation for sickle cell disease: the changing landscape. Hematol Oncol Stem Cell Ther. 2017;10(4):259–66.
52. Patton PE, Battaglia DE. Office andrology. Cham: Springer; 2007.
53. Amer M, Fakhry E. Fresh vs frozen testicular sperm for assisted reproductive technology in patients with non-obstructive azoospermia: a systematic review. Arab J Urol. 2021;19(3):247–54.
54. Critser JK, Huse-Benda AR, Aaker DV, Arneson BW, Ball GD. Cryopreservation of human spermatozoa. III. The effect of cryoprotectants on motility. Fertil Steril. 1988;50(2):314–20.
55. Tournaye H, Goossens E, Verheyen G, et al. Preserving the reproductive potential of men and boys with cancer: current concepts and future prospects. Hum Reprod Update. 2004;10(6):525–32.
56. Mossad H, Morshedi M, Toner JP, Oehninger S. Impact of cryopreservation on spermatozoa from infertile men: implications for artificial insemination. Arch Androl. 1994;33(1):51–7.
57. Morris GJ, Acton E, Avery S. A novel approach to sperm cryopreservation. Hum Reprod. 1999;14(4):1013–21.
58. WHO, editor. WHO laboratory manual for the examination and processing of human semen. 6th ed. Geneva: WHO; 2021.
59. Yeste M. Sperm cryopreservation update: cryodamage, markers, and factors affecting the sperm freezability in pigs. Theriogenology. 2016;85(1):47–64.
60. Hammadeh ME, Askari AS, Georg T, Rosenbaum P, Schmidt W. Effect of freeze-thawing procedure on chromatin stability, morphological alteration and membrane integrity of human spermatozoa in fertile and subfertile men. Int J Androl. 1999;22(3):155–62.
61. Gilmore JA, Liu J, Gao DY, Critser JK. Determination of optimal cryoprotectants and procedures for their addition and removal from human spermatozoa. Hum Reprod. 1997;12(1):112–8.
62. Desrosiers P, Legare C, Leclerc P, Sullivan R. Membranous and structural damage that occur during cryopreservation of human sperm may be time-related events. Fertil Steril. 2006;85(6):1744–52.
63. Isachenko E, Isachenko V, Katkov II, et al. DNA integrity and motility of human spermatozoa after standard slow freezing versus cryoprotectant-free vitrification. Hum Reprod. 2004;19(4):932–9.
64. O'Connell M, McClure N, Lewis SE. The effects of cryopreservation on sperm morphology, motility and mitochondrial function. Hum Reprod. 2002;17(3):704–9.
65. Ozkavukcu S, Erdemli E, Isik A, Oztuna D, Karahuseyinoglu S. Effects of cryopreservation on sperm parameters and ultrastructural morphology of human spermatozoa. J Assist Reprod Genet. 2008;25(8):403–11.
66. Morris GJ. Rapidly cooled human sperm: no evidence of intracellular ice formation. Hum Reprod. 2006;21(8):2075–83.
67. Verza S Jr, Feijo CM, Esteves SC. Resistance of human spermatozoa to cryoinjury in repeated cycles of thaw-refreezing. Int Braz J Urol. 2009;35(5):581–90; discussion 591.
68. Schuster TG, Keller LM, Dunn RL, Ohl DA, Smith GD. Ultra-rapid freezing of very low numbers of sperm using cryoloops. Hum Reprod. 2003;18(4):788–95.
69. Li YX, Zhou L, Lv MQ, Ge P, Liu YC, Zhou DX. Vitrification and conventional freezing methods in sperm cryopreservation: a systematic review and meta-analysis. Eur J Obstet Gynecol Reprod Biol. 2019;233:84–92.
70. Riva NS, Ruhlmann C, Iaizzo RS, Marcial Lopez CA, Martinez AG. Comparative analysis between slow freezing and ultra-rapid freezing for human sperm cryopreservation. JBRA Assist Reprod. 2018;22(4):331–7.
71. Zhou D, Wang XM, Li RX, et al. Improving native human sperm freezing protection by using a modified vitrification method. Asian J Androl. 2021;23(1):91–6.

72. Herbemont C, Mnallah S, Grynberg M, Sifer C. Prospective comparison of different techniques for cryopreservation of small numbers of human spermatozoa. Gynecol Obstet Fertil Senol. 2019;47(11):797–801.
73. Karthikeyan M, Arakkal D, Mangalaraj AM, Kamath MS. Comparison of conventional slow freeze versus permeable cryoprotectant-free vitrification of abnormal semen sample: a randomized controlled trial. J Hum Reprod Sci. 2019;12(2):150–5.
74. Slabbert M, du Plessis SS, Huyser C. Large volume cryoprotectant-free vitrification: an alternative to conventional cryopreservation for human spermatozoa. Andrologia. 2015;47(5):594–9.
75. Kalludi SN, Kalthur G, Benjamin S, Kumar P, Adiga SK. Controlled cooling versus rapid freezing of teratozoospermic semen samples: Impact on sperm chromatin integrity. J Hum Reprod Sci. 2011;4(3):121–4.
76. Chen Y, Li L, Qian Y, et al. Small-volume vitrification for human spermatozoa in the absence of cryoprotectants by using Cryotop. Andrologia. 2015;47(6):694–9.
77. Ali Mohamed MS. Slow cryopreservation is not superior to vitrification in human spermatozoa; an experimental controlled study. Iran J Reprod Med. 2015;13(10):633–44.
78. Tongdee P, Sukprasert M, Satirapod C, Wongkularb A, Choktanasiri W. Comparison of cryopreserved human sperm between ultra rapid freezing and slow programmable freezing: effect on motility, morphology and DNA integrity. J Formos Med Assoc. 2015;98(4):33–42.
79. Jarow JP, Espeland MA, Lipshultz LI. Evaluation of the azoospermic patient. J Urol. 1989;142(1):62–5.
80. Mazzilli F, Rossi T, Delfino M, Sarandrea N, Dondero F. Azoospermia: incidence, and biochemical evaluation of seminal plasma by the differential pH method. Panminerva Med. 2000;42(1):27–31.
81. Schlegel PN, Palermo GD, Goldstein M, et al. Testicular sperm extraction with intracytoplasmic sperm injection for nonobstructive azoospermia. Urology. 1997;49(3):435–40.
82. Tsujimura A, Matsumiya K, Miyagawa Y, et al. Conventional multiple or microdissection testicular sperm extraction: a comparative study. Hum Reprod. 2002;17(11):2924–9.
83. Ramasamy R, Padilla WO, Osterberg EC, et al. A comparison of models for predicting sperm retrieval before microdissection testicular sperm extraction in men with nonobstructive azoospermia. J Urol. 2013;189(2):638–42.
84. Ramasamy R, Reifsnyder JE, Husseini J, Eid PA, Bryson C, Schlegel PN. Localization of sperm during microdissection testicular sperm extraction in men with nonobstructive azoospermia. J Urol. 2013;189(2):643–6.
85. Yu Z, Wei Z, Yang J, et al. Comparison of intracytoplasmic sperm injection outcome with fresh versus frozen-thawed testicular sperm in men with nonobstructive azoospermia: a systematic review and meta-analysis. J Assist Reprod Genet. 2018;35(7):1247–57.
86. Ohlander S, Hotaling J, Kirshenbaum E, Niederberger C, Eisenberg ML. Impact of fresh versus cryopreserved testicular sperm upon intracytoplasmic sperm injection pregnancy outcomes in men with azoospermia due to spermatogenic dysfunction: a meta-analysis. Fertil Steril. 2014;101(2):344–9.
87. Schlegel PN, Sigman M, Collura B, et al. Diagnosis and treatment of infertility in men: AUA/ASRM guideline part II. Fertil Steril. 2021;115(1):62–9.

Part VII

Future Directions

On the Way to the 7th Edition

19

Rupin Shah, Ramadan Saleh, Florence Boitrelle,
and Ashok Agarwal

Introduction

Interestingly, the 6th edition of the World Health Organization (WHO) manual of human semen analysis unequivocally states that semen analysis reference ranges, which were the cornerstone of previous editions, cannot be used to label a man as fertile or infertile. This may create a confusion among clinicians about how to interpret a semen report and how to plan further treatment [1]. Additionally, while many new tests have been introduced in the 6th edition, their indications, interpretation, and clinical implications have not been discussed.

This book has been an attempt to bridge that gap between the 6th edition as a laboratory manual and its utility as a clinical guide. It is hoped that the preceding chapters will serve as a guide to clinical decision-making based on the results of semen analyses conducted as per the 6th edition of the manual.

R. Shah (✉)
Department of Urology, Lilavati Hospital & Research Centre, Mumbai, India

R. Saleh
Dermatology, Venereology & Andrology, Sohag University, Sohag, Egypt

F. Boitrelle
ART and Andrology Center, Centre Hospitalier Intercommunal de Pois, Poissy, France

A. Agarwal
Global Andrology Forum, Moreland Hills, OH, USA

Cleveland Clinic, Cleveland, OH, USA

Yet, questions do remain and these will need to be addressed in the seventh edition of the manual. In this concluding chapter we will peep into the future to predict what may be added to the seventh edition.

SWOT Analysis of the 6th Edition

SWOT stands for "strengths" (S), "weaknesses" (W), "opportunities" (O), and "threats" (T). Through this analysis, we summarize the key strengths and weaknesses of the 6th edition. Additionally, we highlight potential threats that could impede the global use of the 6th edition in clinical practice, and also provide an overview of available opportunities that can be used to maximize the benefits of this manual as a global reference in the field of human reproduction.

Strengths

This 6th edition is a robust laboratory technical guide and includes detailed step-by-step procedures. It provides detailed information on quality control and quality assurance that can help optimize laboratory performance.

The 6th edition includes results of semen samples of 3589 fertile men (1800 subjects from the 5th Edition and 1789 new subjects). The newly added data originate from two countries in Southern Europe, which were under-represented in the previous 5th edition, along with two countries from Asia and one country from Africa that lacked representation in the previous 5th edition. These additions addressed the criticism of unbalanced geographic representation in the previous 5th edition.

The 6th edition has included many specialized tests like sperm DNA fragmentation (SDF), and others, that may be recommended for certain clinical indications. This is important in light of the extensive research on new ways of assessing sperm function that has been done over the past decade.

Furthermore, this edition recognizes that 5th percentile values of semen parameters are not sufficient to make an accurate diagnosis of male infertility. It emphasizes the multifactorial nature of infertility, and highlights the importance of thorough clinical evaluation of the infertile men.

Weaknesses

Nevertheless, some weaknesses persist in this 6th edition. Data on fertile men from certain geographic areas, such as South America and sub-Saharan Africa, are still under-represented.

In addition, the manual does not provide clinical decision cut-offs, or describe the clinical indications for the sperm tests described. The clinician is therefore faced with a paradox: on the one hand, semen analysis is technically reliable and precise if the laboratory follows the recommendations of the WHO manual, but on the other hand, the values obtained from these tests are not analyzable in themselves.

Opportunities

To address these weaknesses, future research could help determine globally accepted reference ranges and thresholds that would be useful in the management of male infertility. If such studies are conducted, they would allow WHO to refine the upcoming 7th edition of its manual. Additionally, future research could contribute to the development of updated guidelines on important sperm tests such as SDF, and help incorporate advanced diagnostic tests such as sperm epigenetics and seminal oxidative stress (OS) into clinical practice. In light of the growing literature on the subject, some of the latter tests can be moved to the section of "extended tests of semen" in the next edition.

Threats

The abundance of technical detail in the manual may diminish clinicians' interest in reading and adopting it.

What Is Expected in the 7th Edition?

The SWOT analysis of the current edition of the WHO manual of human semen analysis may provide insights to the changes that are expected in the next edition. In this section, we summarize some of our predictions for the 7th edition of the WHO manual of human semen analysis.

Integration of Computer-Assisted Semen Analyzer and AI

Currently, majority of the semen tests are done without rigorous validation and lack critical data documenting their sensitivity, specificity, positive and negative predictive values, and cut-off values. Use of this data in research and publications often leads to a lack of reproducible findings and erratic conclusions. Thus, the results of these tests are unreliable from a diagnostic point of view. Computer-assisted semen analyzer (CASA) was introduced with the aim of overcoming these limitations. However, due to the high cost of these systems, and the need for training to operate these systems correctly, they are still listed as "advanced tests" in the 6th edition. This may change in the 7th edition.

Recently introduced artificial intelligence (AI)-based systems for semen analysis [2] are compact, rapid, operator-independent, and affordable. Already, cell phone-based home testing of semen is available [3]. As cell phones evolve with more processing power and the incorporation of AI, it is possible that the 7th edition will include cell phone-based evaluation in the standard protocol for semen examination. This should prove to be particularly useful in the conduct of those aspects of semen analysis which are difficult to perform by mere visual inspection such as the differentiation of rapid progressive and slow progressive motility [4], or those which are time-consuming and subjective such as sperm morphology assessment.

Elaboration of the Role of SDF Testing

The relationship between Sperm SDF and men's fertility potential has been extensively investigated over the last few decades with over 1500 research papers on the topic. Evidence suggests a significant negative impact of high SDF on both natural fertility [5, 6] and assisted reproductive outcomes [7–9]. The 6th edition of the WHO laboratory manual of human semen analysis has endorsed SDF assay as an extended test of semen that can be ordered in certain clinical indications [1] and provides detailed descriptions of four assays for SDF testing. However, the manual neither provides guidance as to the indication for testing nor addresses the variability of test results with different SDF assays [10]. The 6th edition recommends that each laboratory determine and validate its own diagnostic thresholds based on the assay used [1]. Recent guidelines by the European Society of Human Reproduction and Embryology [11] and the European Association of Urology (EAU) [12] recommend SDF testing for explanatory purposes in couples with recurrent pregnancy loss. Additionally, the EAU recommends SDF test in couples with unexplained infertility [12]. However, the clinical utility of SDF testing remains limited due to lack of clarity on which technique is best, indications for testing and reference values for further clinical decisions. It can be expected that 7th edition will incorporate the conclusions of new research to standardize the currently available SDF assays and provide reliable reference values for practitioners. It may also include new tools for assessment of SDF in clinical practice such as those involving cell-free DNA (cfDNA) [13–15].

Elaboration of the Role of Oxidative Stress Testing

Oxidative stress (OS) has been established as a major contributing cause of male infertility [16, 17]. In the 6th Edition of the WHO manual, seminal OS is described as an emerging technology under "Advanced examinations of semen," indicating that it is not currently usable in routine clinical practice [10]. Additionally, the manual provides a brief description of oxidation–reduction potential (ORP) using the male infertility oxidative system (MiOXSYS) for seminal OS assessment [1]. However, the current manual does not provide a clear guidance on the predictive potential of seminal OS testing for natural or assisted conception. Also, given the availability of different methodologies for assessment of seminal OS it is not clear which technique would best diagnose male infertility [10]. Recent studies highlight the predictive power and significance of seminal ORP in the context of male infertility [18–21]. With the availability of additional robust studies that provide reliable cut-off values of seminal OS in infertile men, it is likely that the test will be included in the basic or extended semen analysis in the 7th edition.

Alternative to Reference Range of Semen Parameters

Semen analysis is a complex test with significant intra-individual variations over time, lack of consistency between laboratories, and a complex interaction between various sperm-related factors. Additionally, there is a marked overlap between the semen parameters of fertile versus infertile men [22], thus limiting the predictive value of basic semen analysis. Furthermore, the chance of pregnancy is significantly affected by the female partner's fertility status. Despite these limitations, all previous editions of the WHO manual provided a reference range of basic semen parameters above which a man was considered normal and therefore did not require therapy. However, the 6th edition states that "The lower fifth percentile of data from men in the reference population does not represent a limit between fertile and infertile men" [1]. The editors of the 6th edition also indicate that "a better prognostic value of semen examination can be obtained from using the combination of several parameters." However, the 6th edition acknowledges that such combined reference parameters are still to be developed.

Hence, it can be expected that a major advancement in the 7th edition would be greater clarity on how to use the various parameters of the semen examination to predict male fertility potential, and the probability of pregnancy (if the female factors are normal). It is likely that the semen analysis report would include diagnostic entities such as "Lower limit of fertility," below which probability of pregnancy is low [23], and "Optimal limit of fertility," beyond which further improvement in semen parameters do not increase the chances of pregnancy [24]. The range of semen parameters between these two limits would constitute a gray zone of indeterminate fertility [22] in which pregnancy is possible but there is scope for improvement of fertility potential. Despite the abandonment of the reference range in the 6th edition, the editors suggest that "decision limits" for various semen parameters could help guide specific clinical decisions for further investigations or therapy, and possibly these will be elaborated upon in the 7th edition. It is hoped that the 7th edition will provide a reliable fertility measure that takes into account the relative weight of different conventional and extended semen parameters, as well as clinical variables such as age and duration of infertility.

Elaboration of the Role of Genetic, molecular, and Toxicological Biomarkers

The 7th edition may include more tests that assess genomic and epigenetic aspects of the sperm [25]. Various molecular biomarkers may also be included in extended or advanced tests since they can add to the predictive value of the semen examination [26]. With an increased recognition of the environmental impact on semen [27], perhaps toxicological measurements may become part of the extended tests.

Conclusions

The WHO manual for semen examination remains the standard method for evaluation of semen. Its strength has been its ability to change and adapt to new developments, and these are reflected as continuing changes in each new edition of the manual. An important note in the 6th edition has been the acknowledgement that reference ranges alone cannot be used to distinguish between fertile and infertile men. The 7th edition is expected to introduce a new way of interpreting semen parameters to accurately determine male fertility potential. Additionally, the 7th edition is expected to standardize newer tests such as SDF and seminal OS. There may be an expansion in the utility of CASA systems integrated with AI, and elaboration of the role of genetic, molecular and toxicological factors in the assessment of male fertility.

References

1. WHO. WHO laboratory manual for the examination and processing of human semen. 6th ed. Geneva: World Health Organization; 2021.
2. Agarwal A, Panner Selvam MK, Ambar RF. Validation of LensHooke® X1 PRO and computer-assisted semen analyzer compared with laboratory-based manual semen analysis. World J Men's Health. 2021;39(3):496–505.
3. Onofre J, Geenen L, Cox A, Van Der Auwera I, Willendrup F, Andersen E, et al. Simplified sperm testing devices: a possible tool to overcome lack of accessibility and inconsistency in male factor infertility diagnosis. An opportunity for low- and middle-income countries. Facts Views Vis Obgyn. 2021;13(1):79–93.
4. Tsai VF, Zhuang B, Pong YH, Hsieh JT, Chang HC. Web- and artificial intelligence-based image recognition for sperm motility analysis: verification study. JMIR Med Inform. 2020;8(11):e20031.
5. Evenson DP, Jost LK, Zinaman MJ, Clegg E, Purvis K, de Angelis P, Clausen OP. Utility of the sperm chromatin structure assay (SCSA) as a diagnostic and prognostic tool in the human fertility clinic. Hum Reprod. 1999;14(4):1039–49.
6. Evenson DP, Wixon R. Clinical aspects of sperm DNA fragmentation detection and male infertility. Theriogenology. 2006;65:979–91.
7. Larson-Cook K, Brannian JD, Hansen KA, Kasperson K, Aamoldt ET, Evenson DP. Relationship between assisted reproductive techniques (ART) outcomes and DNA fragmentation (DFI) as measured by the sperm chromatin structure assay (SCSA). Fertil Steril. 2003;80:895–902.

8. Deng C, Li T, Xie Y, Guo Y, Yang Q, Liang X, Deng C, Liu G. Sperm DNA fragmentation index influences assisted reproductive technology outcome: a systematic review and meta-analysis combined with a retrospective cohort study. Andrologia. 2019;51:e13263.

9. Zhao J, Zhang Q, Wang Y, Li Y. Whether sperm deoxyribonucleic acid fragmentation has an effect on pregnancy and miscarriage after in vitro fertilization/intracytoplasmic sperm injection: a systematic review and meta-analysis. Fertil Steril. 2014;102:998–1005.

10. Boitrelle F, Shah R, Saleh R, Henkel R, Kandil H, Chung E, Vogiatzi P, Zini A, Arafa M, Agarwal A. The sixth edition of the WHO manual for human semen analysis: a critical review and SWOT analysis. Life. 2021;11(12):1368. https://doi.org/10.3390/life11121368.

11. Bender Atik R, Christiansen OB, Elson J, et al. ESHRE guideline: recurrent pregnancy loss. Hum Reprod Open. 2018;2018:4.

12. Minhas S, Bettocchi C, Boeri L, et al. European association of urology guidelines on male sexual and reproductive health: 2021 update on male infertility. Eur Urol. 2021;80(5):603–20.

13. Aitken RJ, Whiting S, Connaughton H, Curry B, Reinheimer T, van Duin M. A novel pathway for the induction of DNA damage in human spermatozoa involving extracellular cell-free DNA. Mutat Res. 2020;821:111722.

14. Ranucci R. Cell-free DNA: applications in different diseases. Methods Mol Biol. 2019;1909:3–12.

15. Bartolome-Nebreda J, Vargas-Baquero E, Lopez-Fernandez C, Fernandez JL, Johnston S, Gosalvez J. Free circulating DNA and DNase activity in the ejaculates of men with spinal cord injury. Spinal Cord. 2021;59:167–74.

16. Agarwal A, Saleh RA, Bedaiwy MA. The role of reactive oxygen species in the pathophysiology of human reproduction. Fertil Steril. 2003;79(4):829–43.

17. Agarwal A, Said T. Oxidative stress, DNA damage and apoptosis in male infertility: a clinical approach. BJU Int. 2005;95:503–7. https://doi.org/10.1111/j.1464-410x.2005.05328.x.

18. Karabulut S, Korkmaz O, Yılmaz E, Keskin I. Seminal oxidation–reduction potential as a possible indicator of impaired sperm parameters in Turkish population. Andrology. 2021;53:e13956. https://doi.org/10.1111/and.13956.

19. Garcia-Segura S, Ribas-Maynou J, Lara-Cerrillo S, Garcia-Peiró A, Castel A, Benet J, Oliver-Bonet M. Relationship of seminal oxidation-reduction potential with sperm DNA integrity and pH in idiopathic infertile patients. Biology. 2020;9:262. https://doi.org/10.3390/biology9090262.

20. Agarwal A, Arafa M, Chandrakumar R, Majzoub A, Alsaid S, ElBardisi H. A multicenter study to evaluate oxidative stress by oxidation-reduction potential, a reliable and reproducible method. Andrology. 2017;5:939–45. https://doi.org/10.1111/andr.12395.

21. Agarwal A, Roychoudhury S, Sharma R, Gupta S, Majzoub A, Sabanegh E. Diagnostic application of oxidation-reduction potential assay for measurement of oxidative stress: clinical utility in male factor infertility. Reprod Biomed Online. 2017;34:48–57. https://doi.org/10.1016/j.rbmo.2016.10.008.

22. Guzick DS, Overstreet JW, Factor-Litvak P, Brazil CK, Nakajima ST, Coutifaris C, Carson SA, Cisneros P, Steinkampf MP, Hill JA, Xu D, Vogel DL, National Cooperative Reproductive Medicine Network. Sperm morphology, motility, and concentration in fertile and infertile men. N Engl J Med. 2001;345(19):1388–93. https://doi.org/10.1056/NEJMoa003005.

23. van der Merwe FH, Kruger TF, Oehninger SC, Lombard CJ. The use of semen parameters to identify the subfertile male in the general population. Gynecol Obstet Investig. 2005;59(2):86–91. https://doi.org/10.1159/000082368. Epub 2004 Nov 29.

24. Romero Herrera JA, Bang AK, Priskorn L, Izarzugaza JMG, Brunak S, Jørgensen N. Semen quality and waiting time to pregnancy explored using association mining. Andrology. 2021;9(2):577–87. https://doi.org/10.1111/andr.12924. Epub 2020 Nov 14.

25. Ghieh F, Barbotin AL, Leroy C, Marcelli F, Swierkowsky-Blanchard N, Serazin V, et al. Will whole-genome sequencing become the first-line genetic analysis for male infertility in the near future? Basic Clin Androl. 2021;31(1):21.

26. Llavanera M, Delgado-Bermúdez A, Ribas-Maynou J, Salas-Huetos A, Yeste M. A systematic review identifying fertility biomarkers in semen: a clinical approach through omics to

diagnose male infertility. Fertil Steril. 2022;118(2):291–313. https://doi.org/10.1016/j.fertnstert.2022.04.028. Epub 2022 Jun 17.

27. Bonde JP. Male reproductive organs are at risk from environmental hazards. Asian J Androl. 2010;12(2):152–6. https://doi.org/10.1038/aja.2009.83. Epub 2009 Dec 7. PMID: 19966832; PMCID: PMC3739096.

Index

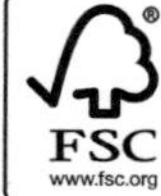